Alternative Medicine Guide to

Women's Health 1

BURTON GOLDBERG *and the Editors of*

ALTERNATIVE MEDICINE

 FUTURE MEDICINE PUBLISHING

TIBURON, CALIFORNIA

Future Medicine Publishing, Inc.
1640 Tiburon Blvd., Suite 2
Tiburon, CA 94920

Editor: Richard Leviton
Senior Editor: Stephanie Marohn
Writers: Richard Leviton & Stephanie Marohn
Research Editor: Keri Brenner
Associate Editor: John Anderson
Assistant Editor: Emily Rabin

Art Director/Cover Design: Janine White
Art Assistant: Jennifer Snipes
Production Assistant: Gail Gongoll

Interior design: Amparo Del Rio Design

Manufactured in the United States of America.

10   9   8   7   6   5   4   3   2   1

Library of Congress Cataloging-in-Publication Data
Goldberg, Burton, 1926-
    Alternative Medicine Guide to Women's Health 1 / Burton Goldberg and
the Editors of Alternative Medicine.
        p.   cm.
    Includes bibliographical references and index.
    ISBN 1-887299-12-2 (paperback) ISBN 1-887299-31-9 (hardcover)
    1. Women—Health and Hygiene—Alternative treatment. 2. Women—
Diseases—Alternative treatment. 3. Self-care, Health.
I. Alternative Medicine. II. Title.
RA778.G682   1998
616.5'082--dc21   98-3598
                                                            CIP

Portions of this book were previously published,
in a different form, in *Alternative Medicine:
The Definitive Guide* and *Alternative Medicine.*

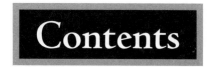
Contents

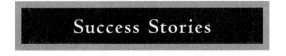

Success Stories

Throughout this book, we illustrate the effectiveness of alternative medicine therapies for women's health problems with actual patient cases. Use this handy guide to quickly locate these "success stories."

Important Information

URTON GOLDBERG and the editors of *Alternative Medicine* are proud of the public and professional praise accorded Future Medicine Publishing's series of books. This latest book continues the groundbreaking tradition of its predecessors.

The health of you and your loved ones is important. Treat this book as an educational tool that will enable you to better understand, assess, and choose the best course of treatment when women's health problems strike, and how to prevent these problems from striking in the first place. It could save your life.

Remember that this book on women's health is different. It is not another catalog of mainstream medicine's conventional treatments and drugs used to treat these problems. This book is about *alternative* approaches to women's health–approaches generally not understood and, at this time, not endorsed by the medical establishment. We urge you to discuss the treatments described in this book with your doctor. If your doctor is open-minded, you may actually educate him or her. We have been gratified to learn that many of our readers have found their physicians to be open to new ideas.

Use this book wisely. Because many of the treatments described in this book are, by definition, alternative, they have not been investigated, approved or endorsed by any government or regulatory agency. National, state, and local laws may vary regarding the use and application of many of the treatments that are discussed. Accordingly, this book should not be substituted for the advice and care of a physician or other licensed health-care professional. Pregnant women, in particular, are especially urged to consult with a physician before commencing any therapy. Ultimately, you, the reader, must take responsibility for your health and how you use the information in this book.

Future Medicine Publishing and the authors have no financial interest in any of the products or services discussed in this book, other than the citations to Future Medicine's other publications. All of the factual information in this book has been drawn from the scientific literature.

User's Guide

One of the features of this book is that it is interactive, thanks to the following 8 icons:

This means you can turn to the listed pages elsewhere in this book for more information on the topic.

This tells you where to contact a physician, group, or publication, or how to obtain substances mentioned in the text. This is an editorial service to our readers. Most importantly, the use of this icon empowers you right now, by giving you a source to acquire something vital to your health, quickly and easily. Whenever possible, we give you complete contact information for all substances mentioned in the text. All items are based on recommendations from the clinical practice of physicians in this book. The publisher has no financial interest in any clinic, physician, or product discussed in this book.

Many times the text mentions a medical term that requires explanation. We don't want to interrupt the text, so instead we put the explanation in the margins under this icon. This gives you the option of proceeding with the text or taking a moment to learn more about an important term. You will find some of the key definitions repeated at different places in the book so you don't have to search for the definition.

This sign tells you there may be some risks, uncertainties, side effects, or special contraindications regarding a procedure or substance.

This icon will alert you to an article published in our bimonthly magazine, *Alternative Medicine*, that is relevant to the topic under discussion.

This icon asks you to give a particular point special attention in your thinking. It is important to the overall discussion at hand.

Here we refer you to our book, *An Alternative Medicine Definitive Guide to Cancer*, for more information on a particular topic.

Here we refer you to our book, *An Alternative Medicine Definitive Guide to Headaches*, for more information on a particular topic.

You Don't Have to "Put Up" With Your Health Problems

MANY PEOPLE HAVE COME to understand that illness and disease are not something you have to live with, that alternative medicine has practical solutions for identifying and treating the underlying causes and thus can reverse the illness itself. Many have learned this the hard way, living with discomfort and pain for years before discovering that there is another option.

While you may be one of those who knows this when it comes to disease, you may not apply the principle to women's health problems. Conventional medicine tends to place these problems in a separate category from illness and disease, viewing them as something that goes with being a woman and must therefore just be endured. This is particularly true of menstrual disorders. Is it any surprise that many women don't seek help for premenstrual syndrome or excessively heavy menstrual periods? Even when a condition is regarded as serious, as in the case of endometriosis, the woman is often considered—by conventional physicians—to have brought the problem on herself by delaying childbearing or by some other lifestyle choice.

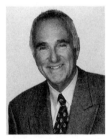

Alternative medicine, on the other hand, places the health problems covered in this book in the same category as any other disease or illness: they are *signs* of underlying imbalances or deficiencies and should be attended to as the warning signals they are. This applies equally to recurrent vaginitis and ovarian cysts as it does to menstrual disorders. As the late William Ghent, M.D., so aptly summarized it, "Premenstrual breast pain and tenderness is not normal. If it's painful, premenstrually, it's sick. I am sure that males would not accept sore testicles for seven to ten days of each month as normal."

If the warning signals are not heeded, the problem will deepen and eventually show up in other body systems as well. As with any other disorder, once you identify the hidden and usually multiple factors which are combining to produce the problem, you can systematically treat each one and permanently eliminate the condition. Alternative medicine has discovered that a core group of factors often underlies problems related to the female reproductive system. You will encounter them in the chapters of this book.

Two of the most prominent are hormonal imbalances and an underactive thyroid gland. These two causal factors are notoriously overlooked by conventional medicine. While doctors frequently prescribe estrogen for women's reproductive ailments, insufficient estrogen in the body is not always the problem. Often, too *much* estrogen in relation to the level of progesterone is behind the hormonal havoc occurring in the body. Unfortunately, conventional medicine does not usually consider the ratio of the hormones. The role of the thyroid in hormonal imbalance and a host of health disorders is similarly ignored, even though research has shown how it interacts with the hormonal status of the body.

The conventional medical establishment has an investment—both intellectual and financial—in relying on prescriptive palliatives rather than in addressing the underlying causes for long-lasting health conditions. To them, for a woman in menopause, the answer is synthetic estrogen. In 1997 alone, American women bought 33.6 million prescriptions of Premarin (a synthetic estrogen derived from the urine of female horses), making it the nation's best-selling drug. For that matter, the answer to all female dysfunction is a pill—not cures. Women now account for 59% of prescription drug purchases overall. Pharmaceutical companies, recognizing the potential of the women's market, are currently developing 372 medicines to treat a range of women's health conditions—up from only 263 experimental drugs in 1991. Drugmakers are also expanding the clinical testing of their products to include more women participants. The drug companies are doing a great business, though we aren't any healthier.

While reaping huge cash benefits for the drug industry, these drugs are not going to solve your health concerns. At best, they may temporarily relieve your symptoms, but between the side effects they invariably create and a tendency to worsen the original problem by masking it and driving it deeper into the body, it's hardly worth it—especially when you have a choice. That choice is alternative medicine.

Alternative medicine physicians focus on finding the *root* causes, rather than merely trying to alleviate symptoms so you can "live with the problem." In this book, you will learn how hormonal imbalances, an underactive thyroid gland, and a range of other contributing factors can be reversed with natural therapies that don't cause even more uncomfortable symptoms in the form of side effects.

This approach to health has particular significance for a diagnosis such as infertility which is represented as a "static" condition—that is, unfixable—and therefore brings such sadness and loss to so many women. Through investigating the deep causes contributing to a present inability to conceive and then treating them, the seemingly permanent state becomes temporary imbalance in many cases. Once the imbalances are corrected, the infertility is transformed into fertility. Traditional Chinese medicine, for example, has had remarkable success using acupuncture and herbs to reverse even long-term, so-called infertility—and all without the nightmare roller-coaster ride of conventional fertility drugs.

Our message is simple: you don't have to live with your health problems and you owe it to yourself not to. By treating what is actually causing the condition, be it severe menstrual cramps or uterine fibroids, not only can the original disorder be eliminated, but further health problems which might otherwise emerge from the same source can be prevented. With your overall health improved, taking care of the cramps or fibroids you're suffering from today is good preventive medicine for your future. God bless.

—Burton Goldberg

CHAPTER

1

Despite common belief, PMS and
other menstrual cycle disorders are not normal;
they are warning signals of an
underlying imbalance. This means you don't have
to endure these uncomfortable
to extremely painful conditions, but can eliminate
them permanently using natural
therapies that restore your body's innate balance.

CHAPTER

1

Menstrual Problems

A WOMAN MENSTRUATES an average of 500 times during her life. Yet there are many misconceptions about menstruation, and some have been repeated so often that they are considered fact. Most notable is the assumption that the normal menstrual cycle is 28 days, neatly paralleling the cycles of the moon. While women's bodies do have an observable rhythm, the menstrual cycle actually has a wide range of lengths that can be considered normal.

"The 28-day cycle is a complete myth," says Toni Weschler, M.P.H., of Seattle, Washington. "Cycles vary anywhere from about 24 to 37 days. If a woman uses the 28-day cycle as a point of reference and her cycle is different, she may think there's something wrong with her," Weschler notes.[1]

While two or three generations ago women began to menstruate at around 15 or 16 years of age, today puberty begins at age 12 or 13. Menstruation begins when body estrogen (see sidebar: "A Woman's Hormone Glossary," pp. 18-19) reaches a certain level, and aspects of modern life may be pushing that date ever earlier. These include: a diet high in estrogenic foods (meat, eggs, and dairy products, to name a few); eating meat and poultry products with residues of hormones and other drugs (fed to cattle and poultry to fatten them or increase their milk or egg output); and exposure to estrogen-mimicking chemicals that are increasingly prevalent both in our food and in our environment which, once in the body, act like estrogen.

The result of this estrogen onslaught is a *relative* excess of estrogen, meaning there is too much estrogen in relation to the level of progesterone, the other primary female hormone. Also known as estrogen dominance, this condition underlies many of the health problems discussed in this book. According to enzyme therapist and biochemist Lita Lee, Ph.D., of Lowell, Oregon, estrogen excess is a primary cause in almost all female conditions, including PMS, mood swings, excessive bleeding, endometriosis, fibroids, infertility, ovarian cysts, and fibrocystic breast disease. Women's health specialist Jesse Lynn Hanley, M.D., of Malibu, California, concurs. "A relative estrogen excess is a significant cause of female reproductive problems in the Western world," she states.

In the early years following puberty, it is common for menstrual periods to vary due to hormonal imbalances. However, if symptoms such as irregular bleeding, midcycle spotting, bleeding with a lot of clots, or bleeding too much or too little persist, they are signs that a woman's reproductive system needs attention. If untreated (that is, if the underlying imbalances producing them, such as estrogen dominance, are not addressed), they can develop into full-blown conditions such as menorrhagia (excess menstrual bleeding) or amenorrhea (lack of menses). New symptoms or previously only annoying symptoms may become the more serious dysmenorrhea (cramping pains with menstruation) or premenstrual syndrome (PMS) and make a woman's menstrual life miserable.

Menstrual Problems Covered in This Chapter

- Premenstrual syndrome (PMS): Uncomfortable symptoms such as bloating, cramping, achiness, headaches, short temper, irritability, sudden mood swings, depression, frustration, breast tenderness, crying spells, and abdominal discomfort occurring one to two days before a woman's period to the onset of bleeding

- Dysmenorrhea: Pain and cramping during menstruation

- Menorrhagia: Excessive bleeding during menstruation

- Amenorrhea: Absence of menstrual cycle for at least three months, not due to pregnancy or menopause

Such problems are not unusual among adult women; in fact, they could be said to be epidemic. As just one example of the scope of these menstrual conditions, abnormal uterine bleeding is the fourth most common gynecologic cause for hospitalization, and 89% of those hospitalized undergo surgery.[2] From 1980 through 1992, abnormal uterine bleeding led to more than five million hospitalizations, two million hysterectomies, and 20 million hospital days.[3]

Fortunately, there are alternatives to life-changing surgeries such as hysterectomy and conventional drugs with their disturbing side effects. This chapter tells you how you can treat four common menstrual disorders—PMS, dysmenorrhea, menorrhagia, and amenorrhea—using natural, safe, and effective therapies.

How the Monthly Cycle Works

The monthly menstrual cycle, which typically occurs in the years from age 12 to 51 in a woman's life, results from coordinated hormonal interplay among the hypothalamus, the pituitary gland, and the ovaries. The menstrual cycle contains three phases: the follicular or preovulatory, the ovulatory, and the luteal or postovulatory.

The Follicular or Preovulatory Phase—This phase begins with the first day of menstrual bleeding and extends to one day before luteinizing hormone (LH) surges, about day 13 or 14, just before ovulation. The purpose of this phase is to grow and mature a group of follicles (sac containing a developing egg), one of which will be selected for ovulation.

During this phase, the levels of LH gradually rise, while follicle-stimulating hormone (FSH) levels, which were high prior to menstruation, gradually fall off. (See the graph "Hormone Levels During the Menstrual Cycle," p. 18.) A hormone called inhibin or folliculostatin, blocks the release of further FSH. Around seven to eight days before ovulation (soon after bleeding has stopped), levels of estradiol and estrone (two of the body's three forms of estrogen) begin climbing. In the early days of the follicular phase, secretion levels of both estradiol and estrone are about equal at 60-170 mcg per day. Once the dominant follicle has been selected, estradiol secretion increases to 800 mcg per day, and most (90%) of this is produced in the follicle and corpus luteum.

Around this time, levels of two other hormones, androgens called androstenedine and testosterone, and some progestins (types of progesterone) rise as well. Their levels peak when LH surges, around day 13 or 14. During this phase, the body prepares the uterus to accept a fertilized egg.

Estrogen is released to trigger the thickening of the lining of the uterus

The Female Reproductive System

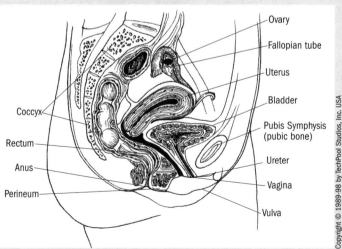

Ovary
Fallopian tube
Uterus
Bladder
Pubis Symphysis (pubic bone)
Ureter
Vagina
Vulva
Coccyx
Rectum
Anus
Perineum

(the endometrium) with blood vessels, glands, and cells in anticipation of the egg, and causes a fertile cervical fluid to be produced, which eases the sperm's passage through the cervix and enhances sperm survival. Once the mature egg has left the ovaries, it can be fertilized.

The Ovulatory Phase—The purpose of this phase is to release an egg capable of being fertilized by sperm. The ovum (egg or oocyte) is released by the mature graafian follicle (about 1-2 cm in diameter) approximately 32 to 34 hours after the surge of LH precipitated by the pituitary gland. Ovulation lasts from about one day before to one day after the LH surge, and is sometimes accompanied by pelvic pain, called "mittelschmerz." When LH levels peak, the levels of estradiol drop.

The Luteal or Postovulatory Phase—This phase lasts about 14 days, or up until the time of the next bleeding. The term *luteal* refers to the corpus luteum, the "yellow body" that lines the ovary; this phase represents its lifespan. The corpus luteum secretes progesterone to support the released egg; progesterone levels peak typically six to eight days after the LH surge. Progesterone helps form a thick mucous plug in the cervix to prevent sperm or bacteria from entering, and maintains the endometrium in a nutritious, blood-rich stage in anticipation of the egg's fertilization by the sperm (conception).

To a lesser extent, levels of estradiol and estrone also increase during this phase. If conception does not occur, the corpus luteum stops secreting progesterone, all hormone levels drop, and the endometrium sheds its intermediate layer—this is menstruation. The cycle then starts over. If fertilization does occur, progesterone secretion continues to increase, maintaining the uterine lining and pregnancy, until the placenta takes over secreting progesterone and other hormones at about three months' gestation.

The Uterus, Ovaries, and Fallopian Tubes

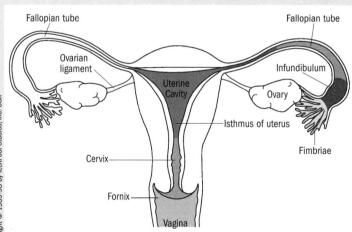

A Woman's Hormone Glossary

Estrogen is one of the female "sex" hormones, produced mainly in the ovaries (some in the fat cells), that regulates the menstrual cycle. Estrogen is important for adolescent sexual development, prepares the uterus for receiving the fertilized egg by stimulating the uterine lining to grow, and affects all the body's cells; its levels decline after menopause. Estrogen slows down bone loss, which leads to osteoporosis, and it can help reduce the incidence of heart attacks; estrogen also improves skin tone, reduces vaginal dryness, and can act as an antiaging factor. For the first ten to 14 days in a woman's cycle, the uterus is mainly under the influence of estrogen. Estrogen levels begin to climb right before menstruation, from about days seven to 14, and peak at ovulation. There are three natural types of estrogen: estradiol (produced directly in the ovary), estrone (produced from estradiol), and estriol (formed in smaller amounts in the ovary). Estradiol is the most potent of the three. It prepares the uterus for the implantation of a fertilized egg and also helps mature and maintain the sex characteristics of the female organs.

Luteinizing hormone (LH), produced by the pituitary gland in the brain, is primarily responsible for ovulation in women. Its name comes from lutein, the yellowish fluid which fills the corpus luteum. This is a hormone-secreting body of endocrine tissues which forms the follicle or sac containing a developing egg. The corpus luteum controls the production of the key female hormones estrogen and progesterone during the second half

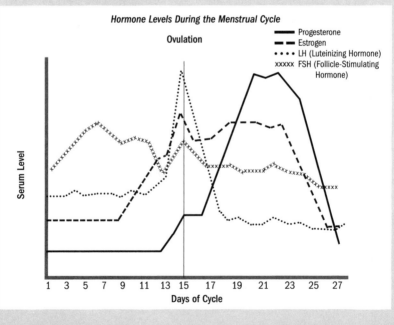

Hormone Levels During the Menstrual Cycle

Ovulation

— Progesterone
--- Estrogen
•••• LH (Luteinizing Hormone)
xxxxx FSH (Follicle-Stimulating Hormone)

Serum Level

Days of Cycle

1 3 5 7 9 11 13 15 17 19 21 23 25 27

of the menstrual cycle (called the luteal phase). At mid-cycle, the body secretes increasing amounts of estrogen, which triggers a dramatic surge of LH and another hormone, called follicle-stimulating hormone (FSH). This usually occurs between days 12 and 16 of the cycle, with ovulation (the release of the egg) at day 14. The sudden increase in LH/FSH causes the corpus luteum (also called the follicular cyst) to burst, allowing the mature egg to travel down into the fallopian tubes. Following ovulation, the corpus luteum gradually shrinks, producing less estrogen and progesterone. The steady decline of these hormones ends in the shedding of the uterine lining (menstruation) and the beginning of a new cycle.

Follicle-stimulating hormone (FSH) regulates the release of a mature egg from its follicle, or protective sac. At mid-cycle, the body secretes increasing amounts of estrogen, which triggers a dramatic surge of FSH and LH (see above).

Progesterone is a female "sex" hormone (produced in the corpus luteum of the ovaries) which prepares the uterus for a fertilized egg and then stops the cell proliferation in the uterus if pregnancy does not occur. When estrogen is high, during days seven to 14 of a woman's cycle, the level of progesterone is at its lowest. Its levels climb to a peak around days 14 to 24 and then dramatically drop off again just before the start of menstruation. When the cells stop producing progesterone, it's a signal to the uterus to let go of all the new cells produced during the month and to start afresh. In a sense, menstruation is progesterone withdrawal. Starting at age 35, a woman's progesterone production begins to decline.

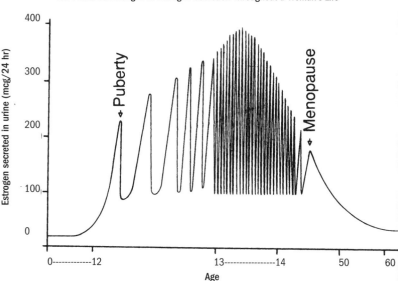

The Peaks and Troughs of Estrogen Secretion Throughout a Woman's Life

Causes of PMS

- Poor diet
- Estrogen dominance
- Underactive thyroid gland
- Exhausted adrenal glands
- *Candida albicans* overgrowth
- Parasites
- Nutritional deficiencies
- Food sensitivities or allergies
- Environmental sensitivities
- Mercury dental fillings
- Stress
- Sleep disorders
- Caffeine
- Lack of light
- Lack of exercise
- Unresolved physical or sexual abuse

Alternative Medicine Therapies for PMS

- Acupressure
- Aromatherapy
- Ayurvedic medicine
- Castor oil packs
- Detoxification
- Dietary recommendations
- Herbal medicine
- Natural progesterone therapy
- Nutritional supplements
- Probiotic therapy
- Reflexology

Premenstrual Syndrome

At least 150 different symptoms are believed to be related to premenstrual syndrome. With the incidence of PMS varying widely, medical researchers estimate that it affects anywhere from 25% to 100% of women, for whom the majority experience PMS as "annoying," while 5% to 10% of women experience serious difficulties as a result of PMS.[4] According to Christiane Northrup, M.D., of Yarmouth, Maine, "Sixty percent of women have enough symptoms due to PMS to suffer. This is far too many women to be suffering from a normal physiological function."

The symptoms of PMS may be divided into body-based (somatic) and emotional. In the first category, a woman may experience abdominal bloating, pimples, intolerance to alcohol, tenderness or enlargement of the breasts, clumsiness, intestinal disturbances (constipation or diarrhea), headaches, swelling and water retention in the hands and feet, and weight gain, among many other symptoms. In the second category, typical PMS symptoms include anxiety, a shift in sexual interest, depression, fatigue, food cravings (notably for salt and sugar), hostility, concentration difficulties, insomnia, irritability, lethargy, mood swings, panic attacks (even paranoia), violence towards self or others, and a desire to withdraw from the company of other people.

Understanding the Four Types of PMS

Clinical research suggests that there are various types of PMS, each characterized by different nutritional needs and hormonal imbalances, although many women's PMS is a combination. Conventional medicine

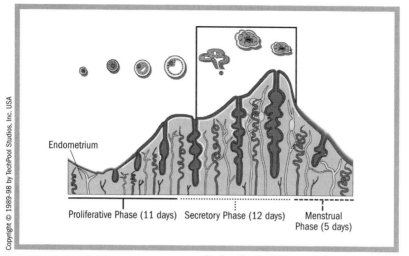

Endometrium

Proliferative Phase (11 days)   Secretory Phase (12 days)   Menstrual Phase (5 days)

THE STAGES OF THE MONTHLY MENSTRUAL CYCLE. During the first three weeks of the cycle, following menstruation, the lining of the uterus (endometrium) is built up. During the five days of bleeding, this lining is shed. In the Proliferative Phase, estrogen is dominant, while in the Secretory Phase, progesterone is dominant.

classifies PMS according to the following four basic types:

■ PMS-A (for anxiety): This type of PMS is characterized by anxiety, irritability, and insomnia, and, late in the menstrual cycle, depression. PMS-A affects about 65% to 75% of sufferers and usually involves a hormonal imbalance in which the body produces a disproportionate amount of estrogen relative to progesterone. Estrogen is a central nervous system stimulant, hence the tendency to anxiety. Progesterone is a central nervous system depressant.

■ PMS-C (for cravings): Symptoms include cravings for sweets, increased appetite, headaches, and fatigue. (High ingestion of sugar can lead to headache, palpitations, fatigue, or fainting.) This form of PMS affects about 33% of PMS sufferers and is caused primarily by an inability to adequately process sugar (glucose intolerance). That is, in the weeks between ovulation and menstruation, the body craves sweet foods, but is unable to properly digest all of the extra sugar it takes in.

■ PMS-D (for depression): Typical symptoms are depression, forgetfulness, confusion, and lethargy or sluggishness. It affects between 25% and 35% of PMS sufferers. According to clinical research, one cause of PMS-D might be a disproportionately high amount of progesterone in the body, although some sufferers with normal progesterone and estrogen levels may be experiencing some form of lead toxicity. Much like clinical depression, PMS-D has proven to be the most diffi-

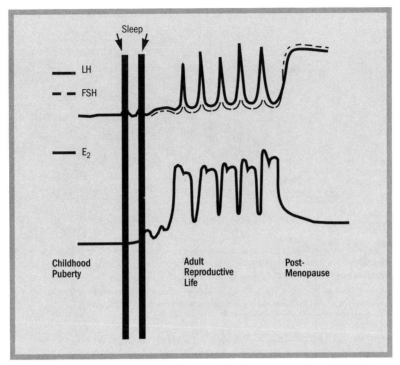

HORMONAL CHANGES THROUGHOUT A WOMAN'S LIFETIME. Key hormones, such as luteinizing hormone (LH), follicle-stimulating hormone (FSH), and estradiol (E_2, one of the estrogens), are present in differing amounts in puberty, adult life, and after menopause.

cult to treat, because effective treatment varies so widely according to the individual.

■ PMS-H (for "hyperhydration" or water retention): With symptoms of hyperhydration, weight gain above three pounds, breast congestion and tenderness, abdominal bloating, and swelling (edema) of face and extremities, PMS-H is associated with the body's retention of too much water and salt. Although PMS-H symptoms can range from slight bloating to severe edema, over 50% of PMS sufferers experience PMS-H to some degree.

Sixteen Causes of PMS

There are a host of dietary and lifestyle issues that are proven causal factors in PMS and many other women's health problems. When these factors are identified and addressed, the presenting health condition can be resolved. "The key to solving the PMS puzzle is to identify the possible causes and eliminate or correct them," says nutritionist Linaya Hayn,

L.N.C., of the PMS Holistic Center in Buffalo Grove, Illinois. She cites 16 imbalances and deficiencies as potential causes of PMS.[5] You will encounter many of these throughout the book in discussions of the causal factors involved in other health conditions.

1) Poor Diet—Researchers have shown that the typical woman with PMS consumes 275% more sugar, 62% more refined carbohydrates, 78% more sodium, 79% more dairy products, 52% less zinc, 77% less magnesium, and 53% less iron than non-PMS women. Low levels of magnesium and a higher percentage of total dietary calories derived from fat have both been linked with PMS symptoms.[6]

2) Estrogen Dominance—As stated earlier, estrogen dominance, or an excess of estrogen relative to progesterone, is behind many women's health conditions, including PMS. All of the most common PMS symptoms, such as bloating, weight gain, headaches, and backache are also symptoms of a relative estrogen excess, according to women's health expert John R. Lee, M.D., of Sebastopol, California, who coined the term estrogen dominance.[7] "The healthy ratio of progesterone to estrogen is ten to one," states Dr. Lita Lee (no relation). "The lower the ratio, the more health problems."

Estrogen dominance can be created by numerous factors. Eating a diet high in estrogenic foods is often double exposure because many of the foods that naturally contain estrogen are from animals which have also been pumped full of synthetic hormones to increase their weight or egg or milk production. Estrogen-mimicking chemicals, also known as environmental estrogens or xenoestrogens, are found in our food, air, and water. Herbicides, pesticides, by-products of plastics manufacture, and many other poisons mimic estrogen once they enter the body. The body responds as if it is real estrogen and the result is estrogen dominance and all the problems that imbalance carries with it.

For more about **estrogen dominance,** see Chapter 2: Endometriosis, p. 73. For more about **environmental estrogens,** see Chapter 2: Endometriosis, pp. 74-75. For more on ***Candida* overgrowth,** see Chapter 6: Cystitis, p. 211, and Chapter 7: Vaginitis, pp. 244-245.

If the woman has chronic constipation or toxic buildup in her intestines, the excess estrogen is reabsorbed by the body instead of being eliminated, further adding to the imbalance of the hormonal ratio. Other contributing factors to estrogen dominance are chronic stress and perimenopause (the ten to 15 years before the actual cessation of menses) which deplete progesterone supplies, thus skewing the estrogen-progesterone ratio. Finally, an underactive thyroid gland can lead to a relative estrogen excess as

"Sixty percent of women have enough symptoms due to PMS to suffer. This is far too many women to be suffering from a normal physiological function," states Christiane Northrup, M.D.

well (see the next causal factor of PMS, below).

Estrogen dominance has many unpleasant results, including: heavy menstrual bleeding; PMS symptoms such as cramps, migraines, and water retention; breast, uterine, or ovarian pathology; increased fat storage; tissue damage; bruising and pigment discoloration on the face; and aging of the skin. Estrogen dominance can also damage the pituitary gland and put stress on liver function, reports Dr. Lita Lee. The liver is required to detoxify estrogen and to convert thyroid hormone to its active form. If the liver is not working properly, it will perpetuate the estrogen excess cycle by allowing estrogen to build up.

Rather than artificially manipulating your estrogen levels with synthetic hormones and ignoring the reasons behind the imbalance, it is more valuable to determine why you have the estrogen buildup or progesterone deficiency in the first place. Depending on the source of the relative excess estrogen, restoring hormonal balance can be more effectively achieved with dietary changes, nutritional supplements, natural progesterone cream, bowel detoxification, and eliminating exposure to environmental toxins.

3) Underactive Thyroid Gland—This condition, known as hypothyroidism (see sidebar: "A Primer on the Thyroid," p. 25), can lead to estrogen dominance which, as noted above, is often a factor in PMS. It does so because an underfunctioning thyroid results in a decreased production of progesterone, explains Dr. Lita Lee. There is then an insufficient quantity of progesterone to balance (or oppose) the toxic effects of too much estrogen, and PMS can be the seemingly unrelated consequence.

One study found that of 54 women with PMS (defined as irritability, moodiness, bloating, fatigue, and cravings for sweets at least one week before menstruation), 51 (or 94%) of participants showed evidence of poor thyroid function.[8] In a later study at the same clinic, 34 of the original 54 women were treated with a synthetic thyroid supplement (levothyroxine sodium). After raising the dosage from 0.025 mg to 0.1 mg over a period of four weeks, all 34 women reported complete relief from PMS symptoms.[9]

As this study shows, reversing hypothyroidism and its influence on PMS can be relatively easy once the problem is identified.

A Primer on the Thyroid

The thyroid gland, one of the body's seven endocrine glands, is located just below the larynx in the throat, with interconnecting lobes on either side of the trachea. The thyroid is the body's metabolic thermostat, controlling body temperature, energy use, and, for children, the body's growth rate. The thyroid controls the rate at which organs function and the speed with which the body uses food; it affects the operation of all body processes and organs. Of the hormones synthesized in and released by the thyroid, T3 (triiodothyronine) represents 7% and T4 (thyroxine) accounts for almost 93% of

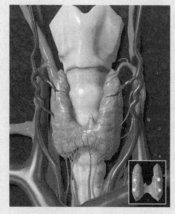

the thyroid's hormones active in all of the body's processes. Iodine is essential to forming normal amounts of thyroxine. The secretion of both these hormones is regulated by thyroid-stimulating hormone, or TSH, secreted by the pituitary gland in the brain. The thyroid also secretes calcitonin, a hormone required for calcium metabolism.

Hypothyroidism is a condition of low or underactive thyroid gland function that can produce numerous symptoms. Among the 47 clinically recognized symptoms: fatigue, depression, lethargy, weakness, weight gain, low body temperature, chills, cold extremities, general inappropriate sensation of cold, infertility, rheumatic pain, menstrual disorders (excessive flow, cramps), repeated infections, colds, upper respiratory infections, skin problems (itching, eczema, psoriasis, acne, dry, coarse, or scaly skin, skin pallor), memory disturbances, concentration difficulties, paranoia, migraines, oversleep, "laziness," muscle aches and weakness, hearing disturbances, burning/prickling sensations, anemia, slow reaction time and mental sluggishness, swelling of the eyelids, constipation, labored or difficult breathing, hoarseness, brittle nails, and poor vision. A resting body temperature (measured in the armpit) *below* 97.8° F indicates hypothyroidism; menstruating women should take the underarm temperature only on the second and third days of menstruation.

Unfortunately, many patients fall through the cracks of medicine's obliviousness to thyroid function or, if they're fortunate enough to have a thyroid test, they may get "normal" results because most standard tests are not sensitive enough to identify hypothyroidism. The TRH (thyrotrophin-releasing hormone) test is a far more sensitive

For more about the **TRH test,** contact: Raphael Kellman, M.D., The Center for Progressive Medicine, 140 West 69th Street, New York, NY 10023; tel: 212-721-6633; fax: 212-721-6714.

laboratory measure than routine thyroid blood tests and can show conclusively that a patient is suffering from an underactive thyroid, states Raphael Kellman, M.D., a New York City physician who specializes in thyroid-related cases and uses the test regularly in his clinical practice.

For the TRH test, the physician measures the patient's level of TSH (thyroid-stimulating hormone) through a simple blood test, then gives an injection of TRH (a completely harmless synthetic hormone modeled after the TRH secreted by the hypothalamus gland in the brain), and finally draws blood 25 minutes later to remeasure the TSH. The TRH injection stimulates the pituitary gland which produces TSH; if the thyroid is underfunctioning, the pituitary gland will secrete excess TSH upon stimulation. If the second TSH blood test measures are high (above 10), it means the patient's thyroid is underactive. A TSH reading of 15 is suspicious, while 20 strongly points to hypothyroidism.

4) Exhausted Adrenal Glands—Chronic stress or hypothyroidism can exhaust your adrenal glands (two small glands nestled atop your kidneys) and lead to PMS. The adrenal glands respond to stress by producing the hormones adrenaline and noradrenaline. Progesterone is the primary raw material the glands use for producing the adrenal hormones. The more adrenaline produced, the more progesterone needed. Thus, chronic stress can lead to a state of estrogen dominance as supplies of progesterone become depleted. As stated earlier, estrogen dominance is a major causal factor in PMS.

In the case of hypothyroidism, the adrenals work overtime attempting to compensate for the malfunctioning thyroid gland. This produces the same situation as above. In both instances, the adrenal glands become exhausted and the fatigue associated with PMS is one of the results.[10]

5) *Candida albicans* Overgrowth—Increased progesterone levels in the second half of the menstrual cycle tend to feed the yeast-like fungus *Candida albicans* (SEE QUICK DEFINITION), says nutritionist Linaya Hayn of Buffalo Grove, Illinois. An overgrowth (a condition called candidiasis) releases more toxins into the system and produces PMS symptoms. Women often have both PMS and candidiasis at the same time, she says.[11]

6) Parasites—Intestinal parasites (SEE QUICK DEFINITION) can trigger digestive symptoms such as bloating, gas, weight gain, and water retention and also cause a buildup of estrogen which stimulates classic PMS symptoms.

7) Nutritional Deficiencies—Many PMS symptoms have been traced to a lack of specific nutrients. For example, a lack of vitamin B6 can hinder the liver's ability to metabolize estrogen, resulting in estrogen dominance. As mentioned previously, estrogen dominance symptoms include fluid retention, bloating, tender breasts, and weight gain—also symptoms of PMS.[12]

8) Food Sensitivities or Allergies—Allergic reactions to certain foods can trigger PMS symptoms such as intestinal disturbances, headaches, depression, and fatigue.

9) Environmental Sensitivities—Women with other toxicities, such as *Candida* overgrowth, can become overly sensitive to chemicals in their environment, such as perfume, car exhaust, and chemically treated building and furniture materials. As with food allergies, exposures can also trigger PMS symptoms.

10) Mercury Dental Fillings—Every year, more than 100 million mercury amalgam fillings are put into the mouths of U.S. dental patients, despite the negative health effects and the fact that, in 1988, the Environmental Protection Agency (EPA) declared scrap dental amalgam a *hazardous waste*. Studies have found a link between mercury amalgam dental fillings and PMS; symptoms improved after filling removal.[13] In addition to PMS, these negative effects include anorexia, depression, fatigue, headaches, nausea, arthritis, and multiple sclerosis.

Electrodermal screening (SEE QUICK DEFINITION) and hair analysis can determine the level of mercury in your body. If you have mercury dental fillings and testing reveals a high mercury level, you might want to consider having your fillings replaced with composite fillings which contain no mercury. Mercury detoxification methods can only provide temporary relief of symptoms if the source of mercury exposure is not eliminated. Once the mercury has been removed from your mouth, you can proceed with detoxification protocols to remove the mercury stored in your tissues.

Chelation therapy (SEE QUICK DEFINITION) is an effective method for accomplishing this. Here, DMPS, the chelating

QUICK DEFINITION

Candida albicans is a yeast-like fungus found widely in nature, in the soil, on vegetables and fruits, and in the human body. It is frequently present in small quantities in the intestines and in a woman's vagina. When its numbers are few, *Candida* is generally not harmful to the human body. A *Candida* overgrowth, a condition called candidiasis, can become pathogenic and cause allergic reactions throughout the body. These reactions can lead to a wide range of symptoms, including depression, fatigue, weight gain, anxiety, rashes, headaches, and muscle cramping.

A **parasite** is any organism that lives off another organism (called a host), and draws nourishment from it. Specifically, parasites are the protozoa (single-cell organisms), arthropods (insects), and worms that infect the body and cause serious damage to tissues and organs. Common forms of the protozoan parasites are *Giardia lamblia*, which causes giardiasis; *Entamoeba histolytica*, which causes dysentery; and *Cryptosporidium*, which causes diarrhea, particularly in people with immunologic diseases such as AIDS. The most common arthropod parasites are lice, mites, ticks, and fleas. Worm parasites include pinworms, roundworms, tapeworms, whipworms, *Trichinella spiralis* (worms usually acquired from eating tainted pork), hookworms, Guinea worms, and filaria (threadlike worms that inhabit the blood and tissues).

agent for mercury, is delivered intravenously. It binds with the mercury in your body and both are then eliminated through the urine and feces. Garlic and chlorella (blue-green algae) also aid in chelation and can be taken as oral supplements to support the intravenous program.

11) Stress—Stress raises adrenaline levels, which increases agitation and hyperactivitiy, both PMS symptoms. Chronic stress leads to adrenal exhaustion (see above) and estrogen dominance.

12) Sleep Disorders—Disturbances in sleep are linked to abnormal production of melatonin, a brain chemical that is a precursor of serotonin. Serotonin, a brain neurotransmitter (SEE QUICK DEFINITION), is stimulated by full-spectrum light (as in sunlight) and improves mood, alertness, and energy levels.[14]

13) Caffeine—Researchers have found that caffeine inhibits the brain neurotransmitter adenosine, which calms the nerve receptors in the body's cells. Without adenosine, the nerve receptors become overly reactive, leading to possible mood swings, agitation, and a general magnification of existing symptoms.[15]

14) Lack of Light—Sunlight and other full-spectrum light sources stimulate serotonin production. A lack of this kind of light produces a deficiency of serotonin which can create lethargy and depression—both PMS symptoms.

15) Lack of Exercise—Exercise promotes the elimination of toxins from the body and improves blood and lymph circulation, important since toxic accumulation tends to worsen PMS symptoms. It also raises the level of endorphins, hormones that have a relaxing, mood-elevating effect, a benefit for PMS mood swings. Finally, exercise relieves stress and anxiety by lowering adrenaline levels.[16]

16) Unresolved Physical or Sexual Abuse—Professionals in the field of treating victims of physical or sexual abuse observe that their patients' PMS symptoms often improve after these issues are resolved in some way.[17]

Understanding all the causal factors which can be involved in PMS enables you to identify what is operating in your particular case. You can then treat the origins of the syndrome, rather than throwing antidepressants and other drugs at the symptoms. In her own words, **Jesse Hanley, M.D.**, explores the emotional components of PMS, explains in more detail the physiological factors, and offers successful natural solutions for eliminating the disorder:

> A **neurotransmitter** is a brain chemical with the specific function of enabling communications to happen between brain cells. Chief among the 100 identified to date are acetylcholine, gamma-aminobutyric acid (GABA), serotonin, dopamine, and norepinephrine. Acetylcholine is required for short-term memory and all muscle contractions. GABA works to stop excess nerve signals and thus keeps brain firings from getting out of control; serotonin does the same and helps produce sleep, regulate pain, and influence mood, although too much serotonin can produce depression. Norepinephrine is an excitatory neurotransmitter.

Hormonal Balancing and Self-Awareness are Keys to Reversing PMS

PMS is an opportunity for women to look at their lives and see how much they are in rhythm or out of rhythm with their own body. Premenstrual syndrome and menopause are generally viewed as "curses," but in my practice, I help women discover their "gifts." PMS is a valuable opportunity to become more attuned to what's going on inside yourself. When women can transform their relationship to their cycle, the hardship melts into increased sensitivity and clarity of direction and purpose.

In my consultations with women who have PMS symptoms, I suggest they honor their feelings and appreciate that there is a purpose to these symptoms. PMS is actually valuable because it opens a window of increased sensitivity to pain and helps women to remember their wisdom. Technically, PMS is a sign that something is not working right, whether nutritionally, hormonally, or psychologically. By taking us to the brink each month, PMS becomes a wake-up call to correct these imbalances. When we attend to them, the result is a healthier life and deeper self-respect, as well as a preparation for a smooth transition through menopause (cessation of menstrual periods).

I strive to empower women to develop self-respect for their normal biological processes and womanhood. I encourage women to ask questions, to evaluate the possible effects of trading a little comfort now for a long-term risk. Regrettably, we're a culture that doesn't deal with things until they're an emergency, especially the health of a woman's body. Too often we wait until it's a dreadful problem, such as fibroids, endometriosis, or cancer that might require surgery.

Many women work in mainstream jobs where it is uncomfortable and unsafe for them to be fully, biologically, a woman. Birth control pills keep their hormones so even they barely have a noticeable monthly

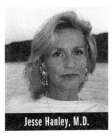

Jesse Hanley, M.D.

"PMS is a sign that something is not working right, whether nutritionally, hormonally, or psychologically," says Dr. Hanley. "By taking us to the brink each month, PMS becomes a wake-up call to correct these imbalances."

cycle except for minimal bleeding. Many women become almost addicted to not being a woman, to not understanding the natural cycling of hormones and the feelings, increased sensitivity, intuition, and creativity this evokes. It's a kind of medical self-destruction that will surely create health problems.

There is an old concept that the uterus, the *hyster*, is the cause of "hysteria" in a woman, and that by removing it through a hysterectomy a woman will become less emotional, more like a man and thus easier to control. Approximately 33% of American women will have a hysterectomy by age 60; about 600,000 are performed every year, but many of these are medically unnecessary. Chinese medicine describes the uterus as the place where a woman's energy and essence reside, so we need to rethink our approach to uterine health.

PMS is a clustering of symptoms magnified by a hormonal imbalance. If you are truly healthy, the experience of menstruation will not be so upsetting, biochemically or psychologically. But to get to this kind of health, you need to undo the effects of a series of obstacles. There are many human-made environmental chemicals, pesticides, and herbicides that masquerade as estrogen once they're inside your body and thereby upset the delicate hormonal balance. The message is this: heed what your premenstrual symptoms are telling you before you get sick from them.

Hold the Estrogen—Many of the reproductive problems women experience, including PMS and many menopausal symptoms, are not a deficiency of estrogen, but instead an excess of estrogen relative to the level of progesterone [the estrogen dominance discussed earlier]. There is a dramatic lack of understanding in mainstream medicine of this progesterone/estrogen imbalance and its significance and dangerous effect on female tissues. Consequently, women are not getting the help they need.

A perfect example is the way so many physicians immediately put women on estrogen replacement therapy the minute they start complaining about perimenopausal (nearing menopause) symptoms. It's the wrong thing to do because it's the wrong hormone; for women who suffer from PMS, it will make their symptoms worse. Physicians do this with no hormonal monitoring. I've only met one patient in my years of practice whose physician actually measured her hormone levels after giving female hormones to her.

There are natural, safe, and healthy alternatives to birth control pills, hysterectomies, and estrogen replacement therapy as a way of making a healthy transition from being a menstruating woman to being a menopausal woman. Estrogen rarely declines until the onset of menopause and hot flashes and declines much less than progesterone. Taking Premarin, Estraderm, or Estrase (the three estrogens most commonly prescribed) further upsets your estrogen/progesterone imbalance and only invites more problems.

The idea that if a woman takes estrogen she'll look young forever is a dangerous illusion. Estrogen causes her to retain fluids which plump up her skin and produce weight gain. Excess water can be retained in the brain, causing irritability; or it can be retained in the breasts, making them swollen, lumpy, tender, and crampy; or it can stimulate excessive, potentially dangerous glandular growth in the colon, breast, and uterus.

Restoring Progesterone Naturally—We're seeing declining levels of progesterone starting at age 30 all through the Western world. Mainstream medicine doesn't understand the importance of progesterone. It focuses on progestin in the form of products such as Provera, Agest, and DepoProvera. These progesterone-like synthetic chemicals don't have all the good effects and benefits, such as stimulating bone growth and preempting osteoporosis, that you get from natural progesterone. Instead, they have many negative side effects including water retention, depression, and the increased risk of blood clots.

Progesterone cream delivered through the skin (transdermally) is the best form of delivery. When you take female hormones orally, 90% are destroyed by the liver and only 10% get into your blood. The burden on the liver and gallbladder is known to increase the risk of gallstones, gallbladder disease, and liver cancer.

The doses and periods of application vary according to what it's being used for (PMS, fibroids, or menopause) and the strength of the product. Generally, women should apply a half-teaspoon twice a day from ovulation to the day before bleeding. I recommend that you rub it on your abdomen below the navel, over your uterus, on your breasts, and perhaps a tiny amount on your arms and face. For about 80% of the women I've treated with progesterone cream, the

Acupressure First Aid for PMS

Acupressure applied to your pelvic and sacral areas can be a quick and potent emergency strategy to relieve the pain, cramping, and other symptoms of PMS and dysmenorrhea. Consult the accompanying charts to determine which are the best points to press for your condition.

Once you have selected the points, lie down and relax on a treatment table or bed, and apply firm, but not painful pressure (thumbs work the best) on one or two points (a friend may have to do the sacral points) for ten seconds to one minute, until the application feels complete, or until you feel a relaxation of the underlying muscles or organs. Then move to another set of points. Continue until you feel relief, repeating the points if necessary. Rest quietly afterward for at least a few minutes.

QUICK DEFINITION

Acupressure is an ancient Chinese massage technique, based on acupuncture, which uses gentle pressure of the fingers instead of needles on the meridian points to clear these energy pathways and stimulate the organs. Many acupressure techniques can be self-administered. Finger pressure should be steady and firm and may be applied to a point for 10 seconds to one minute, depending on the individual.

According to acupressure educator Michael Gach, treating the following points can provide relief for PMS symptoms:[18]

Point	Benefits and Uses (Location on the body)
CV 6	Relieves PMS, menstrual cramps, reproductive problems, abnormal vaginal discharge, irregular periods, and constipation that increases menstrual pain. (Two finger widths below belly button)
CV 4	Relieves menstrual cramps, uroreproductive problems, abnormal vaginal discharge, irregular menstrual periods, and incontinence. (Four finger widths below the belly button)
Sp 12, Sp 13	Relieves menstrual cramps and abdominal discomfort. (In the pelvic area, in the middle of the crease where the leg joins the trunk of the body)
B 27, B 28	Relieves hip pain, menstrual cramps, urine retention, and reproductive problems. (On the sacrum—the large bony area at the base of the spine)
B 29, B 30	Relieves lower back pain, sciatica, and sacral pain due to menstruation. (On the sacrum)
B 31, B 32	Relieves PMS and menstrual tension. (On the sacrum)
B 33, B 34	Relieves back problems, genital pain, impotency, and sterility. (On the sacrum)
B 48	Relieves pelvic tension, PMS, menstrual cramps, and urinary problems. (One or two finger widths outside the sacrum and midway between the top of the hipbone and the base of the buttocks)

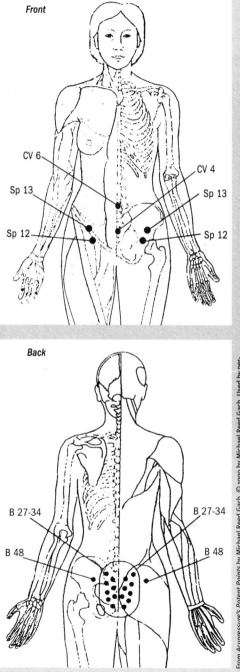

Front

CV 6
Sp 13
Sp 12
CV 4
Sp 13
Sp 12

Back

B 27-34
B 48
B 27-34
B 48

"I've observed that the Norplant contraceptive tends to upset women," says Dr. Hanley. "It contains a synthetic progesterone that interferes with the monthly hormonal cycle and makes women more miserable."

hormones are efficiently absorbed and reduce symptoms.

In addition to using progesterone cream if that is appropriate for your age and hormonal level, the following are useful steps to take in eliminating your PMS:

Run From Norplant—I've observed that the Norplant contraceptive tends to upset women. It contains a synthetic progesterone that interferes with the monthly hormonal cycle and makes women more miserable. This product, like all synthetic progesterones, is associated with an increased risk of cardiovascular disease and blood clots, can produce water retention, weight gain, irregular bleeding, and depression, and interfere with thyroid function. Some patients tell me that using this form of contraception makes them feel as if a black cloud has settled over them.

Have a Hormone Fast—I recommend that a woman "cycle" her hormones in a way that resembles how her body has always done this. Constant hormonal stimulation (as in hormone replacement therapy) may be convenient; unfortunately, it is also probably dangerous. Previous to this generation, women have always "cycled," meaning they've had four to seven days off every month (during menstruation when estrogen and progesterone levels are at their lowest) so their body gets a break. Discontinue all hormone treatments during this "fast." Let your tissues and organs have four to seven days off monthly to detoxify from the hormonal effects.

Change Your Diet and Take Supplements—Choose foods that are low in fat, high in fiber, unprocessed, and unrefined. Sugar, fats, alcohol, and white flour are notorious for increasing the symptoms of hormonal imbalances, from the mood swings and irritability of PMS to uterine fibroids and fibrocystic breasts. The greater your discomfort, the cleaner your diet must be. Milk products, however, should be completely eliminated, regardless of your symptom status. According to research from Frank Oski, M.D., of Johns Hopkins University School of Medicine, milk products can help cause osteoporosis, heart disease, and allergies. Milk is probably one of the most concentrated sources of harmful pesticides and environmental estrogen-like chemicals. These mimic and exaggerate the activity of natural estrogen in your body.

Taking a vitamin supplement is as important as changing your diet. That's because we get fewer nutrients in our depleted standard American diet; the soil our food is grown in is gravely deficient in nutrients, so even healthy foods have fewer nutrients than they used to; and our absorption and digestion become less efficient as we age. I recommend multiple vitamin formulas that are taken with meals. A good supplement for women should contain, specifically, 600 mg of calcium and 500-600 mg of magnesium.

Detoxify Your Liver—Many of the problems women experience can be alleviated by cleansing the liver. The liver is the largest filter in the body, responsible for processing all hormones and toxins; it must also deal with thousands of toxic substances that routinely enter the human body. First, take the pressure off your liver by lowering the amounts of oils (except olive oil) and fats in your diet, especially fried fats because these do more damage to the liver than any other single food.

Second, start a liver-cleansing program using a preformulated blend, such as Eclectic Institute's Opti-Lipotropic and Prevail's Metabolic Liver Formula. The purpose of Opti-Lipotropic (containing vitamin B6, choline, inositol, dandelion, celandine, beet leaf, Oregon grape, and milk thistle, among others) is to remove fats and other poisons from the liver. Metabolic Liver Formula also contains herbs and natural plant enzymes that help detoxify and strengthen the liver. These ingredients work best when used together, so do not take them singly.

I recommend doing a two-month (even better, three-month) course of this at least once a year. For women with severe PMS, the course can be for longer periods of time and more often. All women should start doing this by age 35 to 40, and it wouldn't hurt to begin this preventive-

Magnesium Can Ease PMS Symptoms

Taking magnesium supplements the next time you experience the various symptoms of PMS may be the solution, advises Melvyn Werbach, M.D. Recent studies showed that of 192 women taking 400 mg of magnesium daily during PMS, 95% experienced less breast pain and had less weight gain; 89% suffered less nervous tension; and 43% had fewer headaches. Dr. Werbach further advises that women should take 50 mg daily of vitamin B6 with the magnesium, as this helps with magnesium absorption.[19]

Aromatherapy Baths for PMS

The following essential oil baths can help relieve PMS, according to aromatherapy educator Erich Keller.[20] Put drops as directed below into an empty, one-quart container; fill with warm water. For complete dispersion of oil particles in the bath, dribble the mixture slowly into the bath water as it comes out of the tap. Remain in the bath for at least 20 minutes.

- **Menstrual cramps and pain:** 4 drops clary sage, 3 marjoram, 2 peppermint

- **Muscle tension:** 4 drops rosemary, 2 marjoram, 3 lavender

- **Shock:** 4 drops clary sage, 2 marjoram, 2 rose, 2 ylang-ylang

- **Toxicity:** 2 drops geranium, 2 rosemary, 2 juniper or 3 drops thyme, 2 rosemary, 1 lavender, 1 peppermint

- **Insomnia:** 4 drops neroli, 2 Roman chamomile

- **Mental confusion:** 6 drops lemon, 2 lemongrass, 2 lavender

- **Fatigue:** 6 drops rosemary, 2 bergamot

- **Stress:** 6 drops frankincense, 4 patchouli, 2 bergamot, 3 lavender

- **Irritability:** $1/8$ ounce jojoba oil, 4 drops lavender, 3 chamomile, 2 clary sage, 1 frankincense. Wear this as a body fragrance, inhale directly from the container, or mix in your next bath.

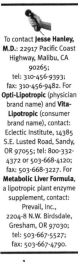

To contact **Jesse Hanley, M.D.**: 22917 Pacific Coast Highway, Malibu, CA 90265; tel: 310-456-9393; fax: 310-456-9482. For **Opti-Lipotropic** (physician brand name) and **Vita-Lipotropic** (consumer brand name), contact: Eclectic Institute, 14385 S.E. Lusted Road, Sandy, OR 97055; tel: 800-332-4372 or 503-668-4120; fax: 503-668-3227. For **Metabolic Liver Formula**, a lipotropic plant enzyme supplement, contact: Prevail, Inc., 2204-8 N.W. Birdsdale, Gresham, OR 97030; tel: 503-667-5527; fax: 503-667-4790.

ly in your twenties. Detoxification with these herbal formulas assists your liver in undoing its part in the body's imbalance. I recommend that you do this in consultation with a health practitioner who will tailor it to your unique needs. ■

Alternative Medicine Therapies for PMS

Once you have established the causal factors of your PMS, alternative medicine has many treatment options to address those issues and assist in rebalancing your body. Included here are lifestyle recommendations, aromatherapy, Ayurvedic medicine, herbal medicine, probiotic supplements, and liver detoxification.

Lifestyle Changes

A few minor lifestyle adjustments are all that stands between you and permanent relief of PMS symptoms, according to Marla Ahlgrimm, R.Ph., a registered pharmacist and co-founder of PMS Access, an organization providing information to women and health-care providers. Ahlgrimm outlines these steps for eliminating PMS:[21]

- **Eat Smart, and Often**—Eating three small meals and three snacks in between meals each day can greatly reduce PMS symptoms. When you don't eat for several hours, your blood sugar drops and your body produces more adrenaline. The increase in adrenaline tends to produce feelings of tension and aggression, making PMS symptoms more severe. Ahlgrimm recommends "holistic" combinations of food for meals and snacks. You will benefit more, for example, by combining a piece of fruit with a small amount of protein (a slice of cheese) or complex carbohydrates (a handful of plain popcorn) than by eating fruit alone.

Eating every few hours may also reduce the food cravings typically reported by PMS sufferers. Avoid sugary and salty foods, caffeine, and alcohol, as these can promote bloating, headaches, tension, and depression.

■ **Exercise Regularly**—Research suggests that even moderate exercise can benefit PMS sufferers. During exercise, the body releases endorphins, substances which reduce tension and anxiety. To further reduce stress, exercise in a pleasant place such as an outdoor park, says Ahlgrimm. Exercise also increases circulation and alleviates bloating and breast tenderness. Walking briskly for 30 minutes, three days a week can significantly decrease PMS symptoms, she says.

■ **Use Nutritional Supplements Wisely**—While many women know that taking supplements can ease PMS, they may not know how to combine them for maximum absorption. For example, while calcium deficiency has been linked to some PMS symptoms, taking calcium alone may not help because the body will not absorb calcium unless it has enough magnesium. Ahlgrimm typically prescribes a combination supplement with a two-to-one ratio of magnesium to calcium.

Vitamin B6: Proven PMS Relief

Vitamin B6 (pyridoxine) may be the "ideal nutrient" for women with PMS, according to Alan Gaby, M.D. In one study, 25 women whose PMS symptoms ranged from moderate to severe took vitamin B6 daily for three months; then they took a placebo (an inactive substance) for three months. Of these women, 84% experienced a far greater improvement in their symptoms with vitamin B6 than with the placebo.

In another study of 70 women with PMS who took vitamin B6, 60% of those who had reported depression with their PMS said they were cured or markedly improved. Among those with headaches, 81% said they felt better; for bloating and swelling, 60%; for irritability, 56%; lethargy, 52%; and breast tenderness, 52%.[22]

A third study involving 434 PMS sufferers showed that taking 25-100 mg of vitamin B6 twice daily (adjusting dosage on an individual basis) contributed to overall symptom relief in 82% of participants.[23]

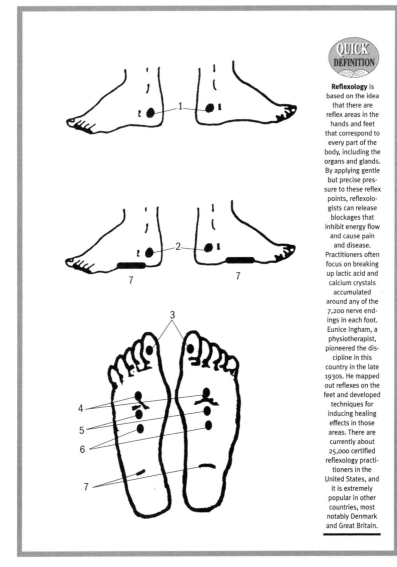

REFLEXOLOGY FOR PMS SYMPTOMS. **Applying pressure to reflexology (SEE QUICK DEFINITION) points on the hands and feet can reduce the symptoms of PMS. After receiving ear, hand, and foot reflexology in 30-minute sessions once weekly for eight weeks, 35 women experienced a 62% reduction in their PMS symptoms.[24] Here's a diagram of the foot points used to help women in the PMS study described above. The numbers indicate what part of the body is influenced: 1—ovary; 2—uterus; 3—pituitary; 4—solar plexus; 5—adrenal glands; 6—kidneys; 7—sympathetic nervous system.[25]**

The body also requires a certain amount of magnesium for effective absoption of vitamin B6. Vitamin B6 helps to reduce premenstrual bloating and depression. If you are not already supplementing with calcium/magnesium, Ahlgrimm suggests taking a B-complex formula which also contains magnesium. The B-complex also helps the body absorb evening primrose oil which lowers the body's production of the hormone prolactin and thus alleviates PMS symptoms. You should also take at least 600 mg of vitamin C daily with the evening primrose oil for optimum absorption of the herb.

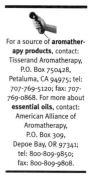

For a source of **aromatherapy products**, contact: Tisserand Aromatherapy, P.O. Box 750428, Petaluma, CA 94975; tel: 707-769-5120; fax: 707-769-0868. For more about **essential oils**, contact: American Alliance of Aromatherapy, P.O. Box 309, Depoe Bay, OR 97341; tel: 800-809-9850; fax: 800-809-9808.

British health authority Lynne McTaggart, editor of the journal *What Doctors Don't Tell You*, culled the clinical research and summarizes proven natural techniques for obtaining relief from PMS symptoms, a number of which concur with those recommended by Marla Ahlgrimm above. They are as follows:[26]

■ Reduce or eliminate the use of dairy products and caffeine from coffee, soft drinks, or chocolate. This can help reduce breast tenderness.

■ Increase your intake of vitamins B6, B12, and the entire B complex as deficiencies in these nutrients are associated with high levels of estrogen. Also helpful for the liver in its job of inactivating estrogen are vitamins C and E and the minerals selenium and magnesium.

■ Expose yourself to at least two hours of bright light treatment to help with symptoms such as weight gain, depression, fatigue, irritability, and social withdrawal.

■ Get 20 minutes of aerobic exercise (such as brisk walking) at least three days a week to improve blood circulation and the secretion of endorphins, brain chemicals known to improve mood.

■ Switch to a vegetarian diet. Studies show that vegetarians excrete two to three times more estrogen in their feces than nonvegetarians; women vegetarians also have 50% less unconjugated estrogen (estrogen after being metabolized) in the blood than meat-eating women.

Along with the lifestyle changes you can implement yourself, there are a number of therapies you can use for further relief and complete reversal of your PMS.

Success Story: Aromatherapy Eliminates PMS Symptoms

Jane, 18, had considerable premenstrual difficulties including abdominal pain, bloating, cold sweats, disturbed sleep, headaches, lethargy, nausea, skin blemishes, and tension—a total of 22 major symptoms—when she consulted British aromatherapy practitioner J. Noel

Hulmston. He designed a six-month treatment program for Jane consisting of body massage with aromatherapy oils (SEE QUICK DEFINITION).

For rubbing on her back, Hulmston selected a blend of chamomile and marjoram essential oils in a sweet almond oil base. For massage on the front of her body, Jane used a blend of lavender and clary sage. On her arms and shoulders, Jane rubbed a rose blend, mixed with lemon grass. For her legs she used a mix of lavender and ylang-ylang, and for her face, a mix of neroli oil. All of these oils were in a base of sweet almond oil.

Jane applied (or had someone else apply) these essential oils on the appropriate body areas on days ten and five before the onset of her period each month. After two months of this, Hulmston changed it to days seven and three before menstruation. After six months of treatment, the most serious of Jane's conditions were "markedly improved," while her problem with skin blemishes had improved by 50%. In all, 89% of her original symptoms had ceased.[27]

Ayurvedic Medicine

Ayurveda's (SEE QUICK DEFINITION) approach to treating PMS relies on basic principles that, once understood, can also shed light on other female health disorders, says Nancy Lonsdorf, M.D., a practitioner of Ayurvedic medicine and medical director of the Maharishi Ayurveda Medical Center in Rockville, Maryland. Dr. Lonsdorf explains: "All female disorders are caused by imbalances that fall into three categories of diagnosis: the balance of the *doshas* or bodily humors—*vata* (responsible for movement), *pitta* (for metabolism), and *kapha* (for structure); biological rhythm; and purification. All treatments address these three areas of body health."

In Ayurveda, the individual can do much for herself through dietary and lifestyle changes. In turn, the practitioner provides the diagnosis and sets the direction of self-care, and can provide herbs to balance the interaction of the *doshas*. Dr. Lonsdorf provides the following guidelines for Ayurvedic self-care based on predominant symptoms:[28]

1) Balance of the *doshas*: *Vata* energy is responsible in

menstruation for the flow of blood and the endometrial lining. An imbalance manifests as mood swings, a tendency to cry, insomnia, anxiety, and constipation. To correct an imbalance, establish regular daily routines, reduce workload, increase rest and sleep, meditate, and add to the diet a little more oil, sweet-tasting foods (but not refined sugars), salt, and cooked warm foods such as cereal and stews.

To contact **Nancy Lonsdorf, M.D.**: Maharishi Ayurveda Medical Center, 4701 Randolph Road, Suite G-11, Rockville, MD 20852; tel: 301-770-5690; fax: 301-770-5694.

Pitta energy is responsible in menstruation for hormonal changes. An imbalance manifests as anger, irritability, skin rashes, and diarrhea. To correct an imbalance, reduce "Type A" behavior or overactivity and overperformance, establish regular daily routines, meditate, and avoid spicy foods, greasy foods, artificial ingredients, chocolate, caffeine, and alcohol.

Kapha energy is responsible in menstruation for the contents of the menstrual flow. An imbalance manifests as fluid retention, swollen breasts, weight gain, and lethargy. To correct an imbalance, increase exercise, avoid sour and sweet foods, and increase spicy foods and legumes.

2) Biological rhythm: Dr. Lonsdorf recommends as a general good habit going to bed at 10 p.m. and rising at 6 a.m., hours at which the earth's energy enhances human energy.

3) Purification: This is used to remove *ama* (waste and impurity) from the body. Dr. Lonsdorf sees a parallel in the notion of removing *ama* and the effects of facilitating menstrual flow since iron, eliminated with the blood, is now being linked to heart disease when in excess in the body.[29] Dietary procedures to improve digestion and elimination include drinking plenty of warm to hot water and avoiding meat, cheese, caffeine, and alcohol. On the 14th or 15th day of the cycle, Dr. Lonsdorf suggests using a laxative of four to five teaspoons of castor oil or senna tea followed by a light diet for the rest of the day.

Here's how to reduce your discomfort during PMS and menstruation, according to Dr. Lonsdorf:[30]

■ On the first day of menstruation, have a liquid diet (blended soups, juices) to aid digestion.

■ Avoid eggs and fermented, spicy, or sour foods.

■ Eat foods that are warm and easy to digest.

■ Eat less than usual, especially in the evening.

■ Avoid cheese, yogurt, red meat, fried foods, and chocolate.

■ Avoid carbonated beverages and cold drinks.

■ If you crave salt, satisfy the desire minimally, but try to resist the sugar craving or find natural substitutes such as whipped cream with

honey rather than ice cream.
- Take a hot shower rather than a bath.
- Budget time for resting.
- Reduce your exercise schedule.
- Spend some time turning inward.

Herbal Medicine

While many herbs can aid in the relief of PMS symptoms, research has shown that grape seed extract and chastetree berry are particularly powerful.

Grape seed extract has been found to help a variety of premenstrual symptoms. When 165 women took a standardized extract of grape seed proanthocyanidin (a bioflavonoid, or vitamin C helper) daily for two months, they experienced a 60.8% improvement in their third cycle; and after a total of four cycles, a 78.8% improvement in abdominal swelling, breast symptoms, pelvic pain, fluctuations in weight, and water retention and swelling in the legs. Researchers believe that the bioflavonoids in grape seed block the synthesis of estrogen and thereby produce their benefits.[31]

Another all-purpose PMS aid is chastetree berry *(Vitex agnus-castus)*. *Vitex* effectively reduces PMS symptoms while producing very few side effects, according to a comprehensive German study. In the study, 551 women with PMS and other menstrual problems were treated with a tincture (fresh herbal essence extracted and preserved in alcohol) of chastetree berry.

Within three months, nearly 84% of the women experienced marked improvement of symptoms, and more than 25% of these reported feeling better after only four weeks of using chastetree. By the end of the study, 25% of the patients discontinued treatment because their symptoms had disappeared entirely. The side effects reported by 28 women (5% of all patients) were mild and harmless. Research indicates that chastetree is so effective in relieving menstrual problems because it lowers the body's production of the hormone prolactin which, as mentioned previously, is commonly linked with PMS symptoms.[32]

Probiotic Therapy

Another nutritional supplement that indirectly helps PMS symptoms are the so-called "friendly" bacteria or probiotics. Noted natural health spokesman Michael Murray, N.D., of Bellevue, Washington, recommends taking one billion to ten billion cells daily of either *L. acidophilus* or *B. bifidum* bacteria. (In most cases, the number of cells per capsule is printed on the bottle. For example, if there are one billion cells per capsule, the dosage would be between one and ten capsules.) These bacteria help establish the proper bacterial flora in the digestive tract, which in turn promotes the elimination of excess estrogens and toxins (both causes of PMS) from the body.

Probiotics not only aid in the elimination of estrogens by improving digestion, but they also support the liver which is the organ responsible for processing excess estrogen and other toxins and excreting them into the bile, where they can be eliminated. An enzyme called beta-glucuronidase can disturb that process. Beta-glucuronidase breaks a bond that is formed between the toxins and glucoronic acid. This bond is important to maintain because the liver needs to have the glucoronic acid attached to the toxins and excess estrogens in order to process them. If the body has a healthy intestinal flora balance (as with probiotics), the beta-glucuronidase won't have the strength to break the glucoronic acid bond and the toxins and excess estrogen can be excreted by the liver.[33]

For more about **probiotics**, see "Two Ways to Support Your Friendly Bacteria," Chapter 6: Cystitis, p. 222, and Chapter 7: Vaginitis, pp. 250-251.

Liver Detoxification

As Dr. Jesse Hanley discussed earlier, detoxification and support of the liver are important elements in restoring reproductive health and eliminating PMS. In addition to probiotics, Dr. Murray recommends that women with PMS further assist their livers in the detoxification process by taking lipotropic supplements. These are substances, such as choline, methionine, betaine, folic acid, and vitamin B12, that increase fat metabolism and so help remove fat and bile in the liver. This, says Dr. Murray, has a "decongesting" effect on the liver and improves its function. Dr. Murray recommends using a lipotropic supplement that supplies at least 1,000 mg daily of choline and 500 mg of methionine and/or cysteine daily.[34]

Try Fish Oils for Relief of Cramps

Taking as little as 6 g of fish oil daily during the time of menstrual cramping can significantly reduce the pain. When 42 young women, 15 to 18 years old, took 6 g of fish oil (omega-3 essential fatty acid) daily for two months for relief of menstrual pain, pain reduction was rated at 37%. The women also managed on 53% less conventional pain medication (ibuprofen) for their cramps.[35]

Practical Tips for Eliminating the Four Types of PMS

The alternative therapies described in the previous sections can be effective for PMS in general. In addition, there are specific remedies you can try for each of the four categories of PMS described at the beginning of this chapter. Following are nutritional treatments for individual variations of premenstrual syndrome.

PMS-A–Taking vitamin B6 (pyridoxine) has been shown to reduce blood estrogen and increase progesterone levels, thereby reducing PMS-A symptoms (see sidebar: "Vitamin B6: Proven PMS Relief," p. 37). Most women respond to 50-100 mg daily of vitamin B6, although increasing the dose in the week before menstruation can be helpful, says Alan R. Gaby, M.D., a professor at Bastyr University, a naturopathic college in Bothell, Washington.[36]

In addition to vitamin B6 supplements, adding more fiber to the diet may lessen PMS-A symptoms. A study comparing the estrogen levels of vegetarian versus meat-eating women documented that the vegetarian women, who tended to eat more fiber, had significantly lower blood estrogen levels than did those who ate meat. The authors of the study speculated that eating more fiber helps the body to eliminate excess estrogen through the feces.[37]

As mentioned frequently in this chapter, reducing your caffeine intake can be helpful in reducing PMS. Clinical studies have shown that women who drink large amounts of caffeine are more likely to suffer from PMS-A. According to a survey of 295 female college students, 61% of women who drank 4.5 to 15 caffeinated beverages per day experienced moderate to severe PMS symptoms, while only 16% of women who consumed no caffeine experienced moderate to severe symptoms. By reducing caffeine intake at least three days before onset of PMS, the research suggests, it is possible to reduce the severity of PMS-A.[38]

Melvyn Werbach, M.D., of Tarzana, California, an assistant clinical professor at the University of California School of Medicine in Los Angeles, adds that women who suffer from PMS-A should reduce their intake of dairy products and refined sugars and limit their fats to 30% of their total caloric intake. "Twice as much vegetable protein as animal protein should be consumed," Dr. Werbach adds. He also concurs with the importance of fiber in alleviating PMS-A, recommending at least 20-40 g of fiber daily.[39]

PMS-C–The glucose intolerance associated with PMS-C has been linked to a magnesium deficiency in the blood. Not surprisingly, in a study of women with low blood sugar (hypoglycemia) and PMS, taking a daily supplement of 430 mg of magnesium returned blood sugar levels to normal in over 33%, and produced relief of PMS symptoms in 50%.[40] Another study found that taking 100 mg of vitamin B6 twice daily also helped to normalize magnesium levels in the blood.[41]

In addition to taking magnesium supplements, dietary changes can help PMS-C. Dr. Werbach recommends completely avoiding refined sugar, limiting refined simple carbohydrates to 15% of your daily intake, and consuming unrefined complex carbohydrates as 40% of your diet. These changes will help regulate blood sugar. Dr. Werbach also suggests limiting salt intake to 1 g daily.[42]

In many women, PMS-C is associated with palpitations, fatigue or fainting, and headaches. Of these, premenstrual headache often generates the most complaints, despite the fact that it can be treated fairly easily. As early as 1960, Scandinavian researchers had established that supplementing with vitamin A (200,000-300,000 IU daily) had a beneficial effect on PMS-C-related headaches. Of the 218 participants in the study, 48% reported a complete relief of symptoms, and another 41% noted partial improvement.[43]

PMS-D—For women suffering from premenstrual depression, 6 g daily of the amino acid L-tryptophan, taken from the day of ovulation through the first three days of menstruation, can reduce moderate to severe PMS-related depression by nearly one-half.[44] Women with PMS-D, like those with PMS-C, tend to eat more carbohydrates during the second half of their cycles. Researchers speculate that because the brain's production of serotonin (a known mood enhancer) increases after carbohydrate intake, PMS-D sufferers may eat too many carbohydrates in an unconscious attempt to improve their emotional state.

Instead of eating more carbohydrates, Dr. Werbach recommends women with PMS-D take 3-6 g of tyrosine, an anti-depressant amino acid, every morning if blood tests show they are low in tyrosine. Also, as with the other types of PMS, vitamin B6 and magnesium, in the same doses, can be helpful, he says.[45]

PMS-H—For weight gain associated with water and salt retention, 40 mg of *Ginkgo biloba* extract, taken three times daily, actually prevents sodium from passing out of the circulatory system and becoming trapped in bodily tissues, leading to water retention.[46]

Alternatively, vitamin A and vitamin B6 can also reduce premenstrual water retention. In a clinical study, all 30 participants consid-

To contact **Alan Gaby, M.D.**: 125 N.E. 61st Street, Seattle, WA 98115; tel: 206-522-3404; fax: 206-517-5584, or c/o Bastyr University, 14500 Juanita Drive Northeast, Bothell, WA 98011; tel: 425-823-1300. To contact **Melvyn Werbach, M.D.**: Third Line Press, 4751 Viviana Drive, Tarzana, CA 91356; tel: 818-996-0076; fax: 818-774-1575. Third Line Press can also provide information on Dr. Werbach's series of health books, including *Nutritional Influences on Illness* (1996) and a CD of his collected works.

ered their conditions "considerably improved" after two to six months of treatment with vitamin A supplements (200,000 IU once daily, taken from day 15 of the menstrual cycle until onset of symptoms).[47] Studies involving the effects of vitamin B6 on weight gain and bloating reveal similar results.

Further, simply eating a low-fat diet can also relieve the uncomfortable effects of fluid retention. In a study of 30 healthy premenopausal women, there were "significant" decreases in reports of premenstrual and menstrual weight gain, bloating and breast tenderness (all symptoms associated with water retention) during a four-month period of eating a low-fat diet (fat was 20% of daily intake) compared to four months on a high-fat diet (40% of daily intake).[48] In addition to the low-fat diet, Dr. Werbach recommends that PMS-H sufferers limit salt to 3 g daily and avoid caffeine products altogther.[49]

Dysmenorrhea

Many women suffer through premenstrual syndrome only to endure dysmenorrhea, or pain and cramping, once their period has started. As many as 30% to 50% of women suffer from pain during menstruation[50] and, as with PMS, this has been considered normal. As stated previously, alternative medicine does not regard dysmenorrhea as normal, but rather as an alarm signaling a hidden imbalance in the body.

There are two conventional classifications of dysmenorrhea: primary and secondary. *Primary dysmenorrhea*, in which the pain itself is the main problem, occurs during the ovulatory cycle and is caused by excess production of prostaglandins (SEE QUICK DEFINITION) by the endometrium (uterine lining, normally shed during the bleeding phase) following a decline in progesterone levels.[51] The release of prostaglandins causes the smooth muscles of the uterus to contract, hence the pain. The pain of the cramping can be intense. At least 10% of younger women (those in their teens and early twenties) have symptoms so severe that they cannot participate in their normal activities.[52] Besides lower abdominal pain, cramp sufferers may also experience backache, pinching, and pain sensations in the inner thighs, as well as many of the symptoms of PMS.

For more about **endometriosis**, see Chapter 2: Endometriosis, pp. 68-99.

Secondary dysmenorrhea is menstrual pain that is caused by an underlying pathological factor, such as endometriosis, pelvic inflammatory disease, or a congenital deformity.

Of the two classifications, primary dysmenorrhea is by far the most common and is divided into two subcategories: *primary spasmodic* or *primary congestive*. According to women's health specialist Susan Lark, M.D., of Los Altos, California, primary spasmodic dysmenorrhea, the type most commonly found in women in their early teens to late twenties, includes "sharp, viselike pains that are caused by a constriction and tightening of the uterine muscle." Adding to the problem, says Dr. Lark, is a slowdown in blood circulation and oxygen delivery to the uterine muscles. As a result, metabolism waste products like carbon dioxide and lactic acid accumulate and tend to make the pain worse.[53]

In contrast, primary congestive dysmenorrhea produces a dull aching in the lower back and pelvic regions, often accompanied by bloating, weight gain, breast tenderness, headaches, and irritability. Women in their thirties and forties tend to have the worst cases of this type of dysmenorrhea, particularly if they have an excess estrogen imbalance, states Dr. Lark.[54]

Causes of Dysmenorrhea

- Excess production of prostaglandins
- Hormonal imbalance
- Fluid retention
- Food sensitivities and allergies
- Liver toxicity
- Bladder infection
- Lack of exercise
- Poor circulation
- Stress
- Intrauterine devices (IUDs)
- Vaginal yeast infection

Alternative Medicine Therapies for Dysmenorrhea

- Acupuncture
- Detoxification
- Dietary recommendations
- Homeopathy
- Nutritional supplements
- Traditional Chinese medicine

Alternative Medicine Therapies for Dysmenorrhea

As with PMS, you do not have to just live through dysmenorrhea. There are natural therapies which can help you with both symptom relief and permanent resolution of primary dysmenorrhea. (This section focuses on the primary category because secondary dysmenorrhea involves treating underlying conditions such as that addressed in the chapter on endometriosis). Primary dysmenorrhea and PMS, along

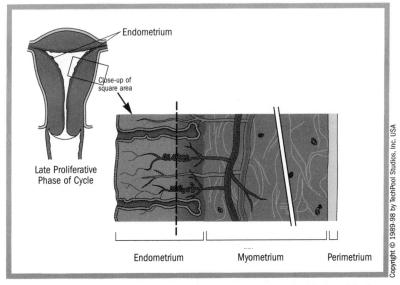

A CLOSE-UP OF THE LAYERS OF THE UTERINE LINING. The endometrium (inside layer) is the uterine layer that builds up during the proliferative phase and then sheds during menstruation. The myometrium, the source of most uterine fibroids, is the "muscle" of the uterus. The perimetrium forms both the outside layer of the uterus *and* part of the inside lining of the abdominal cavity.

with a number of the health conditions included in this book, share many of the same causes. The following case study illustrates the often complex involvement of a number of these causes and demonstrates their successful reversal with natural therapies.

Success Story: Severe Menstrual Problems Cured

Esmé, 36, had serious hormonal disturbances and menstrual problems, including an irregular cycle (from 23 to 31 days), dysmenorrhea, and six years of infertility. In addition, Esmé had endured constipation since the age of five, her hair and skin were overly dry, she had a rash on her hands, and she had a tendency to low blood sugar (hypoglycemia) and yeast infection (candidiasis). Her adrenal glands were under stress and she had sore hips and back pain. Dissatisfied when treatment by conventional physicians failed to bring any relief, Esmé consulted Katrina Marie Kulhay, D.C., of the Kulhay Wellness Centre in Toronto, Ontario, Canada.

Doctors she had consulted prior to seeing Dr. Kulhay had determined that Esmé had an underactive thyroid (hypothyroidism), that all her hormones were at low levels, and that she was already in the earliest stage of menopause. They could find no clinical reason for her infertility and subjected her to three years of hormone injections and artificial insemination, neither of which helped.

Dr. Kulhay used electrodermal screening (EDS—SEE QUICK DEFINITION) to test Esmé for possible allergies. The EDS results indicated that Esmé had food allergies to dairy products, wheat, tea, sugar, honey, shrimp, and bananas. "These were the first clues to her problems that any physician had detected," observes Dr. Kulhay. Esmé subsequently eliminated these foods from her diet.

A second EDS test for the functional status of internal organs showed that her system was infested with parasites (amoebae and ascarids [nematode worms]) and *E. coli*. A hair analysis revealed multiple nutrient deficiencies and high levels of the heavy metals aluminum and copper.

A bone mineral density test showed that osteoporosis (bone embrittlement, leading to easy fractures) was already under way, with a 10% bone loss registered in Esmé's thigh bones (femurs). Darkfield microscopic examination (SEE QUICK DEFINITION) of her blood confirmed the parasite infestation and documented an imbalance of intestinal microflora and the proliferation of bacteria and fungi in her intestines.

Dr. Kulhay, in cooperation with acupuncturists and naturopaths on her staff, put together a treatment program for Esmé. It was a complicated case and required complex prescribing to redress all the symptoms, reports Dr. Kulhay. The complete program to correct Esmé's problems spanned six years; not all components were given simultaneously.

To address the osteoporosis, Esmé took daily dosages of vitamin E (800 IU), vitamin C (3,000 mg), and Formula O.S.X. (a microcrystalline hydroxyapatite form of calcium, 1,000 mg). She also applied natural progesterone cream topically to soft-tissue areas of her body (one teaspoon, twice daily, from days 14 to 28 of her cycle). She did this consistently for two years.

The progesterone and vitamin E also addressed her infertility. In addition, Dr. Kulhay's team started Esmé on wheat germ oil (two tablespoons, twice daily); liquid folic acid (30 drops, twice daily); herbal homeopathic (SEE QUICK DEFINITION) fertility combinations Spectrum

QUICK DEFINITION

Electrodermal screening is a form of computerized information gathering, based on physics, not chemistry. A blunt, noninvasive electric probe is placed at specific points on the patient's hands, face, or feet, corresponding to acupuncture points at the beginning or end of energy meridians. Minute electrical discharges from these points serve as information signals about the condition of the body's organs and systems, useful for the physician in evaluation and developing a treatment plan.

Darkfield microscopy is a way of studying living whole blood cells under a specially adapted microscope that projects the dynamic image, magnified 1,400 times, onto a video screen. With a darkfield light condenser, images of high contrast are projected, so that the object appears bright against a dark background. The skilled physician can detect early signs of illness in the form of microorganisms in the blood known to produce disease. The amount of time the blood cell stays viable and alive indicates the overall health of the individual. Specifically, darkfield microscopy reveals distortions of red blood cells (which in turn indicate nutritional status), possible undesirable bacterial or fungal life forms, and blood ecology patterns indicative of health or illness.

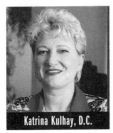

Katrina Kulhay, D.C.

The prescription complexity of Esmé's case highlights how a practitioner in an integrated wellness center such as that of Katrina Marie Kulhay, D.C., must be a master of many fields.

305-E (days one to 14 of her cycle) and Spectrum 305-P (days 14 to 28); *Ovarium compositum* and *Ubiquinone compositum* by ampule injection (three times per week); Sequoia extract from the sequoia tree, a precursor to 17 hormones needed for the female hormonal system (30 drops, twice daily, for one year); and *Folliculinum* (homeopathic organ and tissue extracts, one dose, three times daily).

The sequoia extract is a remedy from gemmotherapy, a homeopathy-based approach, developed in France in the 1960s and involving 56 specific plants (in this case, *Sequoia gigantea*). *Folliculinum* is a homeopathic version of the female ovarian follicle that releases the egg; functionally, it works like a high potency homeopathic estrogen for cases of prolonged and painful menstruation. An excess of estrogen leads to the formation of too much endometrial lining in the uterus, the first stage of growing a fibroid. *Folliculinum* lowers the amount and effects of estrogen in relation to progesterone.

The acupuncturist (SEE QUICK DEFINITION) treated various points on Esmé's body to rebalance the hormone levels while the naturopath prescribed several homeopathic remedies (one at a time) including *Medorrhinum* 10M (one dose for three days), *Natrum muriacticum* 50M (same dose), and *Natrum phosphate* 200K. Esmé was taken off Synthroid, a synthetic thyroid hor-

To contact **Katrina Kulhay, D.C.**: The Kulhay Wellness Centre, 2 St. Clair Avenue, Suite 607, Toronto, Ontario M4V 1L5 Canada; tel: 416-961-1900; fax: 416-961-9578. For more about **Herbotox, H.M.F., Unda 243, 1000, and 16, Juniperus, H-THY Drops, Fucus vesiculosus Combination Drops**, and **Formula O.S.X.**, contact: Seroyal International, Inc., 44 East Beaver Creek Road, Suite 17, Richmond Hill, Ontario L4B 1G8 Canada; tel: 800-263-5861 or 905-764-6355; fax: 905-764-6357. For **Amalgatox, Anti-Stress, Candidiasis, Lymphatic Drainer, Pitui-Plus, Alpha-Ortho-Phos, Hepachol,** and **Fiber Life**, contact: Standard Enzyme Company of North America, P.O. Box 1052, 106 North Buchanan Street, Bremen, GE 30110; tel: 770-537-4445; fax: 770-537-1747. *Ovarium compositum* (called Alviumeel) and *Ubiquinone compositum* (called Ubicoenzyme) are available to physicians only. For more information, contact: Heel, 4001 Cote Vertu, Montreal, Quebec H4R 1R5 Canada; tel: 888-879-4335 or 514-335-2570; fax: 514-335-2463. For *Sequoia gigantea* (and information on 55 other gemmotherapy substances), contact: Dolisos America, Inc., 3014 Rigel Avenue, Las Vegas, NV 89102; tel: 800-365-4767 or 702-871-7153; fax: 702-871-9670.

mone prescribed for her underactive thyroid, and put on several homeopathic formulas including H-THY Drops (ten drops, three times daily), *Fucus vesiculosus* Combination Drops (20 drops, three times daily), and Unda #1000 and #16 for endocrine imbalance.

The constipation and parasite infestation were dealt with through a series of homeopathic formulas, natural liver detoxifying agents, colonics, mustard foot baths, supergreen concentrates, dry skin brushing, and colon cleansing herbs. The low blood sugar, bacterial and fungal overgrowth, and skin rash were addressed with similar multimodal prescribing over several months.

The prescription complexity of this case highlights how a practitioner in an integrated wellness center such as Dr. Kulhay's must be a master of many fields—practicing as a generalist while understanding the specifics of how nutrients, homeopathic remedies, colon cleansing and liver detoxifying protocols, and hormone rebalancing can all work usefully together to restore health to a suffering patient.

The holistic generalist also appreciates the fact that in many cases illness exists in layers and, as it took the patient years to lay down each layer of imbalance, it requires some time (months or sometimes years of treatment) to undo each before the patient's inherent well-being can emerge again.

Esmé remained under Dr. Kulhay's care for six years until her dysmenorrhea and other symptoms, even the early onset of menopause, had been eliminated. Her left and right thigh bones actually regained 10% bone mass, reversing the osteoporosis. Her thyroid and adrenal glands stabilized, requiring no further treatment. Her sugar cravings decreased, the skin rash went away, the constipation disappeared, *Candida* levels returned to normal, and her menstrual cycle became more regular. Although Esmé had still not conceived a child, she reported she felt "fabulous."

The case of Esmé reflects the alternative approach to treating dysmenorrhea. As the result of a comprehensive program addressing each of the underlying causes, not only did Esmé's dysmenorrhea clear up, but her overall health improved tremendously. Following are two more success stories which further illustrate the efficacy of two of the therapies employed in Esmé's case (acupuncture and homeopathy).

QUICK DEFINITION

Acupuncture is an integrated healing system developed by the Chinese over 5,000 years ago and introduced in the United States in the mid-1800s. The treatment is administered by an acupuncturist using hair-thin, stainless-steel needles, generally presterilized and disposable; these are lightly inserted into the skin at any of over 1,000 locations on the body's surface, known as acupoints. Acupoints are places where vital energy, or *qi* (pronounced CHEE), can be accessed by acupuncturists to reduce, enhance, or redirect its flow. These acupoints exist on meridians, which are the body's specific pathways for the flow of energy. In most cases, these energy pathways relate to individual organs or organ systems, designated as Lung, Small Intestine, Heart, and others. There are 12 principal meridians and eight secondary channels. Acupuncture is employed for a wide variety of conditions (the World Health Organization counts 104), including pain relief, asthma, migraines, and arthritis.

Success Story: Dysmenorrhea Reversed With Traditional Chinese Medicine

Janis, 38, had dysmenorrhea which had progressively worsened over the last ten years. The stabbing lower abdominal pains which came on the first day of each period were so severe that Janis had to miss work once a month. Before her periods, Janis experienced bloating and mood swings, and her breasts became lumpy and distended. Her menstrual flow was dark and clotty.

Janis went to Bob Flaws, L.Ac., of Boulder, Colorado, author of more than ten books on traditional Chinese medicine (TCM—SEE QUICK DEFINITION). Based on Janis' symptoms and the appearance of her tongue and quality of her pulses (TCM diagnostic tools), Dr. Flaws determined that she had an energy (*qi*) blockage and accumulation of blood in her liver. In addition, her spleen (involved with the secretion and circulation of bodily fluids) had become weakened.

Janis began treatment one week before her next period. She took herbs through the first day of her period and had one acupuncture treatment every other day for three treatments. When her period came, she experienced no symptoms, except for a few twinges of low back pain. The next month, Janis again took herbs during the week before her period, but this time had no acupuncture treatments. Following this phase of treatment, Janis' menstrual flow was lighter in color and had no clots, clear signals that her blood and energy were moving freely again, notes Dr. Flaws. A few more treatments eliminated the low back pain and Janis has continued to be symptom free.[55]

Success Story: Homeopathy Relieves Painful Menstruation

Although not detailed in Esmé's use of homeopathy, homeopathic remedies can help a woman release the emotions involved in her dysmenorrhea, as the case of Betty illustrates.

Betty, 42, had suffered from painful menstruation since she was 14. In addition, she experienced gas, bloating, and irritability for at least a week before her period began. After a death in the family, her symptoms got worse. In fact, on the second day of menstruation, the pain was so strong and sudden ("like a labor pain," she reported), it made her cry out. She also had a drawing pain down her thighs, occasionally accompanied by prickly skin, which became worse with scratching. Betty was ten pounds overweight and unable to keep to a weight-reducing diet. Her emotions went up and down like a roller coaster and she was often teary.

Betty consulted homeopath Judith A. Lewis, R.N., N.D., of Mill Valley, California. After taking her history and listening to her symptoms, Dr. Lewis gave Betty one dose of homeopathic *Pulsatilla* 10M. Betty cried for three hours, releasing emotional tension. When her next period arrived, there was none of the usual pain (either before or during) and it lasted only three days instead of five. Her next two periods were normal and pain free for the first time in her life. Betty also lost seven pounds, was more focused at work, and more emotionally calm, says Dr. Lewis.[56]

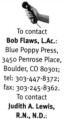

To contact
Bob Flaws, L.Ac.:
Blue Poppy Press,
3450 Penrose Place,
Boulder, CO 80301;
tel: 303-447-8372;
fax: 303-245-8362.
To contact
**Judith A. Lewis,
R.N., N.D.:**
tel: 415-381-4727.

Menorrhagia

Excessive menstruation, or menorrhagia, means that your period is too heavy, flows too fast, or the bleeding is moderate but persists for too long. Mid-cycle spotting (bleeding) may occur as well. Along with a menstrual flow so heavy that it requires changing sanitary pads or tampons every hour, menorrhagia may also involve large blood clots that can be quite painful to pass and further exhaust the already depleted sufferer. In chronic menorrhagia, the blood loss through the excessive flow and blood clots can lead to anemia (a lack of red blood cells).[57]

A common cause of menorrhagia is, again, estrogen dominance. Physical factors such as endometriosis, uterine fibroids, ovarian cysts, or a condition called adenomyosis (endometrial glands lining the uterus grow into the uterine muscle) can also lead to heavy menstruation. Finally, abnormalities of the endometrium, iron and vitamin A deficiencies, hypothyroidism, and intrauterine devices are all considered possible causes of menorrhagia.[58]

In the following section, **Jesse Hanley, M.D.,** explains the hormonal imbalances and the emotional component of menorrhagia, and then presents a case illustrating the successful reversal of this painful and inconvenient malady:

The Hormones and Emotions Behind Menorrhagia

My estimate is that perhaps 16% to 20% of women in their forties have menstrual irregularities in the form of heavy bleeding. According to the *Merck Manual*, about 50% of cases occur in women aged 45 and older. Although it's more common in the forties, it can start showing up in the

Causes of Menorrhagia

In addition to estrogen dominance, other physiological factors can produce heavy bleeding. Some of these are more serious than estrogenic excess and may require a physician's assistance to correct.

- Endometriosis: displaced endometrial cells causing dysfunctional bleeding in 20% to 88% of affected women.
- Fibroids/leiomyomas: benign nodules growing out of uterine smooth muscle occurring in 40% of women by age 40.
- Ovarian cysts: present in 50% of women with menstrual irregularities.
- Adenomyosis: displaced endometrium more likely to occur late in the reproductive years.
- Other causes: blood disorders/abnormal clotting; cervical cancer; thyroid dysfunction; pregnancy complications; vaginal adenosis; intrauterine devices (IUDs).

Alternative Medicine Therapies for Menorrhagia

■ Acupuncture	■ Castor oil packs	■ Chinese herbs
■ Dietary recommendations	■ Herbal medicine	■ Homeopathy
■ Natural hormone therapy	■ Nutritional supplements	■ Psychological counseling

thirties; if it begins when a woman is in her twenties, a genetic predisposition may be involved.

An average healthy menstrual flow lasts from three to seven days. There may be one to two days of heavier bleeding, but each cycle is consistent, much like the preceding period, and the woman does not emerge from menstruation exhausted. With menorrhagia, however, women often cannot get out of bed or leave the house during the heavy flow because they can't be away from a toilet and a tampon for more than an hour. This is abnormal. So, if your flow is heavy enough to make it hard for you to live your life or to contain the flow during menstruation, and if it drains your energy and makes you chronically fatigued and anemic, things have reached the point where you need to take action.

For some, this condition can be resolved easily using natural remedies, especially if a woman doesn't wait ten or 20 years to start dealing with the problem. It is wise not to wait because menorrhagia is a sign of imbalance.

Although birth control pills are often prescribed by conventional physicians to control and reduce the heavy bleeding, I don't regard them as a healthy solution. Some women may not notice the side effects at first, but evidence connects the use of birth control pills with weight gain, water retention, vitamin deficiencies, breast and uterine cancer, blood clots, strokes, and autoimmune diseases.

Remember, oral contraceptives are made of synthetic hormones and these do not match a woman's hormones. However, I would rather a woman use birth control pills temporarily as an emergency measure to control heavy bleeding than have a hysterectomy (surgical removal of the uterus) which is conventional medicine's other solution for severe, health-threatening cases of menorrhagia.

When there is not another organic or physiological factor involved (see sidebar: "Causes of Menorrhagia," p. 54), heavy menstrual bleeding is generally a result of too much estrogen and too little progesterone in a woman's system. Beginning at around age 35, a woman's progesterone production starts to decline. The key to menstrual regularity is achieving the correct balance between estrogen and progesterone.

Progesterone's role in the menstrual cycle is to halt the cells' proliferation in the uterus begun under estrogen and turn on their

"Some women don't know until they search deeply how much pain and terror they are carrying around," says Dr. Hanley. "The terror in their body diminishes the flow of energy to their reproductive organs which means those organs cannot function well."

function of producing a lining in preparation for a fertilized egg. When progesterone levels decline (in the absence of a fertilized egg), it is a signal to the uterus to let go of all the new cells each month and to start afresh. We could say that menstruation is progesterone withdrawal.

If there is excess bleeding, it is usually because there is too much estrogen—literally too much new cell growth in the uterus—and not enough progesterone to help contain it. One major factor that upsets the natural relationship between the two hormones is estrogen-mimicking environmental chemicals (see Chapter 2: Endometriosis, pp. 74-75).

A second factor is that when a woman's liver is not functioning properly, it is unable to eliminate the majority of estrogenic chemicals and natural estrogens from the body as it is meant to do. Then both kinds of estrogen end up being reabsorbed through the intestines back into the bloodstream. The body now has more estrogen than it needs, which causes havoc. In our culture, most men and women age 40 and older probably have some degree of liver dysfunction due to the toxicity in our environment.

If the liver's detoxification systems are working properly, then estrogen levels will decline in the ten days before bleeding starts. But if they are not, that means the uterine (and breast) glands continue under estrogen stimulation; this is often further magnified by too little progesterone being produced.

A third factor that must be considered is the role of suppressed emotions and past sexual trauma. Often, women who have severe menstrual irregularities had some form of sexual abuse or harassment in their childhood or adult life. Their bodies are manifesting their emotional pain. If there is suppressed anger, the liver inevitably is involved because according to Chinese medicine's 5,000-year-old energy model of human physiology, the emotion of anger is directly linked to the liver.

Success Story: Menorrhagia Corrected in Six Months

In this case from my patient files, you can see how heavy menstrual bleeding can be resolved through natural hormone therapies and nutritional and herbal support.

When Fran, 42, came for treatment, she told me that in her last six menstrual cycles she had had midcycle spotting, her period had started three to five days earlier than normal, and when it came, was painful and heavy. A pelvic exam revealed that her uterus was a little swollen and lumpy, probably in the early stages of growing fibroids. A blood test showed that her red blood cell count was 3.75 (normal is at least 4.2); her iron level was also low, suggesting an early stage of anemia. Fran told me that she was under a great deal of stress at work, did not exercise much, drank several cups of coffee every day, was eating a conventional diet, and was not taking any nutritional supplements. I decided to focus first on helping her to make major changes in her diet.

I encouraged Fran to avoid all milk products because they are usually reservoirs of estrogen-mimicking chemicals and synthetic hormones. I asked her to eliminate all red meats for the same reason, and to limit her protein intake to about eight ounces daily of either fish or organically raised poultry. Other recommendations included eating whole grains for their high-fiber content and nutritive value, eliminating all foods made with white flour, and consuming more fresh, organic vegetables. This is pivotal in unburdening the liver and stimulating its function. I also asked Fran to reduce or eliminate her alcohol consumption to further ease the load on the liver.

For additional vegetable fiber, I recommend rice bran (starting at one tablespoon a day and gradually increasing to one ounce) to assist the body to have at least one bowel movement daily. This is particularly important for women with excess estrogen because they need to empty out their intestines which can become a toxic reservoir that keeps recycling toxins through the body. Normal and healthy is two to three bowel movements every day. If the dietary change and rice bran do not produce more bowel movements, then I will prescribe either magnesium citrate or aloe vera capsules to naturally relax the bowels. Usually a good starting dose is 100-200 mg daily at bedtime in a formula that includes a smaller amount of calcium. You may need to increase it to 600 mg if your bowels still do not move more frequently.

Next, I put Fran on a multivitamin/mineral supplement that contained at least 25-50 mg each of the B vitamins, 300-400 mg each of chelated calcium and magnesium, 15 mg of manganese, 20-30 mg of iron, 100-200 mg each of chromium and selenium, 10-20 mg of zinc, 400 IU of vitamin E, and 1,000-2,000 mg of vitamin C. This supplemental package is available under various commercial names (such as Basic Nutrients, Nutrizyme™, and Basic Preventive®). Fran was nutritionally depleted, so I encouraged her to take two capsules of this formula with each meal for at least several months. She took an extra 50 mg daily of vitamin B6 to help her liver process the excess hormones. I also added borage oil (containing 300 mg of gamma linolenic acid) at the rate of two capsules daily .

To help heal Fran's liver and enable it to process the hormones, I prescribed a Chinese herbal formula traditionally called Shao Yao Huan and available in the U.S. as Relaxed Wanderer or PMS Herbal. Fran took ⅔ of a dropperful mixed in ½ cup of water twice daily from midcycle to the start of menstruation. Then to help restore her progesterone deficiency, Fran used a natural progesterone cream starting at 14 days after her period began (at ovulation, when progesterone levels first begin to climb). She applied ¼ teaspoon of 3% ProGest® twice daily (till her next period or for two weeks), rubbing it into the skin on her stomach, breasts, arms, face, and thighs.

Fran followed this program faithfully and, within two months, 50% of her symptoms had abated. Her periods were lighter and much less painful, and she was returning to what was normal for her. But as Fran still had some spotting at midcycle and the day before her period was to start, I increased her progesterone dose to ½ teaspoon twice daily. Within another month, her menstrual problems were resolved. Six months later when I did another pelvic exam, Fran's uterus was no longer swollen and lumpy, but smaller and firmer as it should be.

There was a strong emotional factor in Fran's case. After all, at one point her periods were normal, then they became abnormal, so what caused the shift? About six months before her symptoms appeared, Fran discovered her husband was cheating on her. That left her distraught, feeling betrayed, hurt, and angry. Within a few months, Fran's periods started to become heavier and more irregular. On an energetic level, you could say that her uterus was weeping. I always ask women why they think this is happening now. This gives them an opportunity to open up and talk about the important issues.

Some women don't know until they search deeply how much pain and terror they are carrying around and how much it is affecting their life decisions and physical health. The terror in their body diminishes the flow of energy to their reproductive organs which means those organs cannot function well.

Through counseling Fran realized that she had been shut off sexually and emotionally from her husband for a long time. She recognized that she was carrying old and unresolved anger toward him and also her father. Her father had been verbally abusive and physically threatening to her so she ended up feeling that all men are dangerous. This meant she was always having to protect herself and suppress or sabotage those parts of herself that would make her attractive to men.

Fran had been pushing her husband away for a long time as well as shutting down the energy flow to her sexual organs. In fact, she was doing the same thing both outwardly and inwardly. During counseling, Fran processed her old hurts and anger so that they no longer blocked her body's functioning, or her marriage. Frankly, it was an emotional ride for Fran so she needed to continue with the herbs and progesterone for quite a while. In fact, I kept her on Relaxed Wanderer and progesterone (at $\frac{1}{4}$ teaspoon twice daily) for nearly a year.

For more on **natural progesterone cream**, see Chapter 3: Fibroids, pp. 113-117.

Fran's whole outlook is more positive now and she understands how to take care of herself. She's learned how much of an effect the choices she makes every day at every meal and the choices she makes about feeling safe or unsafe in the world have on her life. Not only did Fran's marriage improve but she went on to better health on all levels.

To contact **Jesse Hanley, M.D.**: 22917 Pacific Coast Highway, Malibu, CA 90265; tel: 310-456-9393; fax: 310-456-9482. For more about **Basic Nutrients**, contact: Thorne Research Inc., P.O. Box 3200, Sandpoint, ID 83864; tel: 208-263-1337 or 800-228-1966; fax: 208-265-2488. For **Nutrizyme™**, contact: Tyler Encapsulations, 2204-8 N.W. Birdsdale, Gresham, OR 97030; tel: 800-869-9705 or 503-661-5401; fax: 503-666-4913. For **Basic Preventive®**, contact: Advanced Medical Nutrition Inc., 2247 National Avenue, P.O. Box 5012, Hayward, CA 94540; tel: 800-437-8888 or 510-783-6969; fax: 510-783-8196. For **PMS Herbal**, contact: McZand Herbal Inc., P.O. Box 5312, Santa Monica, CA 90409; tel: 310-822-0500; fax: 310-822-1050. For **Relaxed Wanderer**, contact: K'an Herb Company, 6001 Butler Lane, Scotts Valley, CA 95066; tel: 800-543-5233 or 408-438-9450; fax: 408-438-9457. For **ProGest® Body Cream Specific**, contact: Transitions for Health, 621 Southwest Alder, Suite 900, Portland, OR 97205; tel: 800-888-6814 or 503-226-1010; fax: 800-944-0168 or 503-226-6455.

Fran's physical problems and the emotional factors which contributed to them are quite common among women in our culture. Nothing in her treatment program was extraordinary either. In general, a woman could do everything in this program on her own without a doctor. Natural progesterone is harmless at the low dose of ¼ teaspoon twice daily. I would expect, in most cases, that a woman following this program will start noticing positive effects within one to two periods. Keep in mind if you are considering self-treating, that you need to first rule out serious organic conditions as the source of menorrhagia. ■

Alternative Medicine Therapies for Menorrhagia

Fran's heavy bleeding responded well to a combination of alternative medicine therapies, including dietary changes, nutritional supplements, natural hormones, Chinese herbal formulas, and psychological counseling. This section includes other useful natural therapies to treat menorrhagia, beginning with a case featuring Chinese herbs, acupuncture, and, like Fran, the resolution of underlying emotional issues as keys to ending heavy bleeding.

Success Story: Acupuncture and Chinese Herbs Stop Menorrhagia

At the age of 45, Claire had an episode of heavy menstrual bleeding so severe that, after six days, she ended up in a hospital. There, after being hooked up to intravenous tubes and given iron supplements, she was told to make an appointment for a D & C (dilatation and curettage, minor surgery to scrape tissue from the uterine lining). However, Claire was terrified of even minor surgery and instead sought help from acupuncturist and herbalist Jason Elias, M.A., L.Ac., of Integral Health Associates in New Paltz, New York.[59]

After feeling Claire's wrist pulses, which were weak, and looking at Claire's tongue, which was pale and bloated, Dr. Elias determined that Claire was deficient in life force energy or *qi*, particularly in the spleen and kidney organ systems. Claire had been experiencing increased stress in recent years. The stress hindered the smooth flow in the energy channels or meridians (SEE QUICK DEFINITION) throughout her body. In particular, the channels that fed her liver, which circulate through the reproductive organs, were blocked or "stagnated," meaning the energy was not flowing freely. This depleted Claire's liver of energy and prevented it from doing its job of regulating blood flow during menses. The liver was unable to contain the blood and it gushed uncontrollably or, as the Chinese would say, "ran recklessly."

Dr. Elias urged Claire to go ahead with the D & C, just to rule out the possibility that the heavy bleeding could be caused by a serious disorder such as cancer, which a tissue sample from the D & C would reveal.

Through herbs and acupuncture, Dr. Elias would work to correct Claire's *qi* deficiency and "liver *qi* stagnation" and stop the heavy bleeding of her current period. In the first acupuncture session, he used eight acupuncture points, mostly on the legs, feet, and belly, to move energy and strengthen the liver, spleen, and kidney channels. He also gave Claire a traditional Chinese herbal formula for heavy bleeding—Yunnan Pai Yao (Yunnan White Powder)—which contains raw pseudoginseng root, among other ingredients.[60]

Dr. Elias also gave Claire an herbal formula of dandelion, nettles, yellowdock, lady's mantle, and agrimony (shepherd's purse)—astringent, blood-coagulating, and iron-rich herbs to nourish the kidneys, liver, and blood. (Nettles are particularly rich in nutrients: vitamins A, C, D, and K, calcium, potassium, sulfur, and iron.)

Finally, Dr. Elias gave Claire the following lifestyle instructions to assist the herbs and acupuncture in rebalancing her body: Avoid caffeine drinks, as the caffeine inhibits absorption of iron; avoid hot showers and baths which dilate blood vessels and encourage bleeding; eliminate alcohol and aspirin which thin the blood; and eat iron-rich foods such as spinach, kale, and seaweed. (Dr. Elias would have recommended calf's liver for its iron, B vitamins, and vitamin A content, but Claire was a vegetarian.)

Although dietary changes and the herbal formulas were adequate to correct Claire's nutritional deficiencies, other women with heavy bleeding may wish to use nutritional supplements. For them, Dr. Elias typically recommends Liquid Floradix Iron (a European herbal formula rich in iron and available at health food stores; follow dosage directions on the bottle), beta carotene (25,000 IU daily), and vitamin C (1-5 g daily).

By the next day, Claire's heavy bleeding had stopped. Dr. Elias continued to work with Claire on the deeper underlying imbalances. He also helped her arrive at an understanding of the emotional significance of the bleeding. In her case, it was her blocked creativity trying to break through. Dr. Elias worked with her on taking steps to nourish herself and unblock her creative energy.

Even without visiting an alternative practitioner, there are some immediate steps you can take to begin reversing heavy menstrual bleeding, says Dr. Christiane Northrup. (However, as other doctors previously cited, Dr. Northrup advises that you first rule out possible pathology by having a physical exam and a Pap smear.) The following are Dr. Northrup's recommendations:[61]

Dietary Changes–You can regulate your hormonal environment through diet, says Dr. Northrup. If you are a carbohydrate-sensitive woman (you crave sugar or salty snacks, are overweight, or have type O blood), it is advisable to reduce your consumption of these foods. They increase insulin levels in the blood and can lead to excess body fat; this in turn is associated with excess circulating estrogen. If necessary, limit your carbohydrate intake to once daily and make sure they are complex, not simple carbohydrates, she says. Specifically, Dr. Northrup recommends soyfoods (miso, tofu, tempeh, soy sauce) and certain green vegetables (broccoli, kale, collard greens, Brussels sprouts).

Exercise–The goal here is to reduce body fat as a way of controlling excess estrogen, says Dr. Northrup. She advises 30 minutes of aerobic exercise three days a week.

Natural Progesterone–Like Dr. Hanley, Dr. Northrup advises using natural progesterone to restore hormonal balance. She usually recommends applying ½ teaspoon of the cream (such as 3% ProGest®) to your palms or other soft skin two times daily beginning two to three weeks before menstruation. Stop at the onset of your period and then begin again one to two weeks later. Results should be apparent within three months, she says. If a stronger dose is required to counteract the estrogen, micronized oral progesterone tablets (by prescription) can be helpful when taken at 100 mg twice daily for the two weeks before menstruation, says Dr. Northrup. Two weeks after the period is finished, resume at this dosage, she adds.

It occasionally may be necessary to use a synthetic progesterone such as Provera, especially if you have a bleeding fibroid and the other natural remedies have failed to stem the heavy flow, she notes. Here Dr. Northrup suggests a dosage of 10 mg Provera one or two times daily for the two weeks preceding the period, followed by two weeks off, then continuing the cycle for a total of three months.

Castor oil packs are often used for relief of menstrual cramps, or at joints to relieve pain. To prepare a castor oil pack, lightly heat enough castor oil to thoroughly wet but not soak a 10" x 12" flannel cloth. Immerse the flannel in the hot oil, then fold to make three to four layers and place against the skin. (The oil helps to draw out toxins, release tension, and improve blood circulation, especially in the lower abdomen.) Wrap a heating pad or hot water bottle in a towel and place this over the pack, then cover pack and bottle with another towel to retain heat. Keep in place for one to two hours. Following the treatment, the oil-soaked flannel may be wrapped in plastic and stored in a refrigerator for later use. After the flannel has been used 20 times, discard it.

Supplemental Iron—If anemia is suspected as a result of heavy flows (and especially in thin women), Dr. Northrup recommends ANR Iron 27+. This provides 27 mg of time-released iron, which comes buffered with 120 mg of vitamin C and 75 mcg of vitamin B12. This iron formulation also contains amino acids and is designed to reach the small intestine before it is digested.

Castor Oil Packs—Castor oil benefits the lymph system and liver and may help balance hormone levels. Dr. Northrup suggests applying a castor oil pack (SEE QUICK DEFINITION) to the lower abdomen for one hour, three times per week. While the packs can be used at any time during your menstrual cycle, they work most effectively during the two weeks before your period, says Dr. Northrup.

NSAIDs—It may be necessary to resort to a nonsteroidal anti-inflammatory drug (NSAID), says Dr. Northrup, beginning one to two days before menstruation and continuing through the days of heaviest flow. She advises using the lowest possible dose (of Advil, Orudis, or Aleve) at which effects are apparent and to take the NSAIDs with bananas to prevent stomach upset.

Homeopathy

In addition to lifestyle changes and nutritional, herbal, and hormonal treatments, homeopathy can be useful in the treatment of menorrhagia. French homeopathic physician Jacques Jouanny, M.D., and his colleagues suggest a series of symptomatic remedies for heavy bleeding, meaning they provide immediate relief of symptoms, but do not effect healing on the constitutional level as in classical homeopathy. Here are a few of Dr. Jouanny's suggestions:[62]

■ *Sabina* 5C—When periods are early, heavy, and last a long time; the blood is bright red, may contain blackish clots, and is aggravated by minor physical movements; there is also pain radiating from the sacrum to the pubic bone. (Dosage: five pellets hourly, until improvement)

■ *Crocus sativus* 5C—When the period is overlong and black blood and long stringy clots are passed. (Dosage: five pellets, 3-4 times daily)

■ *China* 9C—When there is black blood, pallor, low

blood pressure, and weakness, ear ringing, visual disorders, or sweating during or after menstruation. (Dosage: five pellets, 3-4 times daily)

■ *Secale cornutum* 5C—When there is much black blood, the period lasts a long time and is followed by a blackish discharge for a few days or until the next menstruation. There may also be false labor pains. (Dosage: five pellets, 2-4 times daily)

Amenorrhea

Just as some women are troubled by too much menstrual blood, others find that their menstral periods just stop (for a reason other than pregnancy or menopause). In this condition, called amenorrhea, a woman does not have a period for three or more months; a teenage girl who is age 16 and has not started menstruating yet is also judged to have this condition as is a woman whose periods stop when she goes off birth control pills.

Amenorrhea is mainly caused by temporary failure of the ovaries and pituitary gland, according to Ralph Golan, M.D., of Seattle, Washington. An underactive thyroid gland is also frequently a factor. Malfunctions in any of these three organs lead to hormonal imbalance, and lack of menstruation can be the manifestation of the disturbance. As with other reproductive health disorders with similar causality, restoring the function of the organs involved and rebalancing the hormones is essential for a successful treatment outcome. The therapies described in reference to accomplishing this in cases of PMS, dysmenorrhea, and menorrhagia can therefore be effective for amenorrhea as well.

Other causes of amenorrhea include: nutritional deficiencies, often as the result of excess dieting or weight loss; poor adrenal function; and intense, extended exercise, as in marathon training.[63] Diet has a strong influence on menstrual regularity. An insufficient amount of "good" fats (unsaturated fats and essential fatty acids), a lack of protein, and an excess

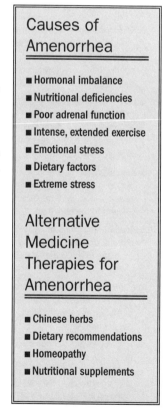

Causes of Amenorrhea

■ Hormonal imbalance
■ Nutritional deficiencies
■ Poor adrenal function
■ Intense, extended exercise
■ Emotional stress
■ Dietary factors
■ Extreme stress

Alternative Medicine Therapies for Amenorrhea

■ Chinese herbs
■ Dietary recommendations
■ Homeopathy
■ Nutritional supplements

of carotene in the blood from drinking carrot juice or taking supplements are all associated with amenorrhea.[64]

Extreme emotional stress or tension can also result in a cessation of menstrual periods. According to Sarah Berga, M.D., at the University of Pittsburgh School of Medicine, stress can interfere with brain's "message" to the reproductive organs to begin ovulation; specifically, the message to begin producing follicle-stimulating hormone (FSH) and luteinizing hormone (LH). (See sidebar: "How the Monthly Cycle Works," pp. 16-17.) "There is no one stressor that is common among women who develop reproductive difficulties," says Dr. Berga. In effect, any stress will do it. For those women for whom stress is the predominant factor in their amenorrhea, improving stress-management skills may be enough to bring about a resumption of menstruation.[65]

The conventional medicine approach of using drugs to induce periods obviously does not address this stress factor or any of the other dysfunctions behind amenorrhea. Thus, the problem will still be there or be worse if the woman discontinues the medication. In the following case, **Dr. Jesse Hanley** highlights the importance of attending to emotional issues and other hidden factors in amenorrhea and demonstrates how simple and safe therapies can resolve both the exhibiting problem and these underlying conditions:

Success Story: Amenorrhea Reversed Naturally

Marie, 28, had periods with so little bleeding they had almost dwindled to nothing. Some months she never had a period at all. A key element in Marie's case was that she was very thin, weighing only 106 pounds, while the normal weight for her height is between 118 and 135 pounds. From her diet, it was clear she wasn't getting enough food, especially fats. With too little bleeding, a woman is often deficient in estrogen. If she is very thin, this is even more likely because she is deprived of those hormones normally produced by fat cells.

Another key factor in Marie's condition was that she was deeply emotionally upset. She had been in a relationship for several years, but recently her mate had become abusive. On an unconscious level, Marie did not feel safe to be feminine. The physical result was that she was losing her womanly curves and her menstrual cycles. She was unaware of how clearly her body received and displayed her emotions as biochemistry. I urged her to begin processing her emotions so she could understand how they were affecting her physiology.

In addressing Marie's diet, I encouraged her to include more whole foods in every meal so that she could put on at least five to eight pounds over the next two to three months. When her body was no longer starving, she would have physiological energy available for her menstruation. Remember, we need fat in our diet because every cell in the body has a surrounding membrane that is made mostly of fat; without fat, the cell cannot survive.

Marie began taking a supplement formula Basic Preventive® (see: "Success Story: Menorrhagia Corrected in Six Months," p. 56) at the rate of four per day along with two capsules daily of borage oil, divided over the day and taken at meals to increase absorption of the nutrients. Marie needed an estrogen precursor to help her body raise its estrogen levels. A Chinese herbal tincture called Woman's Precious is specifically designed to correct estrogenic deficiencies.

For more about **Opti-Borage™ (borage oil)**, contact: Optimal Nutrients, 1163 Chess Drive, Suite F, Foster City, CA 94404; tel: 800-966-8874; fax: 415-349-1686. For **Woman's Precious (Female Formula)**, contact: McZand Herbal, Inc., P.O. Box 5312, Santa Monica, CA 90409; tel: 310-822-0500; fax: 310-822-1050.

Marie took the Zand equivalent (Female Formula), two droppersful in water, three times daily, for two weeks starting two to three days after her period began. In addition, I encouraged her to eat soyfoods, which are high in safe, natural plant estrogens, and other estrogenic vegetables such as bulgur, wheat germ, alfalfa, sesame and sunflower seeds, chickpeas, red beans, green beans, peas, yams, eggplant, tomatoes, potatoes, pumpkin, squash, beets, cabbage, carrots, apples, cherries, plums, garlic, and parsley, among others.

It took two months for Marie's periods to stop being scanty or nonexistent. During this time, she gained six pounds and started the process of healing herself emotionally. In this case, Marie chose to leave her boyfriend and take better care of herself. As soon as she stopped feeling terrorized, she began to have regular periods. After eight months on this simple program of diet, vitamins, herbs, and emotional processing, her menstruation lasted for three days which was normal. ■

At least 25% of American women between the
ages of 30 and 40 have endometriosis and
for most of them the symptoms are both chronic
and severe, including abdominal and
vaginal pain, aggravated PMS, and infertility.
Endometriosis can be decisively reversed when you
correct the underlying hormonal imbalance
and pelvic energy stagnation, and eliminate
the allergies, yeast, and parasite infections.

CHAPTER

2

Endometriosis

WHILE CONVENTIONAL medicine has a poor understanding of the cause of endometriosis, the condition itself is easily described. In endometriosis, small patches of uterine lining tissue (endometrium) migrate to and implant themselves in other parts of the pelvic area such as the ovaries, fallopian tubes, uterine muscles, colon, bladder, and sides of the pelvic cavity.

Endometrial implants, called endometriomas, contain brown blood debris; upon rupturing, they spill into the peritoneum (membrane lining) of the pelvic cavity, creating irritations and peritonitis (inflammation of the peritoneum). During menstruation, these displaced cells swell with blood and bleed, after which fibrous tissue forms in the injured location leading to a buildup of dense tissue adhesions. Inflammation and pain, sometimes so severe as to be debilitating, are the result.

"Once the endometrial cells are transplanted, they still respond

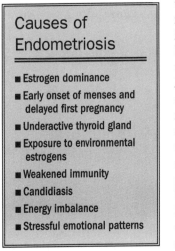

Causes of Endometriosis

- Estrogen dominance
- Early onset of menses and delayed first pregnancy
- Underactive thyroid gland
- Exposure to environmental estrogens
- Weakened immunity
- Candidiasis
- Energy imbalance
- Stressful emotional patterns

to the monthly hormonal (estrogen) messages, just as they would if remaining within the uterus, by filling with blood which is then released at the time of menses," explains John R. Lee, M.D., of Sebastopol, California. "The drops of blood, however, have nowhere to go and can become a focus of excruciating pain and inflammation." Despite their small size (some are no larger than a pinhead), the pelvic pain that results from these blood droplets can be disabling. Symptoms tend to increase gradually over the years as the endometriosis areas slowly increase in size.

Symptoms of endometriosis can appear at any time during the monthly cycle and include pelvic, abdominal, leg, and/or severe lower back pain, and pain during bowel motions and/or urination. However, the most severe pain (called dysmenorrhea) usually begins five to seven days before the peak of menstruation and lasts for two to three days. Additional symptoms or consequences include heavy menstrual bleeding with thick clots; spotting in mid-cycle; pain with intercourse; difficult PMS (premenstrual syndrome); constipation or other bowel problems; and infertility.

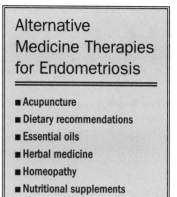

Alternative Medicine Therapies for Endometriosis

- Acupuncture
- Dietary recommendations
- Essential oils
- Herbal medicine
- Homeopathy
- Nutritional supplements

"Once the endometrial cells are transpanted, they still respond to the monthly hormonal (estrogen) messages, just as they would if remaining within the uterus, by filling with blood which is then released at the time of menses," says John R. Lee, M.D.

Endometriosis is widespread. In the United States alone, five million women suffer from the disorder.[1] Of those, an estimated 70% have severe and chronic symptoms, including aggravated PMS, pain on intercourse, and infertility.[2] It is estimated that the fertility rate for women with endometriosis is about 66% compared to 88% for the general population. The condition most commonly affects women between the ages of 30 and 40, and seems especially prominent in women who have postponed childbearing. It is unusual for endometriosis to appear in a woman before age 20, and after age 44 the probability of contracting the condition declines.[3]

Endometriosis erupts variably: sometimes symptoms and related conditions appear abruptly, while in other women they develop over many years. Once in place, symptoms can become progressively worse and are subject to hormonal influences; the role of hormones is made clear by the fact that endometrial implants have been observed in 20% of women undergoing gynecologic surgery. As these surgeries are commonly performed for conditions associated with hormonal imbalance, such as fibroids, the presence of these migrating endometrial tis-

Common Symptoms of Endometriosis

Not all women with endometriosis experience the same assortment of symptoms. The Endometriosis Association of Milwaukee, Wisconsin, gathered data from 3,020 endometriosis case studies to find out how many women are affected by the various symptoms of the disease. The results were:[4]

Dysmenorrhea	96%
Fatigue, exhaustion, or low energy	82%
Diarrhea/gastrointestinal problems	79%
Heavy or irregular bleeding	65%
Dizziness or headaches during menstruation	59%
Dyspareunia (painful sexual intercourse)	59%
Infertility	47%
Nausea	41%
Low resistance to infection	39%
Low-grade fever	29%
No symptoms	3%

QUICK DEFINITION

Laparoscopy is an examination of the contents of the abdominal cavity by means of a specialized endoscope (a tube with a built-in light source and a miniature fiber optic microscope with a magnification of 5X and 50X). During a laparoscopy, the abdomen is inflated with carbon dioxide, an incision is then made in the abdomen, and the laparoscope is passed through this to view the inside of the body, especially the female reproductive organs. This procedure is used when endometriosis or pelvic inflammatory disease is suspected, or when infertility is suspected to be caused by a blockage in the fallopian tubes. The laparoscope is fitted with grasping and cutting tools capable of performing minor surgery and collecting tissue samples and ovarian eggs.

sues indicates a hormonal link as well. In addition, endometriosis tends to subside with menopause, a time when estrogen and progesterone levels typically diminish.

With new developments in medical technology, diagnosis of endometriosis is now done most often through laparoscopy (SEE QUICK DEFINITION). Here, the physician inserts an instrument called a laparoscope through a small incision in the abdomen to search the abdominal cavity for red and clear tissue, which are usually endometrial patches. Although other diagnostic procedures are also used (manual palpation and evaluation of symptoms, for example), most specialists in endometriosis will confirm the diagnosis with a laparoscopy.[5]

In addition to laparoscopy, researchers are exploring new ways of diagnosing endometriosis from a biopsy (removal of tissue samples for laboratory testing). A new test using a sample from an endometrial biopsy is being studied by researchers at the University of North Carolina in Chapel Hill. The test checks for a protein called alpha-v/beta, which is missing in up to 50% of women with endometriosis.[6]

If, after the laparoscopy or biopsy, you are diagnosed

with endometriosis, the physician will present several treatment options. The conventional medical approach to endometriosis generally ignores deeper causes and consists of drugs to dull the pain, synthetic hormones to curb growth of the patches, or surgery to cut out the migrating tissue.

The synthetic hormones (such as danazol) are often effective but can cause disturbing side effects, including masculinization (facial and body hair growth and deepening of the voice), weight gain, acne, decreased sex drive, fluid retention, vaginal dryness, reduction in breast size, liver dysfunction, menstrual disturbances, moodiness, and nervousness.[7] Further, the pain-relieving benefit is often temporary.[8] Another conventional hormone treatment (nafarelin) works by producing a type of artificial menopause, accompanied by all the health disturbances of menopause such as hot flashes, vaginal dryness, and bone loss.[9]

If the endometriosis is severe, or if the case does not respond to hormones, the conventional physician may decide surgery is necessary. The first step is usually to excise only the endometrial tissue patches using a laparoscope (a technique called operative laparoscopy). However, the patches often grow back.

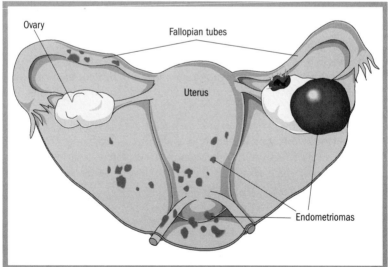

ENDOMETRIAL IMPLANTS. Known as endometriomas, cells from the uterine lining (endometrium) migrate to other areas in the reproductive organs. During menstruation, these cells bleed as if they were still part of the uterine lining.

The conventional medical approach to endometriosis generally ignores deeper causes and consists of drugs to dull the pain, synthetic hormones to curb growth of the patches, or surgery to cut out the migrating tissue.

For information on organ-preserving endometrial surgery, see: "When Surgery is Unavoidable," this chapter, p. 86.

If the pain does not go away after the operative laparoscopy or the location and amount of the errant patches is beyond the scope of such surgery, surgeons may decide they need to remove your uterus (hysterectomy), your ovaries (oophorectomy), or both. Hysterectomy or oophorectomy may result in endometrial pain relief, but have vast consequences for the quality of your post-surgical life. In addition to loss of your female organs, which can be emotionally devastating, if you are premenopausal, oophorectomy will plunge you into premature menopause.

Unfortunately, complete removal of the ovaries, tubes, and uterus is common, particularly if a woman is in her forties," says women's health educator and author Susan Lark, M.D., of Los Altos, California. "This happens even when the disease is entirely treatable by removal of only the implants and scar tissue."[10] Vicki Hufnagel, M.D., an author and surgeon in Beverly Hills, California, says endometriosis has been a major cause of hysterectomy. "From 1965 to 1984, the number of hysterectomies performed for endometriosis has increased by 176%, more than for any other diagnosis, despite the fact that successful surgical techniques and drugs which can conserve organs have been developed over the last 20 years," says Dr. Hufnagel.[11]

Alternative medicine provides a wealth of options for women who would rather not brave the side effects of synthetic hormones or the trauma of surgery. As with the other conditions explored so far in this book, the alternative medical approach is to first determine, through thorough testing, the multilayered, hidden causes of endometriosis. Once those are established, the woman and her alternative practitioner can institute a multifaceted treatment program to address those causes.

Eight Causes of Endometriosis

As in most conditions explored in this book, the cause of endometriosis is a combination of *multiple* factors. You will note that a number of the eight factors listed here appeared in the preceding chapter, and you will encounter them in subsequent chapters as well. The same core group of underlying factors and the imbalances they create in the body can lead to widely divergent health conditions, from menstrual problems and infertility to endometriosis. As you learned in the first chapter, these complex disorders require multimodal treatment to address all the imbalances, deficiencies, and toxicities involved. The treatments covered in case studies throughout this chapter vividly demonstrate that principle.

1) Estrogen Dominance

A relative excess of estrogen (SEE QUICK DEFINITION), is a major contributing cause of endometriosis.

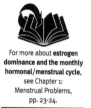

For more about **estrogen dominance and the monthly hormonal/menstrual cycle,** see Chapter 1: Menstrual Problems, pp. 23-24.

Although the balance between estrogen and the other predominant female hormone, progesterone (SEE QUICK DEFINITION), normally fluctuates over the course of a woman's menstrual cycle, a chronic deficiency of progesterone (resulting in a relative excess of estrogen) or a chronic excess of estrogen is linked to endometriosis and thought to worsen it.

2) Early Onset of Menses and Delayed First Pregnancy

Researchers have linked endometriosis to first menstruation at an early age and delayed first pregnancy. Both are more common today than they were two or three generations ago, paralleling a rise in the incidence of endometriosis. In the past, a woman might have had fewer than 40 menstrual cycles before pregnancy, while now many women have 15 years or more of monthly periods before having a child, and many other women never have a child at all.

Pregnancy has long been thought to help the estrogen-progesterone balance by lowering relative estrogen levels. "The fact that many of today's women are putting off childbearing and having more menstrual cycles may explain the increasing incidence of endometriosis,

QUICK DEFINITION

Estrogen is one of the female "sex" hormones, produced mainly in the ovaries (some in the fat cells), that regulates the menstrual cycle. Estrogen is important for adolescent sexual development, prepares the uterus for receiving the fertilized egg by stimulating the uterine lining to grow, and affects all the body's cells; its levels decline after menopause. Estrogen slows down bone loss, which leads to osteoporosis, and it can help reduce the incidence of heart attacks; estrogen also improves skin tone, reduces vaginal dryness, and can act as an antiaging factor. For the first ten to 14 days in a woman's cycle, the uterus is mainly under the influence of estrogen. Estrogen levels begin to climb right before menstruation, from about days seven to 14, and peak at ovulation. There are three natural types of estrogen: estradiol (produced directly in the ovary); estrone (produced from estradiol); and estriol (formed in smaller amounts in the ovary). Estradiol is the most potent of the three. It prepares the uterus for the implantation of a fertilized egg, and also helps mature and maintain the sex characteristics of the female organs.

Progesterone is a female "sex" hormone (produced in the corpus luteum of the ovaries) which prepares the uterus for a fertilized egg and then stops the cell proliferation in the uterus if pregnancy does not occur. When estrogen is high, during days seven to 14 of a woman's cycle, the level of progesterone is at its lowest. Its levels climb to a peak from around days 14 to 24, and then dramatically drop off again just before the start of menstruation. When the cells stop producing progesterone, it's a signal to the uterus to let go of all the new cells produced during the month and to start afresh. In a sense, menstruation is progesterone withdrawal. Starting at age 35, a woman usually starts to make declining amounts of progesterone.

because women who don't get pregnant and nurse have higher circulating estrogen levels," says Alice D. Domar, Ph.D., director of women's health at Harvard Medical School's division of behavioral medicine.[12]

However, the theory that pregnancy is curative for endometriosis is still controversial because medical authorities who object to women in the workplace have used it as an antifeminist argument for women to stay home and bear children. Noted women's health specialist Christiane Northrup, M.D., of Yarmouth, Maine, says some recent studies have found "no difference in the incidence of endometriosis in women who have been pregnant and those who have not."[13] However, a number of physicians, including some alternative practitioners, still subscribe to the belief that pregnancy can improve endometriosis.

3) Underactive Thyroid Gland

An underactive thyroid gland, a condition called hypothyroidism, is often behind relative excess estrogen and many female reproductive problems, including endometriosis, says Dr. Lita Lee. This is because hypothyroidism leads to decreased production of progesterone.

To correct endometriosis in this case, Dr. Lee recommends a program of thyroid glandular support supplements to enhance thyroid function, and natural progesterone cream to restore the hormonal ratio. These strategies are explained later in this chapter.

4) Exposure to Environmental Estrogens

In addition to hypothyroidism, excess estrogen can be the result of exposure to any of a class of estrogen-mimicking chemicals, known as xenoestrogens or environmental estrogens (SEE QUICK DEFINITION), which are increasingly prevalent in our food and in our environment. Once in the body, these chemicals—commonly found in pesticides, herbicides, and certain fuels, as well as in the by-products of incineration of plastics and hazardous wastes—act in the same way as estrogen and, in so doing, throw the estrogen-progesterone ratio off balance.

Researchers have found a possible link between exposure to dioxins (a class of xenoestrogens) and the risk of endometriosis. In a 1993 study, rhesus monkeys developed endometriosis after being fed food containing dioxin over a period of four years.[14] A circumstantial link, but one that certainly bears consideration, is the fact that 70 years ago when the environment was free of the estrogen-mimicking chemicals that pollute it today, there were only 21 report-

For more on **pregnancy as a therapy for endometriosis**, see the case of Dolores, this chapter, pp. 82-87. For more on **women in the workplace and endometriosis**, see this chapter, pp. 77-79. For more on **hypothyroidism and thyroid testing**, see Chapter 1: Menstrual Problems, pp. 24-26, and Chapter 5: Infertility, pp. 163-165. For more about **women's hormones**, see Chapter 1: Menstrual Problems, pp. 18-19.

ed cases of endometriosis versus our current five million in the U.S. alone.[15]

As mentioned earlier, dioxins are found in pesticides and herbicides (and the chemical compounds formed during their manufacture), and therefore in the food we eat; they are present in many manufactured products we use every day; and they pollute the air as a gaseous by-product of incineration. Dioxins, in fact, are all around us; once these estrogen-mimicking compounds enter and are stored in the body, they can seriously upset the delicate hormonal balance necessary for female health.

For more about **detoxification**, see Chapter 1: Menstrual Problems, p. 43, and Chapter 3: Fibroids, pp. 108-111.

For this reason, an effective treatment program for endometriosis in which estrogen-mimicking chemicals are a factor must include eliminating or at least reducing further exposure to these harmful toxins. Women with endometriosis should use only unbleached tampons and sanitary napkins, and make every effort to avoid eating dioxin-containing foods, most notably meats, dairy, and fish. In addition, a detoxification protocol should be implemented to remove those estrogen-mimicking chemicals already lodged in the body.

5) Weakened Immunity

As with all other health conditions, a compromised immune system allows endometriosis to develop when normal immune function might prevent abnormalities from becoming a full-blown disorder. Here's how it works.

A phenomenon called retrograde menstruation is the trigger for endometriosis. Retrograde menstruation means that menstrual blood and endometrial tissues, which normally flow down and out of the body during the menstrual period, instead flow backward through the fallopian tubes to the pelvic tissues. Retrograde menstruation is a normal occurrence; in a healthy woman, the endometrial cells do not attach to pelvic tissues and are naturally eliminated from the body as part of the menstrual cycle. However, in a woman with weakened immunity, the tissues are unable to fend off the cells.

A recent study found that in women with endometriosis, natural killer cells, T-lymphocytes, and other immune system "workers"

Environmental estrogens are foreign compounds and/or chemical toxins that mimic the effects of estrogen. Environmental estrogens, also called xenoestrogens, are present primarily in man-made chemicals ("greenhouse gases," herbicides and pesticides such as DDT) and industrial by-products (from manufacture of plastics and paper, as well as from the incineration of hazardous wastes). Environmental estrogens often cause an imbalance of estrogen relative to progesterone, another key hormone. When a woman's body has too much estrogen (a condition called estrogen dominance), a variety of health problems can result, including breast cancer, fibroids, and endometriosis, among others. According to some researchers, environmental estrogens also affect men, and may contribute to testicular cancer, urinary tract disorders, and low sperm count. Dioxins are one kind of xenoestrogen. The World Health Organization puts the "tolerable" intake of dioxins for a human being at 10 picograms a day; at that rate, one gram of dioxins would provide every person in the United States with their "safe" daily intake for 100 years.

Once dioxins—estrogen-mimicking compounds—enter and are stored in the body, they can seriously upset the delicate hormonal balance necessary for female health.

A **free radical** is an unstable, toxic molecule of oxygen with an unpaired electron that steals an electron from another molecule and produces harmful effects. Free radicals are formed when molecules within cells react with oxygen (oxidize) as part of normal metabolic processes. Free radicals then begin to break down cells, especially the cell membranes, often in a matter of minutes to an hour. A single free radical can destroy a cell. Their work is enhanced if there are not enough free-radical quenching nutrients, such as vitamins C and E, in the cell. While free radicals are normal products of metabolism, uncontrolled free-radical production plays a major role in the development of degenerative disease, including cancer and heart disease. Free radicals harmfully alter important molecules, such as proteins, enzymes, fats, even DNA. Other sources of free radicals include pesticides, industrial pollutants, smoking, alcohol, viruses, most infections, allergies, stress, even certain foods and excessive exercise.

which normally ward off foreign bodies did not function as strongly as in women without endometriosis. (Endometrial cells are treated as "foreign" by tissues in areas where those cells do not belong.) This decreased "surveillance, recognition, and destruction" on the part of the immune system allows the endometrial cells to implant.[16]

Other evidence that immune system function is involved comes from a 1991 study in which researchers blocked the action of destructive free radicals (SEE QUICK DEFINITION) in rabbits. These rabbits showed signficantly less endometriosis than the control group in which free radicals were unrestricted. In a strong immune system, free radicals are counterbalanced by the defense cells of the body. With weakened immunity, free radicals can cause widespread damage to cells and body systems.[17]

A compromised immune system can occur from a wide range of factors: chronic stress, poor diet, chronic or multiple infections, parasites, abuse of drugs or alcohol, antibiotic use, nutritional deficiencies, lack of sleep, and toxic overload, to name a few. Treatment involves eliminating these factors and employing alternative medicine therapies to build up the depleted immune system. Herbal medicine, nutritional supplements, dietary changes, acupuncture, stress reduction, and exercise such as yoga are among the numerous modalities that can effectively accomplish this and help reverse your endometriosis.

6) Candidiasis

Many women with endometriosis also have candidiasis, an overgrowth of the yeast *Candida albicans* (SEE QUICK DEFINITION), states Mary Lou Ballweg, president of the Endometriosis Association in Milwaukee, Wisconsin. *Candida* overgrowth can act to suppress the immune system which, as we said above, can open the door for endometriosis to develop. Ballweg has personal experience with the relationship between candidiasis and endometriosis; she alleviated her own endometriosis by eliminating her *Candida* overgrowth and taking the hormone supplement DHEA.[18]

If testing confirms that yeast is a problem, women with endometriosis should add anti-*Candida* therapies to their alternative treatment program. Such therapies appear in case studies in this chapter and throughout the book.

7) Energy Imbalance

According to traditional Chinese medicine (TCM, see sidebar: "A Glossary of Traditional Chinese Medicine Terms," p. 78), endometriosis may be due to blockages or imbalances in the flow of energy through the meridians, or energy pathways, of your body. Stress, poor diet, overwork, nutrient deficiencies, lack of sleep, or trauma, among other factors, can cause blockages along these channels, leading to what TCM physicians term "stagnation" of energy. Unreleased emotions such as anger or grief can also block the energy pathways.

The stagnation then prevents the flow of energy to organ systems that are supplied by these channels and they become "deficient" or "empty." If allowed to continue, this imbalance can ultimately manifest as conditions such as endometriosis. Imbalances involved in endometriosis are often in the meridians associated with the liver and spleen, as these energy channels circulate through the pelvic region. Such imbalances can be corrected by acupuncture and Chinese herbal medicine.

8) Stressful Emotional Patterns

Endometriosis is an "illness of competition," states Dr. Christiane Northrup. By that, she means that when a woman's emotional needs are in competition with her goals, duties, and ambitions in the outside world, her body attempts to draw attention to the problem by creating endometriosis. Said another way, endometriosis is a product of women who have demanding careers, but who, inside, feel that their emotional selves are not being nurtured. "Many women do not get emotional support in their homes or personal lives," Dr. Northrup says. "Others have abandoned the notion that they even have emotional requirements."

Noting that a Jungian analyst refers to endometriosis as "a blood

---

QUICK DEFINITION

Candida albicans is a yeast-like fungus found widely in nature, in the soil, on vegetables and fruits, and in the human body. It is frequently present in small quantities in the intestines and in a woman's vagina. When its numbers are few, *Candida* is generally not harmful to the human body. A *Candida* overgrowth, a condition called candidiasis, can become pathogenic and cause allergic reactions throughout the body. These reactions can lead to a wide range of symptoms, including depression, fatigue, weight gain, anxiety, rashes, headaches, and muscle cramping.

For more on **anti-yeast treatments**, see Chapter 6: Cystitis, p. 221, and Chapter 7: Vaginitis, pp. 247-254. For more about **acupuncture and TCM treatment of endometriosis**, see the case of Dolores, this chapter, pp. 82-87, and the case of Ida, this chapter, pp. 87-89.

A Glossary of Traditional Chinese Medicine Terms

Traditional Chinese medicine (TCM) originated in China over 5,000 years ago and is a comprehensive system of medical practice that heals the body according to the principles of nature and balance. A Chinese medicine physician considers the flow of vital energy (*qi*—pronounced CHEE) in a patient through close examination of the patient's pulse, tongue, body odor, voice tone and strength, and general demeanor, among other elements. Underlying imbalances and disharmony in the body are described in terminology analogous to the natural world (heat, cold, dryness, or dampness). The concept of balance, or the interrelationship of organs, is central to TCM. In TCM, imbalances are corrected through the use of acupuncture, moxibustion, herbal medicine, dietary therapy, massage, and therapeutic exercise.

Acupuncture is an integrated healing system developed by the Chinese over 5,000 years ago and introduced in the United States in the mid-1800s. The treatment is administered by an acupuncturist using hair-thin, stainless-steel needles, generally presterilized and disposable; these are lightly inserted into the skin at any of over 1,000 locations on the body's surface, known as acupoints. Acupoints are places where *qi* can be accessed by acupuncturists to reduce, enhance, or redirect its flow. Acupuncture is employed for a wide variety of conditions (the World Health Organization counts 104), including pain relief, asthma, migraines, and arthritis.

Acupuncture meridians are specific pathways in the human body for the flow of *qi*. In most cases, these energy pathways run up and down both sides of the body, and correspond to individual organs or organ systems, designated as Lung, Small Intestine, Heart, and others. There are 12 principal meridians and eight secondary channels. Numerous points of heightened energy, or *qi*, exist on the body's surface along the meridians and are called acupoints. There are more than 1,000 acupoints, each of which is potentially a place for acupuncture treatment.

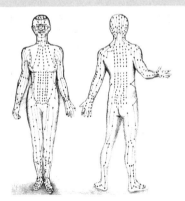

sacrifice to the Goddess," Dr. Northrup sees the disease as reminding women not to forget their feminine natures, their connection to other women, or their need for self-nurturance. This does not necessarily mean, she says, that women should just stay home and have babies, which was the early conventional advice for endometriosis. "What would protect against the disease would be business and personal environments that don't require a mental-emotional split," notes Dr. Northrup.[19]

Alice Domar, Ph.D., concurs with Dr. Northrup regarding the link between endometriosis and work life. She calls endometriosis the "working woman's disease" because she has found it is more prevalent among working women who delay childbearing and that the stress associated with work appears to be an "aggravating factor" in the disorder's symptoms.[20] Neils H. Lauersen, M.D., Ph.D., a clinical professor of obstetrics and gynecology at New York Medical College, reports that 95% of his endometriosis patients are "women under extreme stress who work or have worked [outside the home]."[21]

Energy specialist and author Carolyn Myss, Ph.D., of Chicago, Illinois, whom Dr. Northrup credits with the "competition" concept, observes that endometriosis is one of a handful of conditions that arise due to emotional problems based in the pelvic area. These problems often are connected with negative sexual attitudes, fear of childbirth or guilt about parenting methods, low self-esteem due to lack of financial power, resentment over being controlled by others or feeling so insecure that you need to control others, or fear of never having enough (including fear of poverty), says Dr. Myss.[22]

Dr. Domar notes that chronic pelvic pain, which often accompanies endometriosis, may be linked with early emotional, sexual, or physical abuse. "Even without an abuse history, many women with endometriosis and pelvic pain have stress, sorrow, and anger about circumstances of the past or present," she says.[23]

While emotional patterns play a role in most illnesses and it is always advisable to address this component in treatment, stressful and stored emotions may be particularly integral to the development of endometriosis. Employing mind-body techniques such as relaxation, guided imagery, meditation, and psychotherapy becomes even more important in this disorder.

Alternative Treatments for Endometriosis

Alternative practitioners are successfully reversing endometriosis with-

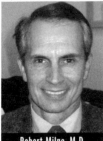

Robert Milne, M.D.

Dr. Milne's therapeutic strategy began with improving Sally's energy levels through dietary changes. He also sought to improve her digestive function and pelvic mobility. "After nine months of treatment, Sally was 90% free of pelvic pain and went on to have a healthy child."

out drugs or surgery by addressing the underlying causes of the disease. The following case studies illustrate many of the causes discussed above and the range of treatments used to address them. In the first case, severe and longstanding endometriosis and infertility were resolved with a multimodal approach of dietary changes, homeopathy (SEE QUICK DEFINITION), herbal and nutritional supplements, and relaxing Epsom salt baths.

Success Story: Endometriosis Reversed in Nine Months With Homeopathy and Supplements

When Sally, 42, consulted Robert Milne, M.D., of the Milne Medical Center in Las Vegas, Nevada, for relief of her endometriosis and chronic pelvic pain, she told him she was trying to have another child. Her health history revealed that she had endured two miscarriages, that her one successful pregnancy had kept her sick during the entire nine months, and that currently she was having difficulty conceiving due to the endometriosis.

Dr. Milne further learned that Sally's mother also suffered from chronic pelvic pain and had sustained multiple miscarriages. Sally started menstruating late, at age 15, and her periods were generally "unbearable," requiring her to retreat to her bed for two to three days a cycle. Her PMS symptoms were intense and included vaginal discharge, weakness, severe irritability, and sometimes rage. "I felt like a rattlesnake ready to strike," Sally commented. At the same time, Sally was concerned that the bulk of her problems might be "in her head" and not physiologically based.

Sally also had a tender neck with a restricted range of motion, back pain between her shoulder blades and around her waist and hips, and a tender abdomen, especially at the pubic bone. In Dr. Milne's view, these symptoms were related to the family history of chronic pelvic pain and her own menstrual problems. A vaginal exam indicated that Sally had severe cervical irritation, which was probably causing the heavy discharges.

Dr. Milne's therapeutic strategy began with improving Sally's energy levels through dietary changes. He also sought to improve her digestive function and pelvic mobility. She was to eat an allergy-free, nutrient-dense diet, omitting sugar, milk, corn, beef, and anything with yeast. She drank fresh vegetable juices in the morning and took frequent Epsom salt baths (see sidebar: "Relax With an Epsom Salt Bath," p. 83) in the afternoon, followed by a rest period.

To treat the vaginal discharge, Sally used vaginal suppositories (containing herbal and homeopathic remedies). In addition, Dr. Milne daubed her cervix with silver nitrate to cauterize (in effect, to burn and shrink) the eroded tissue and to stimulate oxygen and blood flow to the area. Dr. Milne also had Sally insert a tampon "painted" with ichthammol (a thick reddish-brown fluid derived from mineral pitch or tar) into her vagina where it would work as a local skin anti-infective.

In conjunction with these treatments, Sally began a daily multivitamin and mineral supplement program with extra amounts of key antioxidants such as vitamin E (400 IU), selenium (200 mcg), bioflavonoids (500 mg, SEE QUICK DEFINITION), evening primrose oil (4-6 capsules), herbal extracts of blue and black cohosh (25 drops, three times daily), and Tangui-Peony herbal tea powder (1 tsp, three times daily), a traditional Chinese herbal formula for women's problems.

Sally also took several low potency homeopathic remedies: *Lachesis* 12X (bushmaster snake venom), *Magnesium Phosphate* 3X (a mineral used for cramping), and *Thuja* 3X (arbor vitae tree). Finally, Dr. Milne gave Sally special suppositories from Germany called *Latensin* and *Nigersan* which she used three times weekly. These two substances, part of the unique line of Sanum remedies (SEE QUICK

QUICK DEFINITION

A **bioflavonoid** is a pigment within plants and fruits that acts as an antioxidant to protect against damage from free radicals and excess oxygen. In the body, bioflavonoids enhance the beneficial activities of vitamin C, and are often formulated with this vitamin in supplement form. Originally called vitamin P (until 1950), these vitamin C "helper" substances include citrin, hesperidin, rutin, quercetin, epicatechin, flavones, and flavonols. When taken with vitamin C, bioflavonoids increase the absorption of vitamin C into the liver, kidneys, and adrenal glands. Acting as antioxidants, they also protect vitamin C from destruction by free radicals.

Sanum remedies, developed by Guenther Enderlein, M.D., Ph.D. (1872-1968), are produced in the U.S. by Sanum-Enderlein-Pleo™, 5160 West Phelps Road, #B, Glendale, AZ 85306. The line includes about 100 preparations of benign microorganisms or protein particles identified by pleomorphic practice. For example, "Mucokehl" is *Mucor racemosus*, a fungus that regulates microorganisms affecting the thickness of blood. These remedies, when injected, adjust the pH and cellular terrain and help the pathogenic microorganisms revert back to harmless forms. In effect, the Sanum remedies help the body restore the optimal cellular terrain for health.

DEFINITION), would help improve Sally's lymphatic system (*Nigersan*) and immune system (*Latensin*).

"After nine months of treatment, Sally was 90% free of pelvic pain and went on to have a healthy child," reports Dr. Milne.[24]

The key to Sally's recovery was in understanding the many causal factors in her condition and treating each one with an appropriate alternative medicine therapy. The same process worked for Dolores, in the case study below, whose endometriosis involved a number of the causes enumerated above, including energy imbalances, candidiasis, and hypothyroidism.

Success Story: Acupuncture, Herbs, and Supplements Cure Endometriosis

By the time Dolores, 40, first consulted acupuncturist and certified herbalist Rachel Koenig, L.Ac., who practices in Brooklyn, New York, she had been putting up with intestinal discomfort and problems with her reproductive system for about five years.

Dolores lived a fast-paced life in a competitive business climate. In her late thirties, she began having health problems. During the second half of her monthly cycle, from ovulation to menstruation onset, Dolores had bloating, gas, abdominal pain and cramping, and diarrhea. Her PMS included becoming highly irritable and emotionally unbalanced. Once her period began, the pain eased up, but the blood flow was heavy, just short of hemorrhaging, reports Dr. Koenig. Dolores also complained of persistent fatigue, sinus infections, and chronic sore throats.

Under the care of conventionally minded physicians at the time, Dolores had received two laparoscopies, two and four years before coming to Dr. Koenig. In the first laparoscopy, involving laser surgery, doctors removed a large ovarian cyst; in the second, they discovered Dolores had endometriosis. During this second procedure, some of the endometrial patches were excised, but apparently they grew back because Dolores' symptoms, notably the pain—a hallmark of endometriosis—soon returned. The pain was such that she needed a painkiller to endure her periods.

"Neither one of these operations helped her," states Dr. Koenig. "Often with a laparoscopy, there is temporary relief followed by a buildup of the problem again because the underlying, subtle imbalances that cause the stagnation leading to endometriosis are not being eliminated."

During her initial examination of Dolores, Dr. Koenig determined that she was mildly anemic. She lost so much blood during her periods that her system was unable to fully recover in the intervening three weeks and to produce enough replacement blood. As a corollary, Dolores' liver was weak, due both to the heavy bleeding and regular moderate alcohol use (typically, two drinks a day).

Dr. Koenig suspected hypothyroidism was the source of Dolores' chronic sinus and throat infections. Delaying pregnancy can also modulate thyroid function, Dr. Koenig notes. "We are seeing this a lot in older women," she says. "When they postpone childbearing, they don't go through that natural heightening of the female hormonal system and of the metabolism. As a result, many women are developing a condition of subclinical hypothyroidism that isn't caught until it goes out of control." Dr. Koenig points out that often the ovaries will become overactive to compensate for the underactivity of the thyroid or adrenal glands or both. This was probably the case with Dolores, she adds.

Dr. Koenig's first phase of treatment was to suggest major changes in Dolores' diet. As a typical busy New Yorker who tended to eat (nearly anything) on the run, Dolores needed to eliminate caffeine, alcohol, sugar, wheat gluten, dairy products, and cooked or fried fats from her diet. Dr. Koenig recognizes that many people find it hard, or simply undesirable, to immediately jettison major food supports from their diet, so she offers a five-day purified diet.

> ## Relax With an Epsom Salt Bath
>
> Add up to a quart of Epsom salt (magnesium sulfate, available in supermarkets and drug stores) to a bathtub of hot water. Stir until the crystals dissolve, then immerse yourself up to your ears and soak for at least 20 minutes. For best effects, after briefly drying yourself following the bath, lie down on a towel on a bed for another 20 minutes. Epsom salt deeply relaxes muscles and release emotions, thoughts, and stress associated with tight, contracted muscles. Even after you have dried yourself, the Epsom salt is still working, which is why the post-bath relaxation period is important.

For five days once or twice a month, Dolores would follow this streamlined, healthier diet. The goal was to give her internal organs, intestines, and lymphatic system a chance to clean out, detoxify, rest, and get rebalanced. For women with menstrual problems, Dr. Koenig advises staging the five-day diet to run immediately before the expected start of menstruation.

In Dolores' case, Dr. Koenig suspected that her diarrhea was a symptom of irritable bowel syndrome and due to an allergy to wheat

"Often with a laparoscopy, there is temporary relief followed by a buildup of the problem again because the underlying, subtle imbalances that cause the stagnation leading to endometriosis are not being eliminated," says Dr. Rachel Koenig.

To contact **Rachel Koenig, L.Ac., N.C.C.A.C.H.:** 53 Prospect Park West, Brooklyn, NY 11215. Dr. Koenig is not taking any new patients at this writing, but for a list of referrals to other physicians of a similar mind, call 718-390-8898. For **Enterogenic™ Capsules, Glyco-Kinetic™ Complex,** and **Adrenal Complex,** contact: Tyler Encapsulations, 2204-8 N.W. Birdsdale, Gresham, OR 97030; tel: 800-869-9705 or 503-661-5401; fax: 503-666-4913. For **Probioplex™, Lipogen™,** and **FEM Multi™,** contact: Metagenics, Inc., 971 Calle Negocio, San Clemente, CA 92673; tel: 800-692-9400; fax: 714-366-0818. For **Scudders Alterative,** contact: Gaia Garden Herbal Dispensary, 2672 West Broadway, Vancouver, BC, V6K 2G3 Canada; tel: 604-734-4372; fax: 604-734-4376. For **Women's Palace,** contact: Crane Enterprises, 745 Falmouth Rd., Mashpee, MA 02649; tel: 800-227-4118 or 508-539-1700; fax: 508-539-2369. For **Bupleurum** and **Dong quai,** contact: Qualiherb, 13839 Bentley Place, Cerritos, CA 90703; tel: 800-533-5907 or 562-802-0625; fax: 562-802-0035. For **organic essential oils,** contact: PhytoMedicine Company, 6701 Sunset Drive, Suite 100, Miami, FL 33143; tel: 305-662-6396; fax: 305-667-5619.

gluten. Another probable underlying factor for her bloating, gas, and generally loose stools was a yeast overgrowth of *Candida albicans*, said Dr. Koenig. The sugars and simple carbohydrates from Dolores' diet acted as food for the yeast, further complicating the picture. As an additional measure to help balance Dolores' intestines, Dr. Koenig had Dolores undergo a monthly colonic (an intestinal cleansing by irrigation with water or coffee) just before her period.

Dr. Koenig also mapped out a supplement program for Dolores (see sidebar: "Dolores' Supplement Program," p. 85) and gave her instructions on how to apply essential oil packs. For this, she used a mixture of 30 drops of essential ginger oil, 1 oz of organic hazelnut oil, and a pinch of liquid vitamin E to help relax the cervix, reduce inflammation, and move the blood. On the day before the onset of bleeding, preferably in the evening before sleeping, Dolores was to rub this mixture on her stomach, cover with a thin towel, then top with a hot water bottle. If she had back pain as part of her PMS, Dolores could start using the pack one week before menstruation, applying it on her lower back.

With these recommendations in place, Dr. Koenig started acupuncture treatments, spaced four to six weeks apart. Her standard treatment includes placing acupuncture needles in special points on the body known to induce a state of deep relaxation and meditation in the patient. "I feel this is a primary goal, to achieve this empty, peaceful state in which a patient feels *safe*," comments Dr. Koenig. Many women today live in a state of constant overdrive without any down time to relax, she notes. "This creates a lot of hormonal imbalance because these women never get on the *nourishing*, rather than the stressed, side of their nervous system."

After three acupuncture treatments, or about three months into

Dolores' Supplement Program

Here are the highlights of the program Dr. Koenig designed as part of Dolores' endometriosis treatment:

- **Enterogenic Capsules:** highly concentrated mixture of *Lactobacillus acidophilus* and four other friendly bacteria to improve intestinal function; ½ teaspoon twice daily

- **Probioplex Intensive Care:** supplies concentrated whey protein (with protein structures and enzymes intact and biologically active) to promote the growth of beneficial intestinal microflora; one tablespoon twice daily mixed with one tablespoon each of pure organic yogurt and flaxseed oil

- **Lipogen:** combination of amino acids (protein building blocks), vitamins, minerals, and herbs to support and cleanse the liver; two tablets daily

- **Vitamin B complex:** particularly vitamins B6, B12, and folate for general support

- **FEM Multi:** daily multivitamin/mineral formula for nutritional support

- **Scudders Alterative:** herbal tincture to treat Dolores' chronic sore throat; helps build blood, drain the lymph, and nourish the body; one dropperful, two times only

- **Women's Palace:** Chinese herbal formula to relieve conditions of stagnation in the blood, typified by endometriosis; three tablets (500 mg each) daily

the program, Dolores reported a 40% improvement. Her sore throats had disappeared; she had less pain and fatigue and fewer episodes of diarrhea. To address the remaining symptoms, including blood sugar fluctuations, apparent now that Dolores had purified her diet after years of haphazard eating, Dr. Koenig introduced three new supplements and another type of hot pack:

- Glyco-Kinetic Complex: containing glandular extracts (pancreas, liver, adrenal), vitamins, minerals, amino acids, and several herbs to help regulate blood sugar; two capsules, twice daily with meals

- Adrenal Complex: combination of adrenal gland extract, licorice, ginseng, beta carotene, vitamin C, vitamin B5, and zinc to support and gently regulate adrenal gland function and reduce its stress; one capsule, two times daily

- Chinese herbs: a formula containing *Bupleurum radix* and *Dong quai* to ease Dolores' PMS; three capsules, twice daily, taken during the second half of her cycle until menstruation begins

- Castor oil packs (SEE QUICK DEFINITION): castor oil

QUICK DEFINITION

Castor oil packs are often used for relief of menstrual cramps, or at joints to relieve pain. To prepare a castor oil pack, lightly heat enough castor oil to thoroughly wet but not soak a 10" x 12" flannel cloth. Immerse the flannel in the hot oil, then fold to make three to four layers and place against the skin. (The oil helps to draw out toxins, release tension, and improve blood circulation, especially in the lower abdomen.) Wrap a heating pad or hot water bottle in a towel and place this over the pack, then cover pack and bottle with another towel to retain heat. Keep in place for one to two hours. Following the treatment, the oil-soaked flannel may be wrapped in plastic and stored in a refrigerator for later use. After the flannel has been used 20 times, discard it.

When Surgery is Unavoidable

Vicki Hufnagel, M.D., medical director of the Center for Female Reconstructive Surgery in New York and Hawaii, and a surgeon in West Hollywood, California, has been a pioneer in developing an approach to female surgery, called reconstructive surgery, that preserves female organs. "My work puts forth a philosophy that is the complete antithesis of conventional medicine," says Dr. Hufnagel, "a philosophy that views a woman's body as a whole organism that should be conserved and repaired at all times when possible." Dr. Hufnagel performs surgery for endometriosis, fibroids, and other conditions, and in the majority of cases is able to leave the reproductive organs intact.

A preoperation education program and pre-op care involving acupressure, naturopathy, and/or supplements of vitamins and amino acids prepares the patient for the surgery. Dr. Hufnagel uses regional anesthetic for her major surgery, allowing the patient to watch the procedure and talk with the surgery team while the operation is in progress. Family is asked to be present in a neighboring room to watch the operation via camera and talk with the doctor. Dr. Hufnagel states, "This creates a completely different response post-op. The family becomes more involved and gives more assistance to the patient later."

During the procedure, Dr. Hufnagel bathes the exposed tissue in fluids to medicate and cleanse. She says, "In this way I can float a medication that can help prevent future endometriosis." Before closing the incision, she repairs muscle and ligaments so organs have good support and also removes any tissue stretched by a tumor that later would be unsightly. After surgery, Dr. Hufnagel often employs electromagnetic treatments and ultrasound to enhance healing, and she says her patients have better compliance in their post-op care because, as she notes, "A woman takes better care of herself when she doesn't see herself as a victim."

> To contact **Vicki Hufnagel, M.D.:** Los Angeles Her Body Center for Female Reproductive Surgery, 8721 Beverly Blvd., West Hollywood, CA 90048; tel: 310-360-8950; website: http//www.drhufnagel.com.

mixed with essential ginger oil, then applied as a compress (under a hot water bottle) to the abdomen every day for several days before menstruation starts; designed to reduce stagnation and congestion in the uterine area.

Dolores continued to improve. After six months, she said her pelvic pain was "manageable," then after another eight months, it had disappeared. "She was definitely getting more energy and felt she was getting her life back," comments Dr. Koenig. "Her degree of long-term pelvic stagnation took time to clear out and heal."

However, the most impressive and, to all parties concerned, stunning development confirming her recovery was the fact that two years after beginning treatment with Dr. Koenig, Dolores, then 42, got pregnant. Long-term endometriosis is widely believed to render a woman infertile, at least for as long as the condition lasts, says Dr. Koenig. Continuing with the acupuncture and nutrient program (with some alterations), Dolores successfully brought a healthy baby to term. "Her stabbing endometrial pain and low energy never returned. While Dolores would always have to nurture her very sensitive gastrointestinal system, her pregnancy was actually *curative* for her endometriosis."

As Dolores found, acupuncture can be a highly effective treatment for endometriosis. The next case study further illustrates the vital role it can play in eliminating even severe, long-term endometriosis when energy imbalances are one of the underlying causes of the condition.

Success Story: Reversing 33 Years of Endometriosis With Acupuncture

At 47, Ida had suffered from endometriosis for most of her life. The first attacks came when she began menstruating at 14, and four years of painful periods led to an "official" diagnosis of endometriosis after Ida's eighteenth birthday. Over time, the endometriosis flare-ups occurred more frequently, despite the fact that Ida was on danazol (conventional synthetic hormone commonly prescribed for endometriosis) and, during an episode, took various standard anti-inflammatory drugs as well. Nothing relieved the pain and the endometriosis continued for 33 years without a break, except during Ida's only pregnancy at age 30.

Frustrated with her lack of progress and concerned about the effects of long-term hormone treatment (the danazol caused her to stop menstruating), Ida consulted Ken Shifrin, L.Ac., an acupuncturist based in Oxford, England. Ida hoped to find a more effective—and less physically disruptive—resolution of her endometriosis. To choose the best treatment plan, Dr. Shifrin assembled a complete symptom picture for Ida.

Her endometriosis episodes, most frequent during the early spring and late summer, usually began with acute lower back pain, which moved to the pelvic area and then settled on the lower abdomen. Ida's attacks were accompanied by exhaustion and sensations of extreme cold. When she was not suffering an acute episode, Ida had almost uncontrollable food cravings, especially for cheese, and during damp weather she experienced frequent headaches and pain

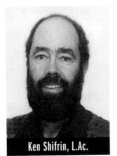

Ken Shifrin, L.Ac.

Dr. Shifrin credits a large part of Ida's recovery to her progress in eliminating the negative emotions which contributed to her endometriosis. "I have no doubt that this emotional change has been a major part of Ida's healing process," says Dr. Shifrin.

and swelling in the joints.

Based on Ida's description of her condition, Dr. Shifrin suspected an imbalance in the flow of vital energy (*qi*) associated with the spleen and liver. Dr. Shifrin also took into consideration the appearance of Ida's tongue and the strength and consistency of her pulse. Her problems with food, sensitivity to damp weather, whitish tongue, and slow, deep pulse all pointed to a spleen imbalance. In addition, Ida's acute abdominal pain and fragile emotional state—built-up frustration and anger about her persistent health problems—indicated an energy blockage or stagnation in her liver.

The concentration of endometriosis attacks during the spring and summer confirmed the involvement of the spleen and liver in causing Ida's condition, Dr. Shifrin explains. An additional energy imbalance in the kidneys (identified by Ida's sensations of extreme cold) also contributed to the problem. This combination of kidney, liver, and spleen distress expressed itself as a problem in the uterus which, according to Chinese medicine, is particularly susceptible to the stagnation of energy and blood.

Dr. Shifrin began treatment by inserting needles at various points along the meridians associated with the spleen. "With this initial treatment, I attempted to accomplish the *greatest* benefit with the *least* amount of intervention," says Dr. Shifrin. "The aim of the Chinese medicine practitioner is to treat only where natural energy cycles are unable to bring about improvement by themselves." To address the emotional aspect of Ida's condition, Dr. Shifrin also used needles and moxibustion (SEE QUICK DEFINITION) on points near the spleen and liver; these treatments lasted for about 30 minutes.

During the course of her first treatment, Ida noted

To contact **Ken Shifrin, L.Ac.:** Oxford Acupuncture Clinic, 40 Walton Crescent, Jericho, Oxford, England OX12JQ; tel: 018-655-4631.

QUICK DEFINITION

In **moxibustion,** a dried herb called moxa (usually mugwort) is burned over the skin at a specific acupuncture point. The moxa may be attached to a special acupuncture needle or in a free-standing cone set on a slice of ginger; its slow burning provides a penetrating heat. The purpose is to warm the blood and *qi* (basic life force energy flowing through energy pathways), particularly when a patient's energy picture is cold or damp.

feeling progressively "calmer, lighter, and more relaxed." Ida returned for her second treatment a week later reporting less pain, reduced swelling and discomfort in her abdomen, and an overall increase in energy level. She described her improvement to Dr. Shifrin as feeling "stronger on the inside."

Dr. Shifrin continued with this approach for the next few weeks, and Ida's symptoms gradually receded. Still, some swelling and discomfort persisted. Dr. Shifrin then shifted the focus of treatment to points on the lower back, in order to encourage more energy movement and blood flow in the area. Over the next few years, Ida's symptoms continued to diminish until they disappeared altogether. The endometriosis has not returned since.

Dr. Shifrin credits a large part of Ida's recovery to her progress in eliminating the negative emotions which contributed to her endometriosis. While she was undergoing treatment, Ida broke off an unsatisfying marriage and successfully dealt with years of accumulated anger and resentment. "I have no doubt that this emotional change has been a major part of Ida's healing process," says Dr. Shifrin. Both practitioner and patient believe that the acupuncture helped set this process in motion.[25]

In the next case, homeopathy rather than acupuncture is the centerpiece of the multimodal treatment needed to heal longstanding endometriosis. Detoxifying the body of estrogen-mimicking chemicals was another important component in finally curing Gail of her painful disorder.

Success Story:
Reversing Endometriosis With Homeopathy

By the time Gail, 40, came to naturopathic physician Andrew Lange, N.D., a board certified homeopath based in Boulder, Colorado, she had pain during her menstrual period that was so severe she sometimes had to stay at home for three days. The pain was in her whole abdominal area, accompanied by strong cramps and heavy menstrual bleeding with thick clots in the blood. Gail had experienced these symptoms since she started menstruating, but they had gotten much worse in the previous four or five years.

Gail also had such severe pain in the lower chest area below her ribs that she would double over. She had tried acupuncture and applied kinesiology (a form of chiropractic using muscle responses to test areas of weakness), and been to numerous gynecologists, but had not gotten any relief. (One doctor did, however, rule out appendicitis,

Dr. Andrew Lange explains that part of the skill involved in homeopathic prescribing is in uncovering the key aspect of a person's personality or symptom picture which will match a specific remedy. "You have to figure out what's unique about the case," he says.

since Gail's appendix had been removed.)

Dr. Lange sent Gail to another gynecologist, who diagnosed her with endometriosis and suggested surgery. Gail went ahead with the surgery, but it did not improve her condition. She came back to Dr. Lange for help. Based on Gail's spasmodic, cramping pain, and on her emotions which she suppressed in her daily life, he prescribed home-opathic copper (*Cuprum*). Although copper isn't a traditional remedy for endometriosis, the homeopathic texts recommend it for severe cramping and severe menstrual periods, he says, adding that "histori-cally, copper has always been associated with female problems."

Dr. Lange explains that part of the skill involved in homepathic prescribing is in uncovering the key aspect of a person's personality or symptom picture that exactly matches a certain remedy. "You have to figure out what's unique about the case," he says. "You don't look up the disease. You *can* look up the disease, but that's misleading because you might not find the medicine that fits your case."

The copper was in the form of an experimental preparation in which the homeopathic copper was mixed in a colloidal suspension primarily made up of water, instead of the traditional remedies, which are usually preserved in alcohol. Gail took the mixture orally, a few drops, once daily for three months. The formula was a 1C dose, or one dilution of the copper tincture mixed with water, a low dose by home-opathic standards.

At the same time, Dr. Lange put Gail on a detoxification regimen to rid Gail's body of xenoestrogens that have an estrogenic effect in the body (see this chapter, pp. 74-75). "The reason we're seeing so much endometriosis is because there are so many pesticides and hor-mones in our food and environment that are mimicking estrogens. So you have this high level of estrogen-like biological substances in our bodies and you have to detoxify those chemicals," Dr. Lange says.

The regimen included a high daily dose (100 mg) of niacin to increase blood circulation so the toxins would move through the body and be eliminated, along with daily doses of vitamin B complex (50 mg), vitamin A (5,000 IU),

To contact **Andrew Lange, N.D.**: 3011 Broadway, Suite 14, Boulder, CO 80304; tel: 303-443-8678; fax: 303-443-8163.

vitamin D (400 units), vitamin C (1,000 mg), and a multimineral tablet. Dr. Lange also told Gail to work up a sweat at least once daily, either by exercise or through saunas, which would further aid detoxification.

By the end of three months, Gail's endometriosis symptoms were gone. She stopped the homeopathic remedy at that point and continued on the detoxification program for another three months. The endometriosis did not return.

Another alternative medicine therapy to counteract the relative excess estrogen often underlying endometriosis is the use of natural progesterone cream, rather than synthetic progestins (progesterone substitutes), such as Provera, which have troubling side effects. The case study below provides an excellent example of how natural progesterone cream (see sidebar: "A Mini-Primer on Natural Progesterone Cream," p. 93) can be combined with other alternative therapies to effect complete recovery. It also highlights another of the causes frequently found in endometriosis: *Candida* overgrowth.

Herbal Medicine for Endometriosis

For endometriosis, medical herbalist Daniel Gagnon, of Santa Fe, New Mexico, recommends an herbal formula called Cycle Balance 2 to help women restore their proper hormonal ratio. The formula promotes progesterone production to offset the toxic effects of excess estrogen characteristic of endometriosis.

Cycle Balance 2 contains wild yam and *vitex* (both of which are hormone regulators), dandelion (to support liver function, important because the liver helps eliminate and detoxify estrogen), reishi (an immune system stimulant), blue cohosh (a hormone balancer), black haw, chickweed, *shatavari*, cinnamon, and orange peel. The dosage is 30 drops twice a day, from days 15 to 28 (the progesterone-dominant phase) of the menstrual cycle.[26]

Success Story: Natural Progesterone Got Her Off Synthetic Hormones

With natural progesterone, Carolyn DeMarco, M.D., began reducing Rosanna's intake of synthetic estrogen and progesterone over a four-week period, and was able to take her completely off Lupron, a powerful hormone drug.

When Rosanna, 30, first came to see Dr. DeMarco in Toronto, Ontario, she had already undergone multiple surgeries for her endometriosis, but with no improvement. Rosanna's pelvic pain was still considerable and she was on Lupron, a synthetic hormone that operates by deliberately

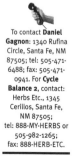

To contact **Daniel Gagnon:** 1340 Rufina Circle, Santa Fe, NM 87505; tel: 505-471-6488; fax: 505-471-0941. For **Cycle Balance 2,** contact: Herbs Etc., 1345 Cerillos, Santa Fe, NM 87505; tel: 888-MY-HERBS or 505-982-1265; fax: 888-HERB-ETC.

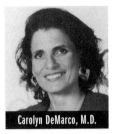

Carolyn DeMarco, M.D.

"*Candida* has a direct effect on hormones, such as estrogen and progesterone, either by binding to the receptor sites or by forming antibodies which can then react against ovarian tissues," says Dr. DeMarco.

To contact **Carolyn DeMarco, M.D.**: 3080 Yonge Street, Suite 2070, Toronto, Ontario M4N3N1, Canada; tel: 416-322-2012. Dr. DeMarco is the author of *Take Charge of Your Body: A Woman's Health Advisor* (Aurora, Ontario: The Well Women Press, 1996; tel: 800-387-4761).

For more about **natural progesterone creams**, and a list of popular brand names and their progesterone content, see Chapter 3: Fibroids, pp. 113-117.

exhausting the brain's pituitary gland (which is responsible for much of the body's hormonal activity). However, Lupron left Rosanna feeling mentally foggy and, at times, mentally dysfunctional.

As a side effect of Lupron, Rosanna went into early menopause with hot flashes and mood swings, for which her conventional physicians prescribed synthetic estrogen and progesterone. These in turn produced many unpleasant side effects and by the time Rosanna came to Dr. DeMarco, she was determined to get off her multiple drug regimen and gain relief for her endometriosis.

Dr. DeMarco started Rosanna on a multifaceted program including castor oil packs placed on her lower abdomen every evening. These would help draw out toxins, release tension, and increase blood circulation to her pelvic area. Next, Dr. DeMarco started Rosanna on a natural progesterone cream, having her apply ½-1 teaspoon daily to different soft tissue sites on her body, on days 10-26 of her menstrual cycle. To avoid saturating a single area, Rosanna rotated the application site from her face to neck, inner arm, back of the wrist, abdomen, inner thigh, and breast. At the same time, Dr. DeMarco began reducing Rosanna's intake of synthetic estrogen and progesterone over a four-week period, and she took Rosanna completely off the Lupron.

Dr. DeMarco prescribed a balanced multivitamin/mineral supplement for Rosanna, an herbal blend (containing milk thistle, dandelion, and celandine) to strengthen her liver, and a lipotropic formula including choline, methionine, and inositol to help her liver break down estrogen. After six to eight weeks on this combined program, Rosanna's pain was reduced and she was better able to cope with what pain there was, says Dr. DeMarco.

At this point Dr. DeMarco began to address Rosanna's diet and possible food allergies. Prior to this, Rosanna had been unwilling to focus attention here. A comprehensive allergy test revealed that Rosanna had a high degree of *Candida albicans* yeast infection and parasites. Although

A Mini-Primer on Natural Progesterone Cream

Natural progesterone can reverse endometriosis by helping to restore proper hormone balance, without side effects, says John Lee, M.D. According to Dr. Lee, natural progesterone can stop the spread of endometrial cells by blocking the activity of estrogen which otherwise stimulates the growth of these aberrant cells.

Dr. Lee suggests using natural progesterone cream from days six to 26 of the monthly cycle, stopping just before menstruation begins. After four to six months of this treatment, the monthly pains and bleeding due to endometriosis will usually subside, he says. Dr. Lee prefers transdermal (absorbed through the skin) natural progesterone in cream or oil formulation, because it is absorbed more efficiently and the effect lasts longer, with-out the emotional highs and lows from oral drops. A woman addressing endometriosis will probably need to use from ⅛ to ½ teaspoon of cream per day or three to ten drops of oil, says Dr. Lee. The cream may be applied to the palms, face, neck, upper chest, breasts, inside of the arms, or behind the knees.

The key criterion is the amount of progesterone (in milligrams) contained in a given natural progesterone product. Under healthy conditions, a premenopausal woman's system produces about 20 mg daily of progesterone between days 15 and 26 of the cycle. While amounts in the range of 20-30 mg daily are often sufficient, relief from the primary symptoms will indicate a woman is taking the appropriate dosage.[27]

the relationship is not yet precisely known, "*Candida* has a direct effect on hormones, such as estrogen and progesterone, either by binding to the receptor sites or by forming antibodies which can then react against ovarian tissues," says Dr. DeMarco. Other physicians have noted that when they eliminated the *Candida* infection in women with endometriosis, it helped to improve this condition as well.

Dr. DeMarco addressed the *Candida* infection with *acidophilus* supplements and dietary changes, emphasizing the avoidance of sugars, fruit juices, yeasted breads, fermented foods, dairy products, dried or over-ripe fruits, and processed, canned, or moldy foods. In addition, Rosanna took caprylic acid (made from coconut oil) tablets, two before each meal; she continued this for three months. She also received desensitization shots for the *Candida*.

To remove the parasites, Dr. DeMarco put Rosanna on a 90-day herbal program including wormwood, black walnut tincture, cloves, and grapefruit seed extract. As Rosanna was low in DHEA (SEE QUICK DEFINITION), a hormone produced by the adrenal glands, Dr. DeMarco put her on DHEA plus adrenal and ovarian glandular

Dr. DeMarco notes that many women with endometriosis are deficient in iodine and that elemental iodine supplementation has benefited some patients in whom it acts "like a natural anti-estrogen."

QUICK DEFINITION

DHEA (dehydroepiandrosterone) is naturally produced by the human adrenal glands and gonads with optimal levels occurring around age 20 for women and age 25 for men. After that, DHEA levels gradually decline so that a person at age 80 produces only a fraction of the DHEA they did when they were 20. As an antioxidant, hormone regulator, and the building block from which estrogen and testosterone are produced, DHEA is vital to health. Low DHEA levels have been associated with cancer, diabetes, multiple sclerosis, hypertension, obesity, AIDS, heart disease, Alzheimer's, and immune dysfunction illnesses. Test subjects using supplemental DHEA reported improved sleeping patterns, better memory, an improved ability to cope with stress, decreased joint pain, increases in lean muscle, and decreases in body fat. No serious side effects have been reported to date, although acne, oily skin, facial hair growth on women, deepening of the voice, irritability, insomnia, and fatigue have been reported with high DHEA doses.

extracts. She took the DHEA and adrenal glandulars on an empty stomach twice daily and the ovarian glandular with meals. "Usually people who have been chronically ill have adrenals that are stressed and under-functioning," says Dr. DeMarco.

In about six months, Rosanna reported a 75% reduction in pain. At this point, Dr. DeMarco added another element to the program in the form of a traditional naturopathic herbal formula called Turska, containing *phytolacca americana* (pokeweed), aconite (*aconitum napellus* or monkshood), *bryony* (tetterberry), and *gelsemium sempervirens* (yellow jessamine). Rosanna took this formula at the dosage of five drops, four times daily, for the next six months.

At the conclusion of 12 months of treatment, Rosanna was pain free. She had to remain vigilant about her diet, stress levels, and exposure to allergenic substances, and remain on the nutritional supplement program and natural progesterone, says Dr. DeMarco.

Dr. DeMarco notes that evidence from animal and human studies indicates that, as mentioned earlier in this chapter, exposure to or ingestion (through foods) of pesticides such as dioxin can lead to an increase in the rate of endometriosis, presumably because these chemicals mimic the action of estrogen. Dr. DeMarco also notes that many women with endometriosis are deficient in iodine and that elemental iodine supplementation has benefited some patients in whom it acts "like a natural anti-estrogen."[28]

In the next case study, we learn about another alternative to synthetic hormones—therapeutic essential plant oils massaged into the skin.

Success Story: Using Aromatherapy to Avoid Synthetic Hormones

Jean, 43, had suffered with endometriosis for three and a half years when she first visited aromatherapist Joanne Hopkins.[29] Her symptoms were typical of an endometriosis sufferer, in particular the "constant dull dragging pain" in her abdomen. This sensation made her physically sick and often confined her to bed, sometimes for days at a time. The continual pain left Jean feeling "washed out," and this affected her concentration, resulting in irritability and occasional depression.

Prior to the visit, Jean had sought help from a conventional physician, who referred her to a gynecologist. The gynecologist told her to continue using birth control pills without breaks until she underwent a laparoscopy to determine the source of her pain. The gynecologist confirmed that Jean had endometriosis, and prescribed Provera (synthetic progesterone substitute).

After doing some research, Jean decided not to take Provera because of its many side effects. Instead, she opted to try aromatherapy (SEE QUICK DEFINITION). At the first session, Hopkins assessed potential weaknesses in Jean's energy patterns, using a form of testing called Touch for Health. (Touch for Health uses changes in large muscle strength as a measure of energy levels). Through this assessment, Hopkins determined that Jean's kidney and large intestine energy pathways were weak.

As treatment, to strengthen those two energy systems and address Jean's other symptoms, Hopkins selected essential oils: bergamot, an immune stimulant; juniper, for menstrual pain; and rose otto, a general tonic, to regulate the menstrual cycle and alleviate the symptoms of depression. Hopkins explains that the oils normally recommended for endometriosis are rose otto, clary sage, frankincense, and lavender, but she tailored the program to Jean's needs.

Hopkins first massaged Jean's abdomen, legs, back, neck, and shoulders with a blend of the essential oils. Hopkins then recommended that Jean take a soothing bath every day after work, using the same mixture. Hopkins also suggested a few pelvic exercises to strengthen the muscles surrounding Jean's reproductive organs.

After the first treatment, Jean reported feeling more enthusiasm and energy than she had in years. Satisfied that Jean's immune system was already improving, at the next weekly session Hopkins applied a warm compress of aromatic oils to Jean's lower abdomen. The compress

QUICK DEFINITION

Aromatherapy uses the essential oils extracted from plants and herbs to treat conditions ranging from infections and skin disorders to immune deficiencies and stress. The volatile constituents of the plant oils (its essence) are extracted through a process of steam distillation or cold-pressing. Although the term "aromatherapy" would seem to suggest an exclusive role for the aroma in the healing process, the oils also exert much of their therapeutic effect through their pharmacological properties and their small molecular size, making them one of the few therapeutic agents to easily penetrate bodily tissues. The benefits of essential oils can be obtained through inhalation, external application, or ingestion. The term aromatherapy was coined in 1937 by the French chemist Rene-Maurice Gattefosse, who observed the healing effect of lavender oil on burns.

For more about **aromatherapy** and **essential oils,** contact: The National Association of Holistic Aromatherapists, (NAHA), 219 Carl Street, San Francisco, CA 94117; tel: 415-564-6785. For another source of essential oils, contact: Phyto Medicine Company, 6701 Sunset Drive, Suite 100, Miami, FL 33143; tel: 305-662-6396; fax: 305-667-5619.

Reduce Your Risk of Endometrial Cancer With Diet

New evidence suggests that the high-fiber, low-fat diet often recommended for weight loss may also reduce your risk of certain types of cancer. According to a study tracking the dietary habits of over 800 women, eating a high-fiber diet can cut your chances of endometrial cancer nearly in half.

The study found that, among 332 women with endometrial cancer and 511 women without the disease, the women who ate the highest quantities of fiber-rich foods reduced their cancer risk by 29%-47%. High-fiber foods such as cereal, vegetables, and fruit provided the most benefit, while soy products and other legumes in the diet similarly reduced cancer risk. On the other hand, eating a diet high in fat may actually increase your chances of endometrial cancer, as obesity is a major risk factor for developing this and other types of cancer.

The study authors believe that a diet high in soy and fiber has an anti-estrogenic effect. In other words, soy- and fiber-rich foods can counteract the negative influence of having too much estrogen in the body, a condition often associated with endometrial cancer, fibroids, and other women's health problems. As these study results suggest, eating a plant-based diet low in calories from fat, high in fiber, and rich in legumes (especially soybeans) may keep you from being counted among the estimated 34,900 new cases of endometrial cancer to be diagnosed in the U.S. this year.[30]

contained clary sage (a menstrual regulator) and lavender (an immune stimulant) blended with a rose otto base. Hopkins also recommended that Jean apply a compress of this mixture at home every day, and that she continue her bath treatments with lavender, geranium, and rose otto.

By her fifth week of treatment, Jean had even more energy and her abdominal pain had significantly decreased. Hopkins extended the treatments to every two weeks, and changed the massage oil blend to rosemary, may chang, bergamot, and rose otto. After that, the treatments were monthly, and then every few months as Jean continued to improve. According to Hopkins, Jean continues to use her oils at home, in her bath and for an abdominal massage. Only once since her treatment began has Jean's endometriosis prevented her from doing what she wanted, and she successfully nursed herself with essential oils. As Hopkins proudly reports, "Jean is happy to have her energy back, to be free of her 'dull dragging pain,' and to be in charge of her life again."

A Dietary and Supplement Program for Endometriosis

As you may have noted in the previous case studies, dietary changes and nutritional supplements were frequently an integral part of the treatment protocols. Even if you use other alternative therapies to cure endometriosis, dietary changes must still be part of the program, says Susan Lark, M.D., of Los Altos, California.

"After years of working with thousands of women patients, I have found that no therapy can be fully effective without including beneficial dietary changes as part of the treatment plan," Dr. Lark says. In addition, nutritional supplements can help reduce the stimulating effect of estrogen on endometrial cell "implants" and speed up a return to health, she states.[31]

The following are Dr. Lark's dietary recommendations:

■ Avoid saturated fats, dairy products, meat, poultry, caffeine, salt, sugar, and chocolate: meat, eggs, and dairy contain arachidonic acid, which promotes inflammation. If you do eat meat, eat only three ounces or less per day.

■ A vegetarian, high-fiber diet is preferable.

■ Eat whole grains such as millet, buckwheat, oats, and rice: these are sources of vitamins B and E (see below); also, the fiber in the grains absorbs estrogen and helps remove it from the body via bowel elimination.

■ Eat soybeans and other legumes: they lower estrogen levels through natural plant estrogens (phytoestrogens) which bind to estrogen receptor sites, taking the place of the estrogen hormone cells, preventing the toxic effects of excess estrogen.

■ Eat plenty of vegetables: many are high in magnesium, potassium, and calcium which can relax tense muscles.

■ Eat fruit: many are high in vitamin C and bioflavonoids, especially the pulp and inner peel of citrus fruits, grape skins, and berries.

■ Use olive, canola, or corn oil: corn oil contains vitamin E (see below); flax oil is also good, but cannot be used for cooking

FOS and Hawthorn for Endometriosis

Shiva Barton, N.D., a naturopathic physician in Brookline, Massachusetts, reports success in clearing endometriosis using a combination of fructo-oligosaccharides (FOS, a supplement that serves as food for bifidobacteria and other beneficial intestinal flora) and hawthorn berry (*Crataegus*) extract, a Chinese herb that is specific for endometriosis. Her recommended twice daily dosage is 1½ tsp of FOS and ¼ tsp of the hawthorn extract.[32]

FOS contributes to combatting *Candida* overgrowth by promoting the growth of healthy intestinal bacteria which naturally keep the yeast in check.

"After years of working with thousands of women patients, I have found that no therapy can be fully effective without including beneficial dietary changes as part of the treatment plan," Dr. Susan Lark says.

QUICK DEFINITION

Essential fatty acids (EFAs) are unsaturated fats required in the diet. Omega-3 and omega-6 oils are the two principal types. The primary omega-3 oil is alpha-linolenic acid (ALA) and is found in flaxseed (58%), canola, pumpkin, walnut, and soybeans. Fish oils, such as salmon, cod, and mackerel, contain the other important omega-3 oils, DHA (docosahexaenoic acid) and EPA (eicosapentaenoic acid). Linoleic acid or cis-linoleic acid is the main omega-6 oil and is found in most plants and vegetable oils, including safflower (73%), corn, peanut, and sesame. The most therapeutic form of omega-6 oil is gamma-linolenic acid (GLA), found in evening primrose, black currant, and borage oils. Once in the body, omega-3 and omega-6 are converted to prostaglandins, hormone-like substances that regulate many metabolic functions, particularly inflammatory processes.

due to its perishability.

■ Make sure you're getting enough essential fatty acids (EFAs, see below and QUICK DEFINITION) in your diet: seeds and nuts are good sources; salmon, tuna, mackerel, and trout contain high amounts of EFAs and help with cramping pain for this reason.[33]

The following are supplements Dr. Lark typically finds useful:

■ Beta carotene (vitamin A precursor): helps reduce the excessive menstrual bleeding associated with endometriosis; 5,000 IU maximum daily.

■ Vitamin B complex: helps regulate estrogen levels by aiding the liver in converting excess estrogen into weaker forms; 50-100 mg of vitamin B complex with up to 300 mg daily of vitamin B6 in addition.

■ Vitamin C: by strengthening blood capillaries, it reduces bleeding and cramps; 1,000-4,000 mg daily.

■ Bioflavonoids: antioxidant that helps regulate estrogen levels; 800 mg daily.

■ Vitamin E: smooths out the disruptive effects of excess estrogen; 400-2,000 IU daily; people with high blood pressure or diabetes should start at 100 IU and increase slowly.

■ Essential Fatty Acids (EFAs): natural anti-inflammatories that help to relax muscles and blood vessels and thus ease cramping; 4 tsp daily is the adult requirement, but the dose for women with menstrual cramps is several tablespoons.[34]

For more about **FOS** and **NutraFlora®**, contact: GTC Nutrition Company, 1400 W. 122nd Avenue, Suite 110, Westminster, CO 80234; tel: 303-254-8012; fax: 303-254-8201; For **hawthorn berry extract** (as mentioned by Dr. Shiva Barton), licensed practitioners may contact: Scientific Botanicals, P.O. Box 31131, Seattle, WA 98103; tel: 206-527-5521. For more about **endometriosis**, contact: The Endometriosis Association, 8585 N. 76th Place, Milwaukee, WI 53223; tel: 800-992-3636 or 414-355-2200; fax: 414-355-6065.

CHAPTER

3

Fibroids growing in the uterus are one of the most

common female health problems

affecting women between the ages of 30 and 50.

It's possible to eliminate fibroids

without surgery when you correct underlying

hormonal, metabolic, or nutritional imbalances,

clear out unresolved emotional issues,

and address hidden toxicities and allergies.

Fibroids

AS WITH A NUMBER of other women's health problems, the incidence of uterine fibroids (benign, fibrous tumors in the uterus) is increasing. By conservative estimates, one in five women in the United States has at least some evidence of fibroids. Among women of childbearing age, the incidence is higher, with estimates ranging from 25% to 50% of women in that age category, with most of those afflicted in their thirties and forties. The incidence is two to three times higher among black women than among white women; the reason for the difference is unknown.[1] Women's health expert and author Susan Lark, M.D., of Los Altos, California, estimates that about 40% of American women have a benign fibroid tumor in the uterus by the time they reach menopause. "Fibroids are one of the most common female health problems affecting women during their reproductive years," she states.

Fibroids are usually firm, spherical lumps occurring in groups. Of varying sizes, they tend to be described in terms of a vegetable or fruit—the size of a pea, lemon, apple, cantaloupe—and can range in size from microscopic to as big as a basketball. If they grow near the outer wall of the uterus, they are easily felt during a pelvic examination, but if they are in the inner uterine lining, ultrasound may be required for detection. If a fibroid grows rapidly, it may outstrip its nutrition supply from nearby blood vessels, resulting in the degeneration and death of the oxygen-deprived tissue; severe abdominal pain may result.

The fibroid itself is composed of hard, fibrous white tissue. One woman, after examining her fibroid following its surgical removal, compared its appearance to "a piece of high-density polyethylene plastic, the stuff cutting boards are made of." Normally, fibroids are encapsulated with another band of tissue.

Sometimes the bulk of a fibroid stops growing and instead it develops a network of fibers, like the feeder roots of a plant. These have the function of bringing nutrients to the fibroid and can change the density of the surrounding tissue; for example, the fibers can actually transform the entire uterine muscle (myometrium) from soft to hard. Due to the interweaving with the surrounding tissue, surgery to remove this kind of fibroid can be very difficult, making it easier for a doctor to recommend hysterectomy (removal of the uterus).[2]

While some women have no symptoms associated with their fibroids, others have symptoms so severe that life becomes nearly unbearable. In more than 50% of the women who have fibroids, the tumor or tumors cause lower abdominal pain, excessive menstrual bleeding, and infertility. Miscarriages and anemia, with weakness and dizziness caused by the heavy bleeding, also result.

Other symptoms include a feeling of fullness and pressure in the lower abdomen, bleeding between periods, increased menstrual cramps, lumps in the abdomen, and a chronic mucus discharge throughout the menstrual cycle. Fibroids, by their very size, frequently cause congestion of nearby areas, resulting in constipation, urinary urgency, and sometimes recurrent bladder infections or irritation.

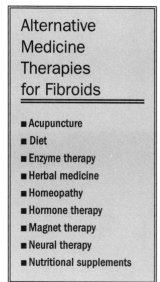

Alternative Medicine Therapies for Fibroids

- Acupuncture
- Diet
- Enzyme therapy
- Herbal medicine
- Homeopathy
- Hormone therapy
- Magnet therapy
- Neural therapy
- Nutritional supplements

If a woman is taking steroidal drugs or is pregnant when a fibroid is removed, a biopsy may wrongfully indicate malignant cellular changes due to the effect of the drugs and elevated estrogen on fibroid cells.

Why Not Hysterectomy?

As in endometriosis and breast lumps, the conventional medical treatment for fibroids is to cut them out, even though almost all cases of fibroids are benign (less than 0.5% of fibroids become cancerous).[3] However, it may be difficult to remove just the fibroid, so the physician may want to perform a hysterectomy, removing the whole uterus through the abdomen or vagina.

Hysterectomy is currently the second most common surgical procedure performed on women in the United States—750,000 hysterectomies (many including ovary removal) every year,[4] at an average

A Primer on Fibroids

Fibroids are classified according to their location and growth characteristics as follows:[10]

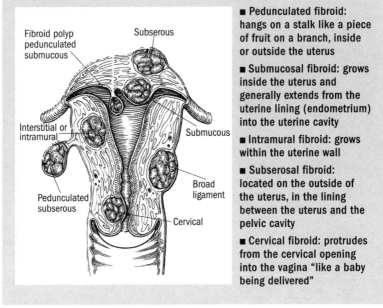

- **Pedunculated fibroid:** hangs on a stalk like a piece of fruit on a branch, inside or outside the uterus

- **Submucosal fibroid:** grows inside the uterus and generally extends from the uterine lining (endometrium) into the uterine cavity

- **Intramural fibroid:** grows within the uterine wall

- **Subserosal fibroid:** located on the outside of the uterus, in the lining between the uterus and the pelvic cavity

- **Cervical fibroid:** protrudes from the cervical opening into the vagina "like a baby being delivered"

Labels on diagram: Fibroid polyp pedunculated submucous; Subserous; Interstitial or intramural; Submucous; Broad ligament; Pedunculated subserous; Cervical

For more about **Dr. Hufnagel's approach to surgery**, see "When Surgery is Unavoidable," Chapter 2: Endometriosis, p. 86.

cost of $4,710 each. Of female surgeries, it is surpassed only by Caesarian section.[5]

Surgeon Vicki Hufnagel, M.D., of West Hollywood, California, estimates that about 90% of hysterectomies are unnecessary.[6] For example, despite the fact that nearly all fibroids are benign, 551,752 hysterectomies to cut out fibroids were performed between 1982 and 1984, according to Dr. Hufnagel.[7] "What is even more astounding is that many of these hysterectomies are carried out on women in their twenties and thirties who have no children," says Dr. Hufnagel. "They are not told that they have options."[8]

In addition to the loss of childbearing ability and the emotional trauma of such surgery, recovery from a hysterectomy takes an average of one year. Further, studies show that for a 35-year-old woman who has had a hysterectomy, the risk of heart attack or angina increases by seven times.[9] Premenopausal women who have a hysterectomy without ovary removal begin menopause typically five years

Ultrasound: Detecting the Fibroid Noninvasively

The standard diagnostic tool for determining if a woman has a fibroid is called ultrasound or ultrasonography. The state of deep structures within the body, in this case, the uterus, can be visualized by way of recording the reflections made from pulsing ultrasonic waves directly into the targeted tissues. The ultrasound reflections are then displayed on a computer monitor and are interpreted by a trained medical technician. Generally, the technician is able to accurately identify a fibroid, assess its approximate size and extent, and determine whether it is benign or cancerous. However, an ultrasound diagnosis is not infallible. Cases have been reported of a prolapsed uterus, prolapsed colon, or ballooned-out, impacted small intestine being misread as a fibroid.

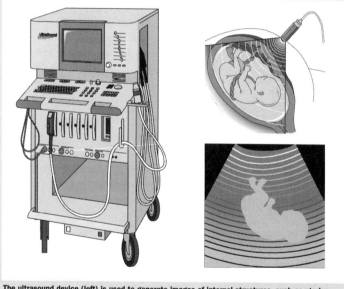

The ultrasound device (left) is used to generate images of internal structures, such as uterine fibroids and the status of fetuses (right).

earlier because one long-term effect of the surgery is accelerated aging of the ovaries. This may be due to the fact that the blood supply to the ovaries is compromised by removal of the uterus.[11]

A hysterectomy that includes removal of the ovaries causes immediate complications. "When menopause is created surgically within a short time, as is the case with hysterectomy, many problems arise," states Lita Lee, Ph.D. "The sudden shock of the surgery causes the remaining organs to try frantically to take over some of the functions

A Glossary of Surgical Procedures for Fibroids

While it is the intent of this chapter to suggest successful ways of avoiding surgery, it is helpful to understand the types of procedures, other than hysterectomy (removal of the uterus), offered by conventional medicine.

Laparoscopy: During laparoscopy, a slender telescopic instrument is inserted through a small incision in the navel to view the uterus and fibroids. One to three more incisions are then made in the abdomen through which the fibroids are removed. This relatively new procedure can also be used for large tumors.

Myomectomy: For large tumors (the size of a grapefruit), myomectomy can be used to remove just the tumor, preserving the uterus. This operation is difficult and takes longer to perform, however, and runs the risk of hemmorrhage and/or infection.

Hysteroscopy: For tumors smaller than a grapefruit, a less invasive operation called hysteroscopy can be performed. This operation involves the use of a small lighted instrument called a hysteroscope which is inserted from the vagina through the cervix and is used to illuminate the inside of the uterus during the operation.

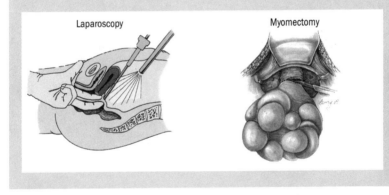

Laparoscopy

Myomectomy

For more about **estrogen dominance**, see Chapter 1: Menstrual Problems, pp. 23-24.

of the ones that were removed." Dr. Lee has observed adrenal and pancreatic problems (including diabetes) along with symptoms of menopause such as vaginal dryness and sudden hot flashes, for which estrogen is commonly prescribed. "This is ironic since relative estrogen excess is one of the primary causes of problems (fibroids, excessive bleeding, endometriosis, and cancer) that lead to hysterectomy in the first place," Dr. Lee says.

The deleterious effects of hysterectomy have obviously not prevented its widespread use. During a Congressional investigation in

1977, the American Medical Association (AMA), testifying on the reasons for the high rate of hysterectomy, stated that the operation was used for sterilization and as a preventative method to forestall cancer of the uterus in later years.[12] The truth is the operation is a big moneymaker. That aside, the AMA's justifications are unconscionable, given the serious consequences of the procedure as enumerated above.

The statistics on who is getting all these hysterectomies reveal that the high rate has little to do with medical need. Research has found that:[13]

■ Hysterectomy appears to be associated with education level. Women who had completed only nine to 11 years of education were more likely to have undergone a hysterectomy than were women with more education. The women with less education were also more likely to have undergone a hysterectomy because of menstrual problems.

■ A history of multiple miscarriages—three or more, especially due to uterine prolapse—increases the probability of hysterectomies.

■ Women who have their first child before age 20 increase their probability of hysterectomy due to endometriosis.

■ Uterine fibroids are the most common reason for hysterectomy, followed by menstrual problems in second place.

While hysterectomy is often the conventional medicine approach to fibroids, the alternative medicine model of treating the causes provides a long-lasting solution that does not require the sacrifice of organs. Here, women's health specialist **Jesse Hanley, M.D.,** of

Fibroids More Common in Black Women

Black women are more likely to develop uterine fibroids, according to researchers at the Harvard School of Public Health. A four-month study of over 95,000 female nurses between the ages of 25 and 44 found that the black nurses had a two to three times higher incidence of fibroids than their white, Asian, and Hispanic colleagues.

Although study results were adjusted for additional factors such as body mass index, history of infertility, oral contraceptive use, and current alcohol consumption, the black participants still showed a significantly greater risk of developing the condition. Researchers have a few theories about why black women are at increased risk for fibroids (such as possible hormonal differences), but the author of the Harvard study notes that "the biology of uterine [fibroids] is not well understood."

Additional factors that increase a woman's risk of fibroids include obesity, smoking, and advancing age.[14]

Malibu, California, recounts how she uses a combination of therapies, from natural hormones to magnets, to treat even advanced fibroids and enable patients to escape surgery:

Success Story: Hysterectomy Avoided

Elizabeth had a fibroid so large she looked six months pregnant. It had been growing for at least ten years, but somehow none of her doctors addressed the problem, other than to recommend a hysterectomy, the standard gynecological procedure for fibroids. As a result of the fibroid, Elizabeth experienced severe PMS and heavy menstrual flow. Despite her pain and discomfort, Elizabeth wanted to avoid surgery, so she came to me for an alternative approach to treating her condition.

Most uterine fibroids are caused by an imbalance in female hormones, specifically the overproduction of estrogen relative to progesterone (estrogen dominance). What most people don't know is that the highly processed foods in our diet can sometimes act as exogenous or "outside" estrogens, and these can artificially increase the amount of estrogen in a woman's body, putting her at risk for developing fibroids and other estrogen-related problems.

In Elizabeth's case, these outside estrogens from processed foods were encouraging her existing fibroid to grow bigger, so the first thing I did was change her diet. Elizabeth began eating a predominantly whole foods, high-fiber, low-fat diet, which was mostly vegetarian, but included twice-weekly servings of organic poultry or low-fat fish. To round out her nutritional program, I encouraged Elizabeth to supplement with a multivitamin and multimineral. Evidence indicates that vitamin A can help shrink fibroids, so I also put Elizabeth on a daily dose of 50,000 IU of vitamin A, derived from fish oil. Elizabeth took this in cycles of six weeks on, then three weeks off, as too much vitamin A can be toxic for the liver.

To help Elizabeth's digestive system process the outside estrogens and eliminate them from her body, I prescribed SymBiotics™, a formula containing *acidophilus*, *bifidus*, and other "friendly" intestinal microflora, at the rate of ¹/₂ teaspoon, twice daily. These beneficial bacteria not only "tag" excess estrogen for elimination but also help flush toxic chemicals from the colon. I also prescribed a commercially available product called UltraClear™, a metabolic detoxification and food-based clearing formula which contains lipotropics (substances which remove and prevent fatty deposits in the liver), liver-supporting herbs, and other nutrients in powder form made primarily from high-protein white rice and safflower oil.

Unfortunately, it's usually not enough simply to flush excess estrogen from the body; you have to offset the effects of estrogen dominance as well. For this, I prescribed 3 mg of the hormone melatonin (SEE QUICK DEFINITION) at bedtime, as research suggests it helps to balance the effects of excess estrogen. For the same reason, I typically recommend using progesterone throughout most of the menstrual cycle, especially if the fibroid is very large. Natural progesterone is useful because even if it doesn't shrink the fibroid, it stops or at least slows down the growth by balancing against the estrogen. I had Elizabeth use natural progesterone twice daily on the days between menstrual periods, at a dosage of ¼ teaspoon applied to her abdomen and other soft tissue areas such as the inside of the legs and arms.

Finally, I gave Elizabeth a Chinese herbal blend called Bupleurum Entangled Qi Formula™ (three pills, three times daily). This formula contains 26 herbs and is useful in treating uterine fibroids, breast lumps, ovarian or cervical cysts, and other conditions of blood and energy (*qi*) stagnation. In Chinese medicine terms, fibroids are a stagnation of blood which becomes so congested that it forms a toxic solid. To get the blood moving again, I prescribed cayenne (two capsules daily), a spice known for increasing blood circulation and dissolving cold, damp lumps.

Normally, I would also recommend acupuncture to help unblock the energy, but Elizabeth wouldn't go near a needle. We got around this problem by having her wear a magnet over her uterus, with the negative pole facing the skin. This helped her body restore and regenerate its own magnetic field, freeing up the energy to make Elizabeth's uterus healthy again.

At this point, I'd like to mention the therapeutic use of

> **QUICK DEFINITION**
>
> **Melatonin**, a hormone produced by the pea-sized, light-sensitive pineal (pronounced pie-NEEL) gland in the center of the brain, regulates the body's internal clock, or circadian rhythm, which determines the 24-hour sleep-wake cycle. With aging, the peak in melatonin secretion is about one hour later than normal (normal peak secretion time is about 2 a.m.), and the maximum peak of melatonin is only one-half the level of young adults. Low melatonin levels have been associated with sleeping disturbances and light-related disorders such as Seasonal Affective Disorder. Eating vitamin- and mineral-rich foods and increasing your exposure to bright light can improve the body's natural melatonin production.

To contact **Jesse Lynn Hanley, M.D.**: 22917 Pacific Coast Highway, Malibu, CA 90265; tel: 310-456-9393; fax: 310-456-9482. **Bupleurum Entangled Qi Formula™** is available in tablet form (750 mg), for licensed health practitioners only. For more information, contact: Health Concerns, 8001 Capwell Drive, Oakland, CA 94621; tel: 510-639-0280; fax: 510-639-9140. **SymBiotics™**, which contains nine different strains of "friendly" (probiotic) intestinal organisms in a matrix of fructo-oligosaccharides (FOS), is available from: Allergy Research Group, 400 Preda Street, San Leandro, CA 94577; tel: 800-545-9960 (information) or 800-782-4274 (direct order); fax: 510-635-6730. For **ProGest®** natural progesterone cream, contact: Transitions for Health, 621 Southwest Alder, Suite 900, Portland, OR 97205; tel: 503-226-1010; fax: 503-226-6455; or contact: Chelsea Lee Enterprises, P.O. Box 602, 1570 Newbury Road, Newbury Park, CA 91320; tel: 800-823-1144; fax: 805-499-7409. Additional sources of hormones in skin cream form, Cycle Balance/PMS Formula and Ultra Harmony/Menopause Formula (containing wild yam, chastetree berry, and vitamins), are available from: Wise Woman Essentials™, 2101 Kennedy Street NE, #307, Minneapolis, MN 55314; tel: 800-705-9473 or 612-378-8830. For **UltraClear®**, contact: Metagenics, Inc., 971 Calle Negocio, San Clemente, CA 92673; tel: 800-692-9400; fax: 714-366-0818.

visualization. Although I did not use this technique with Elizabeth, visualization—also called guided imagery—is another important step toward healing. Essentially, this process involves seeing the fibroid shrinking and investing that image with some energy every day. I had a patient who shrunk five fibroids this way, having each fibroid represent the five unresolved and painful past love affairs in her life.

For a uterine fibroid the size of Elizabeth's, it might take a few years of treatment to completely resolve the problem. However, within one month Elizabeth stopped having PMS pain and heavy periods and, after four months, the fibroid stopped growing, whereas it had been growing consistently for the previous ten years. As Elizabeth continues on the program, the fibroid will begin to shrink and eventually will disappear. Her case demonstrates that even uterine fibroids of considerable size can be treated without surgery. ■

Success Story: Eliminating the Toxicity That Grew the Fibroid

In addition to hormonal imbalance, a buildup of toxins in the body may also contribute to the development of fibroids. According to **Bruce Shelton, M.D., M.D.(H), Di.Hom.**, director of the Allergy Center in Phoenix, Arizona, an effective approach to treating fibroids without surgery is to root out deep toxicities in the body. This may be accomplished with detoxifying homeopathic remedies, nutritional supplements, hormonal balancing, and neural therapy. There is often a dental factor as well, which must be resolved for full healing to take place, as demonstrated by the following case. Here, Dr. Shelton uses a complex array of alternative medicine techniques to reverse a fibroid accompanied by dangerously heavy bleeding.

Nicole, 32, had a uterine fibroid the size of a grapefruit. Despite the urgent insistence of her gynecologist, Nicole had already refused a hysterectomy three times. Unfortunately, the fibroid was producing heavy bleeding, even hemorrhaging, during menstruation, so something of a medical nature needed to be done soon, says Dr. Shelton. "The fibroid was so far advanced, she was almost a surgical candidate," he notes, but he was willing to work with her using alternative procedures, telling her he generally has a 50% success rate with fibroids.

Dr. Shelton's course of treatment for Nicole had many facets. He gave her drainage remedies, dietary changes, supplements, and homeopathic hormones; he prescribed a homeopathic remedy called *Calcarea iodatum* (iodide of lime) and detoxified her system of everything indicated by the LISTEN evaluation. LISTEN is the name of a sophisticated computerized device that performs information gathering on the body systems, a procedure known as electrodermal screening (see sidebar "A Glossary of Dr. Shelton's Therapies for Nicole," p. 110, for more information).

Nicole also took Artemisia Forte II (200 mg daily) consisting of citrus seed extract and the herb artemisia to destroy the various forms of *Candida* in her intestines. She took a formula called Chlorella Algae, containing chlorella (a blue-green algae concentrate), garlic, and enzymes, for nutritional support, and a product called Gastro-Cort™ (containing amino acids, bioflavonoids, and vitamin E) to support her gastrointestinal lining.

QUICK DEFINITION

To improve Nicole's nutrient status, he gave her Balance™Plus containing the omega-3, -6, and -9 essential fatty acids (SEE QUICK DEFINITION), derived from marine lipids, olive oil, and borage seed oil, and containing vitamins E, C, B6, and B3. Dr. Shelton gave her Immuno-Gland-Plex containing glandular extracts of thymus, pancreas, adrenal gland, and spleen (from cow, lamb, and pig). Basic Preventive® 5 was also on Nicole's list; this is an iron-free multiple vitamin and mineral supplement.

In addition, Dr. Shelton had Nicole rub Lugol's solution (a form of iodine) directly on her abdomen from the belly button to the pubic bone and on the soles of her feet every night. Typically, this produces an intense itch after application; after two to three weeks of regular application, the itching goes away, and the treatment stops. "For some reason, fibroids seem due, in part, to an iodine deficiency," he says. He paints the whole foot, because all the acupuncture meridians end there so, in effect, the entire body can absorb iodine from them.

Nicole's fibroid also had a dental connection. In a woman, the two front incisor teeth are associated with the uterus, while in a man, it's the prostate. Nicole had a root canal (SEE

Essential fatty acids (EFAs) are unsaturated fats required in the diet. Omega-3 and omega-6 oils are the two principal types. The primary omega-3 oil is alpha-linolenic acid (ALA) and is found in flaxseed (58%), canola, pumpkin, walnut, and soybeans. Fish oils, such as salmon, cod, and mackerel, contain the other important omega-3 oils, DHA (docosahexaenoic acid) and EPA (eicosapentaenoic acid). Linoleic acid or cis-linoleic acid is the main omega-6 oil and is found in most plants and vegetable oils, including safflower (73%), corn, peanut, and sesame. The most therapeutic form of omega-6 oil is gamma-linolenic acid (GLA), found in evening primrose, black currant, and borage oils. Once in the body, omega-3 and omega-6 are converted to prostaglandins, hormone-like substances that regulate many metabolic functions, particularly inflammatory processes.

To contact **Bruce Shelton, M.D., M.D.(H), Di.Hom.:** The Allergy Center, 2525 West Greenway Road, Suite 300, Phoenix, AZ 85023; tel: 602-978-1722; fax: 602-942-3787. For more about **Sanum/Enderlein remedies,** read the book *Hidden Killers: The Revolutionary Medical Discoveries of Professor Guenther Enderlein* (Erik Enby et al., 1990), Sheehan Communications, Box 706, Saratoga, CA 95071; tel: 408-354-4840. For **Artemisia Forte II, GastroCort™,** and **Immuno-Gland Plex,** contact: Allergy Research Group, 400 Preda Street, San Leandro, CA 94577; tel: 800-545-9960 or 510-630-4572; fax 510-635-6730. For **Chlorella Algae,** contact: Nutrihealth, John Brimhall, D.C., 1626 North Country Club Road, Mesa, AZ 85201; tel: 602-964-5107. For **Balance™Plus** and **Basic Preventive® 5,** contact: Amni, 2247 National Avenue, Hayward, CA 94550; tel: 800-437-8888 or 510-783-6969; fax: 510-783-8196.

A Glossary of Dr. Shelton's Therapies for Nicole

Electrodermal Screening—This is a form of computerized information gathering, based on physics, not chemistry. A blunt, noninvasive electric probe is placed at specific points on the patient's hands, face, or feet, corresponding to acupuncture points at the beginning or end of energy meridians. Minute electrical discharges from these points serve as information signals about the condition of the body's organs and systems, useful for the physician in evaluation.

Homeopathic remedies—These include homeopathic drainage remedies, which are low potency homeopathic substances and tinctures to encourage the lymphatic system, liver, kidneys, blood, tissues, intercellular spaces, fat, and skin to eliminate or "drain" their toxins, thus keeping them from circulating in the body or being deposited in other tissues.

Hormone Balancing—Dr. Shelton prepares homeopathic dilutions of the common sex hormones, then gives them (as oral drops) to the patient, based on electrodermal indications for dosage.

Neural Therapy—This approach, in which the anesthetics Novocain, Xylocaine, or Procain are injected into scars or nerve ganglia, was pioneered by two German physicians named Ferdinand and Walter Huneke in 1925 as a way of relieving pain and physical trauma.

Sanum/Enderlein Remedies—This approach is still on the horizon for most U.S. physicians, but in Switzerland and Germany, for example, it is more widely understood and practiced. German physician Guenther Enderlein, M.D., Ph.D. (1872-1968), developed a line of about 40 preparations of benign microorganisms or protein particles; when introduced into the body (seven drops under the tongue per week), these remedies help restore the optimal cellular terrain for health. They're called "Sanum" because they are made by the Sanum-Kehlbeck company in Hoya, Germany.

Dr. Enderlein's theory was that homeopathic preparations of certain harmful bacteria and fungi could cause the harmful ones still in the body to revert back to an earlier, basic form that was not harmful. His approach was founded on a controversial microbiological theory that microbes are capable of changing shape and activity depending on the internal conditions of cells, and that these multiple shape-changes of a single organism can include forms ranging from viruses to bacteria and fungi. In turn, the forms are correlated with different illnesses for which they are believed to be causes.

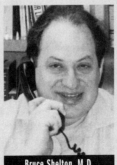

Bruce Shelton, M.D.

QUICK DEFINITION) in one of these teeth and, in Dr. Shelton's assessment, this was creating an energy flow interference that contributed to the growth of her fibroid. At his suggestion, Nicole had this tooth extracted and a false one installed in its place. "That's when her fibroid started to shrink," he reports.

But what produced the most dramatic results in eliminating Nicole's fibroids was a series of neural therapy injections in the Frankenhäuser's nerve plexus surrounding the cervix and uterus. There are two options for this procedure, Dr. Shelton says. First, you can inject the *Nigersan* Sanum remedy with Procain through the abdominal wall, but this runs the risk of perforating the bladder. Second, you can insert a speculum into the vagina, then inject the medicine into the intra-abdominal space next to the cervix.

The speculum procedure takes a minute and the Procain (because it's an anesthetic) eliminates any momentary pain immediately. After the injection, Nicole lay on the treatment table for ten minutes. Thirty days later, her fibroid was 95% gone. Over the next months, it disappeared completely; the ultrasound could find no trace of it and it never came back.

A **root canal** is a dental procedure in which infected bone tissue in the pulp cavity near the root of the tooth (root canal) is removed; the cavity is then filled with a protective substance. While root canals save the tooth from extraction, research indicates that the procedure, for many patients, can be a source of toxicity which can spread to other parts of the body, contributing to illness. During a root canal, bacteria become trapped and sealed within the, literally, three miles of microscopic dentin tubules of the tooth. Unaffected by antibiotics, which cannot reach them, these bacterial toxins can then circulate throughout the body, causing systemic diseases of the heart, kidney, uterus, and nervous and endocrine systems. When the root-canalled teeth are removed, it becomes much easier to reverse these conditions.

Estrogen Dominance: The Main Factor in Fibroids

As the two medical histories above demonstrate, a prominent cause of fibroids, as with many other women's health conditions, is hormonal imbalance, usually a relative excess of estrogen (estrogen dominance, see sidebar: "Ten Reasons Why Your Hormones are Imbalanced," p. 113). As discussed in previous chapters, a relative excess of estrogen means you have too much of that hormone in relation to progesterone.

Estrogen dominance can cause fibroid and other tumor growth because one of the key actions of estrogen is to "create proliferative endometrium (the mucous membrane lining the uterus)," according to John Lee, M.D.[15] Further evidence in support of the estrogen dominance theory is the fact that fibroids develop following the onset of menstruation, enlarge during pregnancy, and shrink after menopause.[16]

"Fibroids are caused by periods of high estrogen production, and our strategy is to level these out so that the fibroids don't grow," says Dr. Susan Lark. In her practice, Dr. Lark employs a conservative approach, using nutrition and lifestyle changes to control estrogen production and reduce bleeding. "A fibroid the size of a 13-week fetus (the size at which Western medicine begins discussing the need for a hysterectomy) and larger can be successfully treated by this approach," she says. "Too many women have hysterectomies."

Until recently, the role of progesterone was overshadowed by a focus, created by the pharmaceutical industry, on estrogen deficiency and synthetic estrogen supplements. In fact, progesterone deficiency is increasing and is much more common than originally thought, according to Dr. John Lee and many other holistic practitioners. Dr. Lita Lee (no relation) states that progesterone deficiency is a factor in virtually every woman's health problem—from PMS and fibroids to ovarian cysts and endometriosis—and can begin quite early in a woman's menstrual life.

As stated in previous chapters, progesterone deficiency can result from an underactive thyroid gland (hypothyroidism). Progesterone is made in the body from cholesterol, if there is adequate thyroid hormone. With hypothyroidism, thyroid hormones are in short supply, so progesterone production declines and a situation of estrogen dominance results. The condition only becomes worse because estrogen inhibits thyroid secretion while progesterone stimulates it, explains Dr. Lita Lee.

You can also develop progesterone deficiency at any age from chronic stress, according to clinical nutritionist Ann Louise Gittleman, M.S., C.N.S., of Bozeman, Montana.[17] As discussed in chapter one, your adrenal glands respond to stress by producing the hormones adrenaline and noradrenaline. Progesterone is the primary raw material the glands use for producing the adrenal hormones. The more adrenaline produced, the more progesterone needed. Gittleman explains that if the adrenals run out of progesterone, they will start using another raw material, androstenedione, to produce their hormones. This can result in a masculinizing syndrome in women, including facial whiskers and thinning scalp hair.

Finally, progesterone deficiency can result from frequent anovulatory cycles (menstrual cycles in which you don't ovulate), according to Dr. John Lee.[18] When you fail to ovulate, the ovarian follicle (sac that holds and matures the egg) fails to enter its normal post-ovulatory stage, the corpus luteum. The corpus luteum produces progesterone during the second half of your menstrual cycle. If it's not doing its job, there is a lack of progesterone. Anovulatory cycles can happen at any age, but they are more common in women athletes undergoing strenuous competition, and in women in the perimenopause phase (the ten to 15 years before actual menopause, or cessation of menstrual periods). The anovulatory cycles can thus create estrogen dominance by causing progesterone deficiency.

Natural Progesterone Therapy

As shown in the case of Elizabeth above and numerous other cases throughout the book, one of the most successful ways to balance an excess of estrogen in the body (or fortify a progesterone deficiency) is to supplement with natural progesterone. Natural progesterone does not cause any of the side effects of synthetic progesterone (progestins) that some women take as part of hormone replacement therapy during menopause or in some birth control pills. Natural progesterone is available as a transdermal (absorbed through the skin) cream, as an oil taken orally, as vaginal suppositories, or as micronized (broken into small fragments) powder placed in a capsule and taken orally.

The cream form is one of the most popular ways of taking natural progesterone. As a result of using the cream, many women are experiencing relief for the first time in their lives from female reproductive problems including fibroids, PMS, ovarian cysts, endometriosis, and others. The usual dosage is $1/8$ to $1/2$ tsp rubbed twice daily on soft tissue, such

Ten Reasons Why Your Hormones are Imbalanced

Estrogen dominance (too much estrogen in relation to progesterone) can be created by both an excess of estrogen and a deficiency of progesterone. Here is how it happens.

Too much estrogen may be caused by:

1) foods that have hormones added to them, such as commercial meat, milk, eggs, and dairy products

2) herbs that have an estrogenic effect in the body, such as licorice, black cohosh, and damiana

3) birth control pills that have high levels of estrogen

4) environmental toxins that mimic the actions of estrogen (known as xenoestrogens); the largest source of xenoestrogens is pesticides

5) exposure to radiation, which increases estrogen levels in the blood

6) chronic constipation, which interferes with the body's ability to eliminate estrogen properly; estrogen then builds up in the colon and can be reabsorbed by the body

7) synthetic estrogen supplements as part of a hormone replacement therapy for menopausal symptoms.

Too little progesterone may be caused by:

8) an underactive thyroid gland (hypothyroidism)

9) chronic stress

10) frequent anovulatory cycles (menstruation without ovulation).

Progesterone Content of Selected Creams/Oils, As Reported By an Independent Laboratory

The following list of natural progesterone products and their progesterone content was compiled by Dr. John Lee, based on laboratory tests conducted for him by Aeron LifeCycles in San Leandro, California (reprinted by permission of John R. Lee, M.D.).

PRODUCT	COMPANY	LOCATION
1,000-1,500 mg progesterone per ounce:		
Progest-E Complex	Kenogen	Eugene, OR
700-800 mg progesterone per ounce		
ProCreme Plus	Health Products	Manassas, VA
Renewed Balance	American Image Mktg.	Nampa, ID
500-700 mg progesterone per ounce		
Femarone-17	Wise Essentials	Hallendale, FL
Pro-Oste-All	Sarati International	Los Fresnos, TX
400-500 mg progesterone per ounce		
Adam's Equalizer	HM Enterprises	Norcross, GA
Angel Care	Angel Care	Atlanta, GA
Bio Balance	Elan Vitale	Scottsdale, AZ
Edenn Cream	SNM	Norcross, GA
E'Pro & Estrol Balance	Sarati International	Los Fresnos, TX
Equilibrium	Equilibrium Labs	Boca Raton, FL
Fair Lady	Village Market	Fond du Lac, WI
Femarone-17	Wise Essentials	Minneapolis, MN
Fem-Gest	Bio-Nutritional Formulas	Mineola, NY
Feminique	Country Life	Hauppauge, NY
Gentle Changes	Easy Way, Int.	Indianapolis, IN
Happy PMS	HM Enterprises	Norcross, GA
Heaven Sent	Answered Prayers, Inc.	Malibu, CA
Kokoro Balance	Kokoro, LLC	Laguna Niguel, CA
NatraGest	Broadmoore Labs	Ventura, CA
Natural Balance	South Market Service	Atlanta, GA
Natural Woman	Products of Nature	Ridgefield, CT
Natural Woman's Formula	Ultra Balance	Savannah, GA
New Woman	Pinnacle Nut, Inc.	Tulsa, OK
Nugest 900	Nutraceutics Corp.	Deerfield Beach, FL
Marpe Wild Yam	Green Pastures	Flat Rock, NC
Osterderm	Bezwecken	Beavertown, OR
PharmWest	PharmWest	Marina Del Ray, CA

PRODUCT	COMPANY	LOCATION
PhytoGest	Karuna	Novato, CA
Pro-Alo	Health Watchers	Scottsdale, AZ
ProBalance	Springboard	Monterey, CA
Progessence	Young Living	Payson, UT
Pro-G	TriMedica	Scottsdale, AZ
Pro-Gest	Transitions for Health	Portland, OR
Progest-DP	Life Enhancement	Petaluma, CA
Progonal	Bezwecken	Beaverton, OR
Serenity	Health & Science	Crawfordvil, FL
Ultimate Total Woman	New Science Nutrition	N. Lauderdale, FL
Wild Yam Cream	Enrich, International	Orem, UT

10-20 mg progesterone per ounce

Endocreme	Wuliton Labs	Palmyra, MO
EFX Wild Yam	Natural Efx, Inc.	Richardson, TX
Life Changes	MW Labs	Atlanta, GA
Novagest	Strata Dermatologics	Concord, CA
Nugestrone	Nutraceuticals	Boca Raton, FL
Phyto-Balance	Transitions for Health	Portland, OR
Progesterone Plus	Prof. Health Products	Sewickley, PA
Woman Wise	Jason Natural Cosmetics	Culver City, CA

Less than 5 mg progesterone per ounce

Born Again	Alvin Last Inc.	Yonkers, NY
Dioscorea Cream	Saroyal Intl. Inc.	Toronto, Canada
Nutrigest	NutriSupplies, Inc.	West Palm Beach, FL
Progerone	Nature's Nutrition	Vero Beach, FL
Progestone 10	Dixie Health, Inc.	Atlanta, GA
Progestone-HP	Dixie Health, Inc.	Atlanta, GA
Yamcon	Phillips Nutrition	Laguna Hills, CA

as the belly, inside thighs, or inside arms. The most common application period is the latter two weeks of your monthly cycle if you are still menstruating or the last two weeks of the month if you are postmenopausal. However, some practitioners may advise applying the cream all month long (except during your period). Consult with your practitioner or try applying the cream starting on day 14 of your cycle (or after ovulation if you know when that occurs) and stopping when menses begins. Lessening of pain from fibroids or reduction of PMS symptoms may happen in a few weeks or it might take two to three menstrual cycles to see results.

To contact **Lita Lee, Ph.D.:** P.O. Box 516, Lowell, OR 97452; tel: 541-937-1123; fax: 541-937-1132. To contact **John R. Lee, M.D.:** BLL Publishing, P.O. Box 2068, Sebastopol, CA. 95473; tel: 707-823-9350. For a **mail order source of ProGest natural progesterone cream,** contact: Transitions for Health, 621 S.W. Alder Street, Suite 900, Portland, OR 97205-3627; tel: 800-888-6814.

Are Your Hormones the Problem?— A Saliva Test Can Tell You

If you want to know if a relative estrogen excess or other hormonal imbalance is a possible factor in your fibroids, you can find out through a simple saliva test. Called the Aeron LifeCycles saliva assay report, the test can be ordered by both laypeople and physicians and measures up to eight different hormones. The results are plotted on graphs for easy interpretation, and changing levels can be plotted over time on the same graph, if supplementation or subsequent testing is done.

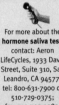

For more about the **hormone saliva test**, contact: Aeron LifeCycles, 1933 Davis Street, Suite 310, San Leandro, CA 94577; tel: 800-631-7900 or 510-729-0375; fax: 510-729-0383.

Although hormones are present in saliva only in fractional amounts compared to the blood, "clinically relevant and highly accurate levels of hormones can be determined in saliva," says John Kells, president of Aeron LifeCycles in San Leandro, California. "Saliva testing provides a means to establish whether or not your hormone levels are within the expected normal range for your age."

Kells says most of the key hormones at play in a man's or woman's body—estrogen, testosterone, DHEA—decline as we age, leaving us more susceptible to reduced physiological functioning and possibly disease. The goal of hormone replacement is to prevent illness and enhance the quality of life, says Kells, but he notes that "there is a fair bit about this that is not yet known."

The saliva assay has several advantages over traditional blood testing for hormones. It is painless and noninvasive, and tests can be performed simply at any time or place. As DHEA, cortisol, estrogen, progesterone, and testosterone levels are highest in the morning, it is far more convenient to be able to test them at home (and then immediately ship the saliva sample to Aeron's laboratory) than to drive to a physician's office possibly at a later time when hormone levels have naturally fallen off a little.

As the test is less expensive than blood testing, you can do frequent testing to monitor changes (brought on by interventions such as diet, exercise, herbs, stress reduction, or acupuncture) and to adjust dosages of over-the-counter hormones such as natural progesterone or melatonin, Kells says. In general, Kells explains that it is best to establish a baseline level of saliva hormones first, then after intervention (which can include hormone supplementation) test a second time to measure the changes.

Various creams are available in health food stores and by mail order. When you purchase a product, there are two things to keep in mind. First, make sure it actually contains natural progesterone, not just wild yam (*Dioscorea villosa*). Don't be misled by claims that wild yam creams are the same as progesterone creams. As an herbal supplement, wild yam can have a mild hormone-balancing effect, but it does not provide natural progesterone. The active ingredient in the yam—diosgenin—is a progesterone precursor that cannot be converted into progesterone by your body. For natural progesterone cream, the diosgenin from wild yam must be converted to progesterone in a laboratory.

Second, make sure you use a brand of cream that has enough natural progesterone in it to make a difference (see sidebar, pp. 114-115). Dr. John Lee advises using only creams that have at least 400 mg of progesterone per ounce. Dr. Lita Lee prefers to use only creams or oils that have more than 1,000 mg of progesterone per ounce, because she believes a lower progesterone content will not be effective for women with serious reproductive problems.

Additional Alternative Medicine Therapies for Fibroids

As is usual in alternative medicine, a wide range of therapies can be effective in treating fibroids. In this section, five case studies illustrate more of your treatment options. The women in these medical histories use acupuncture, enzyme therapy, herbal medicine, and homeopathy, among other therapies, to shrink their fibroids. In several instances, they have decided on surgery and employ the therapies to strengthen their body in preparation or reduce the fibroids to a size that permits safe and minimal surgery, rather than hysterectomy.

Success Story:
Acupuncture Instead of Hysterectomy

Kayla, 32, suffered from multiple fibroids which caused a heavy menstrual flow lasting as long as ten days and occurring twice monthly and accompanied by pain so severe that at one point she had to be hospitalized.[18] In addition, Kayla suffered from PMS, moodiness, cravings for chocolate and salty foods, and bloating in her abdomen, breasts, and ankles before each period. The stress of constant pain and blood loss left Kayla with headaches and fatigue, and she often awoke from a long nap feeling more tired than before.

Kayla underwent a variety of conventional procedures to treat her condition, including two D & Cs (dilatation and curettage, a scraping of the lining from the uterine wall) and a blood transfusion to replace blood loss. Although these procedures helped with the bleeding and pain for a short time, the symptoms always returned. Kayla's gynecologist finally suggested that she have a hysterectomy, but Kayla resisted this idea because she wanted to have children.

To explore other options, Kayla consulted Felicity Moir, L.Ac. Kayla explained her desire to have children and told Dr. Moir that she wanted to have a myomectomy (removal of the fibroids only), though her previous doctors had said her system was too weak to handle the procedure. Dr. Moir suggested that they focus acupuncture treatment on controlling the bleeding which would, in turn, strengthen Kayla's system.

Kayla's symptoms of PMS, food cravings, and stress headaches indicated that the vital energy associated with the liver and its functions was not flowing freely. This blockage of energy also explained her excessive bleeding and abdominal pain. According to Dr. Moir, the pain associated with the onset of bleeding indicated that Kayla's menstrual problems were most likely caused by stagnant blood in the uterus. In Chinese medicine, the free flow of energy in the body can be obstructed by internal or external stressors—including hormonal imbalances, emotional problems, poor diet, and physical trauma. When an obstruction occurs, the liver is unable to do its job of promoting a smooth flow of energy in the body. The result is stagnation, which can lead to pain, more stress, and, if unchecked, compromised functioning of the other organ systems. "Stagnated blood had developed into masses in the abdomen," explains Dr. Moir, "causing an accumulation of energy which manifested as pain."

This blood stagnation suggested to Dr. Moir that a treatment to move the blood out of the uterus would be helpful, but Kayla's already excessive bleeding complicated the situation. Dr. Moir settled on a treatment plan which encouraged blood movement for the first four days of menstruation, but then stopped the bleeding on the fifth day. Moxibustion (SEE QUICK DEFINITION) was a component. Since Kayla's fibroids prevented her from lying comfortably on her stomach, Dr. Moir used slices of ginger to apply the moxa cones at various points on her abdomen.

After one month of twice-weekly visits to Dr. Moir, Kayla's menstrual bleeding had subsided dramatically and then settled into a 27-day cycle with less heavy bleeding and only one day of pain. At the end of three months, the bleeding lasted only four days, followed by four days of spotting. Kayla's fatigue had also reduced considerably. At this point, Dr. Moir suggested that Kayla take a Chinese herbal formula containing cinnamon twig and poria to stimulate more blood movement out and away from the uterus.

QUICK DEFINITION

In **moxibustion**, a dried herb called moxa (usually mugwort) is burned over the skin at a specific acupuncture point. The moxa may be attached to a special acupuncture needle or in a free-standing cone set on a slice of ginger; its slow burning provides a penetrating heat. The purpose is to warm the blood and *qi* (basic life force energy flowing through energy pathways), particularly when a patient's energy picture is cold or damp.

After another three months of treatment, Kayla felt confident enough to approach her gynecologist about the possibility of a myomectomy. Her highly reduced bleeding and regular menstrual cycles indicated remarkable improvement, and the gynecologist agreed to perform the procedure. For the next six months, Kayla received monthly injections of Zoladex (a conventional hormone treatment which affects estrogen levels) to shrink the fibroids prior to surgery.

To contact **Felicity Moir, L.Ac.**: 1-19 South Hill Park, Hampstead, London, England NW32ST; tel: 0171-431-8395.

Kayla's surgery successfully removed her fibroids while preserving her uterus. She still uses moxa daily and takes herbs to regulate her menstrual flow. Dr. Moir sums up the case: "Kayla's acupuncture treatments controlled her bleeding and reduced her pain so she could pursue the operational procedure she wanted—a myomectomy. This meant that she was still able to conceive a child, which is what she desired most."

However, surgical removal of fibroids does not guarantee an end to the disorder; fibroids often grow again. Since problems with liver energy are also associated with emotional trauma or suppressed anger, Dr. Moir had questioned Kayla closely about her emotional history. Three years before, Kayla's menstrual cycle had been a normal 28 days with no pain or excessive bleeding; the onset of her symptoms coincided with a broken engagement and the death of her father.

"The relationship between a 'bleeding heart' and a 'bleeding womb' has long been documented," says Dr. Moir, "and the areas where energy and blood stagnate in women often relate to the specific emotional issues and life confusion being experienced." Dr. Moir advised Kayla to work through her emotional traumas or the symptoms would never entirely disappear.

Success Story: Enzyme Therapy Shrinks Fibroid

In this case, enzymes, thyroid glandular extracts, and natural progesterone resolved multiple problems and enabled Joyce, 45, to give up conventional drugs and naturally shrink her fibroid for surgical removal. She consulted Dr. Lita Lee for help with a melon-sized fibroid in her uterus which did not cause her any pain, but gave her a constant feeling of pressure and heaviness in her pelvic area. She also had digestive disturbances, including gas, bloating, and diarrhea. Joyce's conventional physicians were giving her monthly Lupron (synthetic hormone) shots to shrink the tumor to a size that would yield safely to surgery. She hated the side effects of the shots, which included headaches, depression, and a recurrence of her teenage acne problem. Joyce was also taking a prescription drug for herpes (Acylovir) and had been for ten years; every time she

For more about **underactive thyroid gland and a Barnes underarm temperature test for hypothyroidism,** see Chapter 1: Menstrual Problems, pp. 24-26, and Chapter 5: Infertility, p. 185.

To contact **Lita Lee, Ph.D.:** P.O. Box 516, Lowell, OR 97452; tel: 541-937-1123; fax: 541-937-1132. For more about **Therazyme PAN or Therazyme MSCLR digestive enzymes,** licensed health-care practitioners may contact: 21st Century Nutrition, 6421 Enterprise Lane, Madison, WI 53719; tel: 800-662-2630. For **Nutri-Pak by Atrium,** licensed health-care practitioners may contact: Atrium Nutrition, 2620 Hickory Ridge Road, Tallahassee, FL 32308; tel: 800-522-6461. For **Progest-E Complex,** natural progesterone in vitamin E oil, consumers or practitioners may contact Dr. Lee using her ordering telephone number: 541-746-7621; or contact the manufacturer: Kenogen, P.O. Box 5764, Eugene, OR 97405; tel: 541-345-9855.

stopped taking it, the herpes came back with a vengeance.

Dr. Lee first attempted to determine if Joyce had an underactive thyroid gland. For this, she instructed Joyce to take her temperature, with a digital or basal thermometer, first thing in the morning and a half hour after lunch, for three days in a row during her menstrual period (to avoid the temperature increases at mid-cycle). Joyce's morning and afternoon averages were both below normal (normal is about 98° F in the morning and 98.6° F to 99° F after lunch), which is a common indicator of hypothyroidism.

Based on Joyce's symptoms and the temperature test, Dr. Lee prescribed the following supplements:

■ Thera-zyme PAN (pancreas): a digestive formula for sugar intolerance, to ease Joyce's bloating, diarrhea, and gas; two capsules before each meal. This supplement contains the plant enzymes lactose, maltose, and sucrose, all of which work in the stomach to predigest foods and thus spare the pancreas from doing all the work of digestion.

■ Thera-zyme MSCLR (muscular): a plant enzyme formula used to control herpes and other skin conditions; 3-4 capsules, three times daily. Thera-zyme MSCLR can prevent a herpes attack, relieves muscle pain, and is high in amylase, a digestive enzyme that acts like an antihistamine.

■ Nutri-Pak: a thyroid glandular extract for the hypothyroid condition and for the fibroid. Joyce started with one tablet daily and increased the dose gradually until her body temperature became normal. This supplement contains raw bovine glandular extract and has protein precursors for the two main thyroid hormones, T4 (75%) and T3 (25%).

■ Progest-E Complex: a natural progesterone (10%) in vitamin E oil to help shrink the fibroid; three drops taken orally, five times a day.

After being on the program for several weeks, Joyce discontinued the Lupron shots. The pressure in her pelvis was beginning to ease, indicating the fibroid was shrinking. Her skin cleared up and, with the herpes enzyme formula, she was able to wean herself from the Acylovir. In addition, Joyce's thyroid gland began to improve. Joyce continued on the program and within several months the fibroid had shrunk to the point where it could be successfully removed in a myomectomy, which Joyce had. To prevent a recurrence of the fibroid,

Joyce stayed on the enzyme formulas and made sure she ate a good diet. She has not had any fibroid problems since.

Success Story: Herbal Medicine Reduces Fibroid

For Sandra, 43, herbal medicine provided the key to dissolving her fibroid. When she came to Linda Whitedove, a medical herbalist in Ward, Colorado, she had a uterine fibroid the size of an orange as well as endometriosis (SEE QUICK DEFINITION) in her fallopian tubes. For the past two years, she had been enduring what she described as "periods from hell," with heavy bleeding and severe cramps that sometimes lasted for two weeks. She also suffered from low energy, decreased attention span, severe depression, and a weight problem—only 5'2" tall, she weighed 193 pounds.

In **endometriosis**, the cells of the lining of the uterus (or endometrium) become established elsewhere, such as in the fallopian tubes, uterine muscles, colon, bladder, and sides of the pelvic cavity. During menstruation, these displaced cells swell with blood and bleed, causing pain and inflammation. Symptoms can appear at any time during the monthly cycle and include pelvic, abdominal, leg, and/or severe lower back pain, and pain during bowel motions and/or urination.

Whitedove addressed Sandra's painful menstrual periods by prescribing evening primrose oil, in capsule form, taken throughout her cycle (2,000-3,000 mg daily), and an herbal tincture of shepherd's purse, taken only during menstruation itself (15 drops every 15 minutes until bleeding subsides). After the first month of treatment, Sandra reported much less bleeding and little pain during her period, which had decreased to only four days.

For the fibroid itself, Whitedove prescribed an herbal tea made from yucca tincture, chapparal extract, and chastetree berry (*Vitex agnus-castus*). The yucca tincture functions as an anti-inflammatory, while chaparral helps to reduce the size of the fibroid. Chastetree berry increases progesterone levels to neutralize the effects of excess estrogen in the hormonal ratio.

Do not use chaparral if you have a history of alcoholism or any kind of liver condition or are recovering from a recent bout of hepatitis.

Whitedove also considered the possibility that the fibroid was aggravated by emotional symptoms of depression and anxiety for which she prescribed an herbal formula of passionflower, St. John's wort, wild oats, and skullcap.

"Sandra began to have normal periods after that," Whitedove reports. "After taking this formula every day for nine months, Sandra's fibroid had shrunk to the size of a grape."

To contact **Linda Whitedove, M.H.**: P.O. Box 332, Ward, CO 80481; tel: 303-415-3763. The **herbal tinctures** are available from Linda Whitedove's company; contact: Home Grown Herbals, P.O. Box 251, Hygiene, CO 80533; tel: 303-702-0833; fax: 303-702-0844. **Evening primrose oil capsules** are available at health food stores.

Success Story: Herbs Shrink Fibroids

Chanchal Cabrera, M.N.I.M.H., a clinical herbalist practicing in Vancouver, British Columbia, also uses herbal medicine along with dietary changes, detoxification, and nutritional supplements, to resolve uterine fibroids without surgery.

Lydia, 42, consulted with Cabrera seven months after being diagnosed with several small (1⅓ inches across) uterine fibroids. Lydia complained of progressively heavier menstrual bleeding including passing of clots; the flow was so heavy as to be disabling and tended to last for a week. Lydia also experienced menstrual cramps, mid-cycle bleeding, and pain at ovulation. While Lydia's fibroids were still too small to be noticeable on physical palpation, they were clearly interfering with her menstrual cycle. Her conventional physician had already advocated hysterectomy to remove the fibroids and was waiting for her to book the surgery.

Lydia exercised regularly and followed a mostly vegetarian diet with occasional fish and large amounts of eggs and dairy products and black tea. In addition, she took a prescription iron supplement (presumably to counteract the near anemia caused by the excessive blood loss during menstruation), but this was producing constipation.

A number of factors in Lydia's life were contributing to a condition of relative excess estrogen. Lydia had been on birth control pills from the age of 17 to 23; birth control pills, even when taken a long time ago, contribute to higher estrogen levels, says Cabrera. Her chronic constipation was also an element in the excess estrogen producing her fibroid. "Constipation can be an aggravating factor because when stools are retained in the large intestine longer than six hours, bacterial activity may convert the breakdown products of estrogen metabolism back into an active form which can then be reabsorbed and recirculated through the body, thus stimulating fibroid growth," explains Cabrera. Finally, her high consumption of eggs and dairy products was adding to the estrogen dominance.

Cabrera advised Lydia to start a cleansing diet to remove toxins from her body. This consisted of a fruit or vegetable juice fast for several days or a regimen of only raw foods. Then Lydia was to follow a high-fiber diet, including fresh fruits and vegetables, whole grains, and beans, which would encourage a more complete emptying of her intestines.

In general, all foods that promote estrogen buildup must be avoided, including meats, eggs, and all dairy products, says Cabrera. She usually advises women with fibroids to avoid soyfoods as well because soybeans are slightly estrogenic and could further aggravate the imbalance. In addition, intake of dietary fats (especially of an animal origin) should be reduced, and black tea and coffee should be avoided because they put stress on the liver. "Since hormones are 'deactivated' by the liver before elimination, any liver congestion will lead to raised levels of circulating estrogen and thus aggravate fibroid growth," says Cabrera.

With the dietary changes in place, Cabrera next recommended an herbal tincture of six herbs: dandelion root (*Taraxacum off. radix*), 1 tbsp; stone root (*Collinsonia canadensis*), 1 tbsp; white dead nettle (*Lamium album*), 4 tsp; yarrow (*Achillea millefolium*), 1 tbsp; partridge berry (*Mitchella repens*), 4 tsp; and shepherd's purse (*Capsella bursa-pastoris*), 1 tbsp. Lydia was to

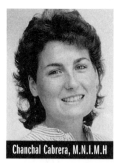

Chanchal Cabrera, M.N.I.M.H

"Since hormones are 'deactivated' by the liver before elimination, any liver congestion will lead to raised levels of circulating estrogen and thus aggravate fibroid growth," says Chanchal Cabrera.

take one teaspoon of this tincture three times daily for six weeks.

Each component of the herbal tincture would focus on an aspect of the fibroid clinical picture, says Cabrera. Dandelion is known to help reduce liver congestion and to have a mild laxative effect. Stone root encourages urination (and the elimination of toxins through the urine) and is given as a pelvic decongestant to help remove unwanted tissue masses from the reproductive organs.

White dead nettle, also a uterine decongestant, helps to relax the uterus and increase the integrity of its endometrial lining. Yarrow increases blood flow to the pelvis, thereby aiding decongestion of the uterus; it also stimulates the liver's ability to remove estrogen from the body. Partridge berry tonifies the uterus and reduces congestion, while shepherd's purse helps stop excessive blood flow, as in hemorrhages, from many organs.

Cabrera also formulated a special tea for Lydia to drink three times daily, mixing one teaspoon of the mixture with one cup of water. Herbs in the tea included equal amounts of yarrow, red raspberry (*Rubus idaeus*), motherwort (*Leonurus cardiaca*), and greater nettle (*Urtica dioica*). "The leaves of red raspberry contain types of condensed tannin which appear to have a tissue specificity for the uterus," Cabrera says. Red raspberry is a rich source of iron; it helps reduce hemorrhaging and tones and strengthens the uterus. Nettle has beneficial effects on the liver, kidneys, and bladder. Cabrera has found other herbs, such as lady's mantle, goldenseal, and ginger, to be beneficial for treating fibroids as well.

According to Cabrera, certain nutrients often play an important role in fibroid reversal. For example, a high potency vitamin B com-

To contact **Chanchal Cabrera, M.N.I.M.H.**: Gaia Garden Herbal Apothecary, 2672 West Broadway, Vancouver, BC, V6K2G3 Canada; tel: 604-734-4372; fax: 604-734-4376. The initials M.N.I.M.H. stand for Member of the National Institute of Medical Herbalists, a British designation used in Canada to indicate professional status as an herbalist.

For more about **intestinal detoxification**, see "Practical Ways to Cleanse Your Colon," Chapter 6: Cystitis, p. 210.

CAUTION

Motherwort contains an alkaloid called L-stachydrine that is "especially stimulating and tonic to the uterine tissues," says Chanchal Cabrera. Therefore, women with fibroids and painful menstruation (dysmenorrhea) should not use it.

plex (containing at least 100 mg of each B vitamin) is recommended because a B-vitamin deficiency can compromise the liver's ability to deactivate inappropriately high estrogen levels; similarly, high estrogen levels deplete the body of B vitamins. Vitamin E (600 IU daily) helps to regulate bleeding and normalize estrogen levels.

High doses of vitamin C and bioflavonoids (vitamin C helpers) taken to bowel tolerance (the amount just short of producing diarrhea, typically around 10 g daily in divided doses) help to minimize bleeding and enhance iron absorption. Iron (20 mg daily) is vital because excessive menstrual bleeding can deplete iron stores and lead to anemia. The amino acid methionine, inositol (an unofficial B vitamin), and the fatty acid phosphatidyl choline can aid the liver in its removal of estrogens.

After six weeks on the dietary, herbal, and supplement program, Lydia reported that the two periods since her first consultation had been much improved. There was less clotting and a lighter flow. She had taken psyllium seed powder as a colon cleanser and was now experiencing more regular bowel movements. Cabrera advised Lydia to continue with the program for another two months.

At that time, Lydia reported that her period was better still, with no mid-cycle bleeding or pain at ovulation. Her physician confirmed that Lydia's uterus felt softer to the touch (as the fibroid grows, it makes the uterus feel hard and solid to the touch when the abdomen is palpated). After another six months, Lydia was symptom free and reported that an ultrasound scan of her uterus revealed that the fibroids had shrunk so considerably that they were no longer a health problem and would not require surgery.

Success Story:
Homeopathy Unravels Emotions Behind Fibroids

John Diamond, M.D., of Reno, Nevada. takes a different approach to fibroids, which is that they are a symbol for unresolved emotional issues. Says Dr. Diamond: "There is a saying in South Africa, where I come from, that 'If you don't cry above, you'll cry below.' As a woman, you either cry tears or you 'cry' blood—through the uterus in the form of heavy menstrual bleeding. The saying means—and I see the truth of it demonstrated frequently in my clinical practice—that strong emotions, if left unresolved, will eventually manifest as symptoms in the body."

This is because the body is metaphorical, Dr. Diamond explains. It always *listens* to the psyche of the individual and responds accordingly, in its own way, translating withheld tears into copious menstrual flow. If you have an unresolved emotional problem, if you have internalized and suppressed emotions, the body has to manifest them somehow.

The body will most often produce a physical symptom in the area relating to the emotional issue, Dr. Diamond adds. Fibroids in the uterus, for example, frequently involve emotional suppression relating to sexuality, and the attendant heavy bleeding may be associated with prolonged internalized sadness and withheld emotions. Homeopathy can help resolve both the physical and emotional aspects of illness. Here, **W. John Diamond, M.D.**, illustrates the connections and homeopathic treatment in a case from his patient files:

Flora, 38, came to me with symptoms of heavy menstrual bleeding and several uterine fibroids about two inches in diameter. Her bleeding was painful and lengthy, extending for six to ten days, involving many large clots, and requiring six to eight tampons daily. Generally, the pain lasted as long as her period. Flora also often had mid-cycle spotting.

The excessive bleeding had made her anemic and her hemoglobin count—the blood molecule made from iron that carries oxygen—was considerably below normal. Flora had seen conventional doctors, undergone ultrasound diagnosis of her uterus, and walked away with a strong recommendation to have a hysterectomy. However, she feared the process of having her uterus removed and decided against the surgery.

As I questioned Flora about her case, I learned that she began menstruating late, at age 15. Flora's mother, who had also begun menstruation late and suffered from fibroids, had undergone a hysterectomy. This told me that the familial medical influence was strong in Flora's condition; in many cases, problems such as these run in families from grandmother to mother to daughter.

With late onset of the menses, a woman will usually develop a reproductive problem at some point. Often, she will have irregular periods; they might stop and start, and any kind of stress will affect menstrual regularity and bleeding. It is as if the woman's body is never quite ready for the start of menstruation; this unpreparedness soon becomes a dysfunctional menstrual cycle.

Flora told me that her menstrual pain and heavy bleeding had begun two years before, around the time her husband began talking

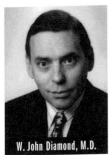

W. John Diamond, M.D.

"As a woman, you either cry tears or you 'cry' blood—through the uterus in the form of heavy menstrual bleeding—meaning that strong emotions, if left unresolved, will eventually manifest as symptoms in the body," says Dr. Diamond.

about divorcing her. They didn't divorce, but Flora, a mother of four (two with her husband and two from his previous marriage), was still nervous, anxious, and fearful about the possibility. Flora "stuffed" her emotions and sadness into her body, and it eventually produced the fibroids and heavy bleeding.

Medically, with fibroids there is an increase in the vascularity of the uterus. This means more blood vessels form to deliver more blood to the uterine tissues. This in turn leads to a thicker endometrial lining of the uterus and thus heavier bleeding at menstruation in an attempt to shed this larger endometrium. Metaphorically, it is as if the fibroid is saying something like this to Flora: "Here I am at last. Now your ugly secret is out. You were trying to hide it, but, look, it's not working, here I am." The ugly secret, of course, is Flora's emotional pain and its suppression.

To start her treatment, I prescribed a single dose of homeopathic *Medorrhinum* 200C (SEE QUICK DEFINITION). This remedy is indicated for conditions in which there is tumor formation—technically, a fibroid is a benign, noncancerous tumor—or any excess growth in the body.

Using an information gathering system called electrodermal screening, I determined that there were energy and functional imbalances in Flora's liver, gallbladder, and kidneys. This finding was consistent with her emotional situation: Flora was in a state of anxiety and fear, which affected her kidneys; she was also angry, which affected her liver and gallbladder, and both organs are usually implicated when there are menstrual abnormalities.

The electrodermal readings also told me that Flora had blood stagnation or what Chinese medicine calls a *qi* deficiency. This means that the energy (*qi*) of her blood circulation was depressed and stagnant. To address this condition, I prescribed a Chinese herbal formula called Women's Precious (with eight herbs including *dong quai*, white peony root, licorice, and ginseng) to be taken three times daily. This remedy would help stop the uterine stagnation and thus the fibroid formation. I told Flora to come back at the end of her next period.

When I saw her again, Flora reported a marked reduction in the amount of menstrual bleeding and that her pain was reduced by half. Next I gave Flora a single dose of homeopathic *Phosphorus* 200C as a constitutional remedy, corresponding to her esssential symptom and personality picture. For example, Flora was easily wounded and made fearful, but able to overcome her fears if she had only a little help and support. This is an aspect of her constitutional type and points to *Phosphorus.*

To complement this remedy, I also gave Flora *Ustilago maydis* 6C (once daily), a homeopathic remedy made from corn smut fungus which is indicated for excessive uterine bleeding and fibroids. Flora stayed on this remedy for one month, then saw me again. She said she had clarified her emotional situation and felt less at risk about her marriage.

Flora also said her last period had been almost normal in terms of bleeding and there had been no spotting in the following weeks. The pain had not receded any more but it had changed its nature; the pain now was occasional cramping, intense during the first few days of the period, then fading off to only a mild sensation by the end. Flora still needed six to eight tampons for the heavy bleeding, but she no longer had large clots and the period lasted for only five days. When she visited her gynecologist for another ultrasound, it revealed that her fibroids had shrunk by about one-third.

I kept Flora on the *Ustilago maydis* for two more months, and gave her homeopathic *Magnesia phosphorica* (from magnesium phosphate), as needed, for the cramping. In addition, I suggested an herbal formula called Crampbark Plus™ (containing crampbark, cinnamon twig, red peony, and four other Chinese herbs) to reduce

W. John Diamond, M.D., is a board certified pathologist; his training in alternative medicine is extensive, including medical acupuncture at the University of California at Los Angeles, classical homeopathy at the Pacific Academy of Homeopathic Medicine in Berkeley, California, and neural therapy at the American Academy of Neural Therapy in Seattle, Washington. Dr. Diamond is coauthor of *An Alternative Medicine Definitive Guide to Cancer* (Future Medicine Publishing, 1997). He may be contacted at: Triad Medical Center, 4600 Kietzke Lane, M-242, Reno, NV 89502; tel: 702-829-2277; fax: 702-829-2365. For **Women's Precious formula**, contact: McZand Herbal, Inc., Zand Herbal Formulas, P.O. Box 5312, Santa Monica, CA 90409; tel: 800-800-0405 or 310-822-0500; fax: 310-822-1050. For **Crampbark Plus™**, contact: Health Concerns, 8001 Capwell Drive, Oakland, CA 94621; tel: 800-233-9355 or 510-639-0280; fax: 510-639-9140. For **homeopathic remedies** *Medorrhinum, Folliculinum, Ustilago Maydis, Phosphorus,* and *Magnesia Phosphorica,* contact: National Homeopathic Products, 518 Tasman Street, Madison, WI 53714; tel: 800-888-4066; fax: 608-221-9533.

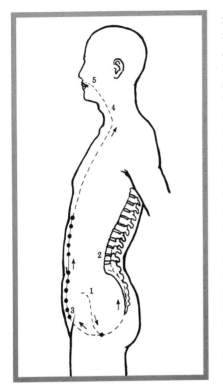

CHONG MO MERIDIAN. **This is a special acupuncture meridian located in the front of the body and primarily affects the pelvic area and reproductive organs.**

menstrual cramping and pain and vitalize blood circulation. Also drawing from Chinese medicine, I gave Flora several special acupuncture treatments to stimulate the energy flow along a pathway in the body called *chong mo*. The *chong mo* flows through the pelvic area and the female reproductive organs, and so the treatments were designed to correct uterine energy and hormonal imbalances.

In cases in which a hormonal imbalance between estrogen and progesterone appears to be the predominant cause of the fibroid (not in Flora's case which was primarily emotional in origin), I use *Folliculinum* to lower the amount and effects of estrogen in relation to progesterone. *Folliculinum* is a homeopathic version of the female ovarian follicle that releases the egg; functionally, it works like a high potency homeopathic estrogen for cases of prolonged and painful menstruation. An excess of estrogen leads to the formation of too much endometrial lining in the uterus, the first stage of growing a fibroid.

Three months after the start of treatment, Flora told me her periods had normalized and that she had resolved her issues with her husband. The menstrual cramping had receded considerably and she no longer needed any *Magnesia phosphorica* as a first aid for the pain.

A hysterectomy would have removed the physical manifestation that she suffered from, but in no way would it have addressed the true pathology of internalized emotional fear and anger that she had harbored for so long. Suppression of her manifestation by hysterectomy would have driven her emotions deeper and resulted in a much more serious physical manifestation such as cancer or mental breakdown. ■

The Autobiography of a Fibroid

What is a fibroid's message to the woman in whose body it has grown? In the following case, a woman discovers a surprising emotional message behind her fibroid.[20]

Alice, 47, had a fibroid the size of a four-month fetus surgically removed. Within a year, however, a new fibroid took its place, soon reaching nearly the same size. Her gynecologist recommended radical surgery to remove most of her reproductive organs. At this point, Alice sought the help of Jason Elias, M.A., L.Ac., a licensed acupuncturist based in New Paltz, New York.

Dr. Elias put Alice on a program of dietary changes, exercise, and acupuncture treatment. However, it was an insight gained during deep inner reflection that gave these remedies the traction they needed to shrink the fibroid.

Six months after starting treatment with Dr. Elias, Alice told him that she felt as if her fibroid were a baby. "It's me as a baby, the person I never allowed myself to be," Alice explained. Throughout her life she had been a rebel, seeking attention, rejecting convention, defying her conformist, well-behaved parents for whom the stiff upper lip was the proper stance toward life. Her parents had taught her to bottle up her feelings and, when she displayed emotion, told her to stop feeling sorry for herself.

Alice's insight was that her fibroid, psychologically—metaphorically—was a growth asking her to "mother it, take care of it, even to love it." She saw she had become attached to it just as it, literally, was attached to her uterine walls. "I feel as if it's the 'me' that never got to grow up and express her feelings," she said. Soon after experiencing this insight, her fibroid shrunk to half its original size, as reported by her gynecologist, and Alice was able to avoid surgery.

To contact **Jason Elias, M.A., L.Ac.:** Integral Health Associates, 3 Paradise Lane, New Paltz, NY 12561; tel: 914-255-2255 or tel/fax: 888-403-5861.

Self-Care Options for Fibroids

Although fibroids are a serious condition and require that you be under the care of a qualified physician, there are certain steps you can take to ease the symptoms and facilitate healing. These include herbal and homeopathic remedies as well as magnetic therapy which you can apply yourself.

Self-Care Herbal Remedies

For fibroids, David Hoffmann, B.Sc., M.N.I.M.H., of Sebastopol, California, past president of the American Herbalist Guild, usually recommends a basic mixture of tinctures of chasteberry, blue cohosh, wild yam, and cranesbill in equal amounts, taken at the rate of ½ teaspoon, three times a day. If there is much cramping pain, he advises taking ¹/₂ teaspoon of crampbark tincture in addition to the basic mixture.

Maitake mushroom, prized for centuries by Japanese herbalists for its ability to strengthen health, has been shown to shrink fibroids. A physician gave maitake to six patients with uterine fibroids at the rate of two tablets, three times daily (3 g). After six months to a year on this program, none of the women required surgery and all of them had substantial reduction in fibroid size.[21]

Herbalist Susun Weed, of Woodstock, New York, advises that to stop heavy bleeding caused by fibroids take ¹/₂ cup of an infusion (a type of strong tea made from dried herbs) of cotton root bark (*gossypium*) every half hour, or a dropperful every 5 to 10 minutes until the bleeding stops.

For a brew to balance the effects of estrogen excess, mix equal parts of tinctures of the following herbs: black currant buds or leaves (*Ribes nigrum*); gromwell herb or seeds (*Lithospermum officinalis*); lady's mantle herb (*Alchemilla vulgaris*); and wild pansy flowers (*Viola tricolor*). Take one teaspoon of the tincture first thing in the morning and you can expect noticeable results in two to four months, says Weed.[22]

To contact herbalist **Susun Weed**: Ash Tree Publishing, P.O. Box 64, Woodstock, NY 12498; tel/fax: 914-246-8081. **Maitake mushroom extract** is available in tablet form as Grifron®. For more information, contact: Maitake Products, P.O. Box 1354, Paramus, NJ 07653; tel: 800-747-7418.

Homeopathic prescribing for fibroids, a fairly serious condition, should be done by a well-trained practitioner. While the homeopathic remedies indicated here can be helpful in a self-care situation, it is best to seek professional consultation for lasting benefit. Misprescribing a homeopathic remedy is not likely to result in any discomfort, but it may also result in no improvement.

Self-Care Homeopathic Remedies

For permanent resolution of the conditions underlying fibroid growth, homeopathic treatment should be constitutional (not based on symptoms but on the person's constitutional type, i.e., body type, appearance, personality, predisposition), according to Andrew Lockie, M.D., and Nicola Geddes, M.D., authors of *The Women's Guide to Homeopathy*. To receive a constitutional remedy, you need to consult a classical homeopath. However, in the short term, for symptom relief, Drs. Lockie and Geddes typically recommend the following:[23]

Specific remedies to be taken four times daily:

■ For small fibroids, profuse yellow or acrid, bloody, copius discharge from vagina; increase of sexual desire or congestion of the uterus; absent, heavy, frequent, irregular, or suppressed periods; pain in ovaries and uterus: *Calcarea iodatum* 6C (calcium iodide)

■ For swollen uterus, urge to bear down, watery brown discharge from vagina, painful cramps during periods; fibroids accompanied by heaviness in the lower abdomen; uterine prolapse, nervousness: *Fraximus americana* 6C (white ash)

■ For heavier than usual menstrual flow, icy cold body feeling, bleeding between periods; especially beneficial for thin women who tire easily, both physically and mentally: *Silicea* 6C (silica)

For instructions on making an **herbal infusion**, see Chapter 6: Cystitis, p. 229.

■ For continuous bleeding; frequent and copious menses, especially alternating periods; bloody and dark vaginal discharge before and after menses; pain in womb on rising; scarcely recovering from one period before another starts: *Thlaspi bursa* 6C (shepherd's purse)

■ For short scanty periods as menopause approaches, great pain eased by menstrual flow, abdomen very sensitive to tight clothing; for fibroids in women who are nervous, restless, somewhat bloated in appearance, and who suffer from PMS: *Lachesis* 6C (bushmaster snake venom)

■ For bright red menstrual blood; this remedy should be added if fibroids have a tendency to bleed: *Phosphorus* 6C (amorphous phosphorus)

■ For sensation of uterus feeling as if it is being squeezed during periods; late and profuse menses; corrosive leukorrhea (vaginal discharge) with subacute inflammatory conditions of the womb in young women: *Kali iodatum* 6C (potassium iodide)

■ For swollen and painful uterus, spasmodic contractions of vagina; this remedy has a consolidating effect on the genital organs: *Aurum muriaticum* 6C (gold chloride)

Self-Care Magnetic Therapy

Therapeutic-quality magnets, worn over the uterus at night while sleeping, can shrink a fibroid tumor over a period of months, according to William H. Philpott, M.D., an author and biomagnetic researcher in Choctaw, Oklahoma. Magnetic fields can stimulate metabolism and increase the amount of oxygen available to cells which will decrease inflammation, he explains.

It could take several months of magnet application before the fibroid starts shrinking and up to a year to eliminate it. However, the magnet will immediately stop the tumor growth process, states Dr. Philpott.

For treatment, he often recommends wearing a magnet over the lower abdomen/pubic area (to cover the uterus) every night while sleeping; specifically a 5" by 12" multi-magnet flexible mat, with a 4" by 6" by ¹/₂" ceramic block booster magnet attached in the center of the mat with

CAUTION
The body's subtle electromagnetic fields can be affected by even the weakest of magnets. Since even minor alterations in the field can cause mild to serious symptoms, magnetic therapy should be practiced only under the supervision of a qualified professional.

Velcro. The mat and booster are kept in place on the body by a wrap cloth with Velcro attachments.

The most important thing to remember about magnetic therapy is that the negative pole is the side that faces the body. The negative magnetic field normalizes the disturbed metabolic functions that cause painful conditions such as cellular edema (swelling of the cells), cellular acidosis (excessive acidity of the cells), lack of oxygen to the cells, and infection. While a negative magnetic field may relieve pain, a positive magnetic field can increase pain due to its interference with normal metabolic function. However, magnetic therapy should not be considered a replacement for local anesthetics or pain relievers.

Dr. Philpott adds the following precautions:

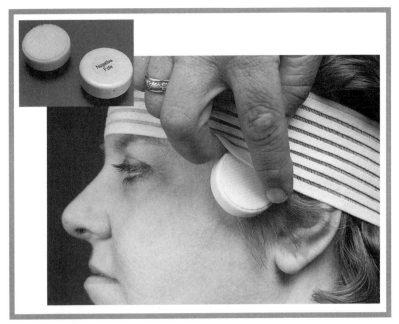

To contact **William H. Philpott, M.D.**: P.O. Box 50655, Midwest City, OK 73140; tel: 405-390-1444.

■ Industrial magnets often have different positive and negative pole identifications than the magnets used in medicine and therapy. Use a magnetometer or compass to confirm proper identification.

■ Don't use magnets on the abdomen during pregnancy.

MAGNETIC THERAPY. Therapeutic-quality magnets (top left), worn over the uterus at night while sleeping, can shrink a fibroid tumor over a period of months, according to William H. Philpott, M.D. These magnets can be strapped to different parts of the body (such as the head for relief of headaches, above), thereby continuously delivering a beneficial magnetic field to that area.

■ Don't use a magnetic bed for more than eight to ten hours.

■ Wait 60 to 90 minutes after meals before applying magnetic therapy to the abdomen, to prevent interference with peristalsis (wavelike contractions of the smooth muscles of the digestive tract).

■ Do not apply the positive magnetic pole unless under medical supervision. It can produce seizures, hallucinations, insomnia, and hyperactivity, stimulate the growth of tumors and microorganisms, and promote addictive behavior.

Dr. Lark's Fibroid Treatment Protocol

Susan Lark, M.D., of Los Altos, California, observes that many women in her practice have reported a noticeable decrease in heavy bleeding and menstrual pain and discomfort within one to two menstrual cycles after starting her program of dietary changes, nutritional and herbal supplements, and lifestyle modifications. The program is typically as follows:[24]

Diet

■ Eat whole grain millet, buckwheat, oats, rice, and rye, but not whole wheat; tofu, black, kidney, pinto, lima, and soybeans, chickpeas; fresh, organic vegetables and fruits, especially dried figs, blackberries, bananas, raisins, and oranges; raw flax, pumpkin, sesame, and sunflower seeds, pistachios, pecans, and almonds

■ Use small amounts of cold-pressed vegetable oils high in vitamin E, such as corn, olive, canola, or flaxseed

■ Keep your consumption of meat, poultry, and fish to a minimum, emphasizing fish and poultry (without the skin) or no more than three ounces of meat daily; avoid these foods altogether if your fibroid is large and uncomfortable

■ Avoid all milk products until the fibroid has dissolved

■ Severely reduce intake of all saturated fats, salt, alcohol, refined sugar, and caffeine

Supplements

■ Beta carotene (vitamin A precursor from vegetable sources): at least 20,000 IU daily

■ Vitamin B complex: 50-100 mg daily, with additional B6 (up to 300 mg daily)

■ Vitamin C: 1,000-4,000 mg daily, plus bioflavonoids (from grape skins, cherries, blackberries, blueberries, pulp and white rind of citrus fruits)

■ Vitamin E (from wheat germ, walnut, or soybean oil): 400-2,000 IU daily

To contact **Susan Lark, M.D.:** 101 First Street, Suite 441, Los Altos, CA 94022; tel: 650-941-5905. To order Dr. Lark's books, contact: Explore Publications; tel: 800-845-7866. Vitamin, mineral and herb supplements endorsed by Dr. Lark are available as the Schiff line of products, sold at health food stores.

A Tomato Poultice for Fibroids

According to acupuncturist Ira J. Golchehreh, L.Ac., O.M.D., of San Rafael, California, a poultice made of green or overly ripe tomatoes can be helpful in reducing the size of a fibroid. It is the acidity in the tomatoes that produces the beneficial effects, says Dr. Golchehreh. Here's how to make a poultice:

1) Mash one large or two medium-sized overly ripe red or green tomatoes (but no tomatoes at an intermediate stage of ripeness) and put them on a piece of cheesecloth. Pull the ends of the cloth together and tie a piece of string around it above the contents to form a compact, round sack.

2) Lie down on a bed on top of a large towel. Place the poultice on the skin over the uterus. Place a thin towel over this and a hot water bottle on top of the towel to provide heat. Keep in place for 30-45 minutes. Repeat 3-4 times weekly. The poultice may be stored in a plastic bag in the refrigerator to be used 2-3 more times before discarding.

To contact **Ira J. Golchehreh, L.Ac., O.M.D.**: Bay Park Business Center, 2175 Suite D, Francisco Blvd., San Rafael, CA 94901; tel: 415-485-4411.

- Calcium: minimum of 800 mg daily during menstruation
- Magnesium: 400 mg daily
- Potassium: 99 mg, 1-3 times daily for one week preceding onset of menstruation
- Iron (the "heme" type from meat sources such as liver): 27 mg (nonheme iron must be accompanied by at least 75 mg vitamin C for absorption)

Herbal Medicine

- To help stop excessive bleeding: goldenseal, shepherd's purse
- For anemia and liver health: yellow dock, pau d'arco, turmeric, silymarin
- For inflammation, pain, and fever: meadowsweet, white willow bark

Lifestyle

- Regular aerobic exercise, slowly performed, at least three times weekly; Hatha yoga exercises to reduce pelvic congestion, improve blood circulation, and relax uterine muscles
- Stress reduction techniques such as meditation, deep-breathing exercises, counseling, psychotherapy, and emotional support from friends and family to ease stressful situations

Dr. Atkins' Anti-Fibroid Program

Robert C. Atkins, M.D., director of the Atkins Center in New York City and editor of the newsletter *Dr. Atkins' Health Revelations*, offers the following tips for both prevention and treatment of fibroids.[25]

To keep fibroids from forming:

- Avoid a high-sugar diet because sugar depletes vitamin B complex, which in turn impedes your ability to process and inactivate estrogen, a fibroid promoter

■ Avoid caffeine and alcohol because they deplete nutrients (especially the B vitamins) and disrupt liver function

To shrink a fibroid, Dr. Atkins usually suggests taking the following daily nutritional supplements:

■ Choline, 1,000-1,500 mg
■ Inositol, 1,000-1,500 mg
■ Methionine, 500-750 mg
■ Beta carotene, 25,000 IU
■ Vitamin C, 1,000-3,000 mg
■ Bioflavonoids, 500-1,500 mg

If you take a multivitamin, it is important to choose one that does not contain folic acid, boron, or PABA, because these otherwise helpful nutrients tend to increase estrogen levels, advises Dr. Atkins.

Dr. Dean's Fibroid-Reducing Plan

Women's health specialist Carolyn Dean, M.D., of New York City, often uses the following protocol in reducing fibroids:[26]

■ Evening primrose oil, four capsules daily
■ Marine lipid capsules, four daily
■ Vitamin E, 400 IU daily
■ Vitamin A, 20,000 IU daily
■ One high-strength multivitamin/mineral tablet daily
■ Foot reflexology massage on the points for the uterus and liver
■ Castor oil packs (SEE QUICK DEFINITION) or bentonite clay poultices over the uterine area
■ Herbal formulas including chasteberry (*Vitex agnus-castus*), *dong quai*, licorice root, wild yam (*Dioscorea*), and sarsaparilla

To contact **Robert C. Atkins, M.D.**: The Atkins Center, 152 East 55th Street, New York, NY 10022; tel: 212-758-2110; fax: 212-754-4284. For **Lipotropic Factors** (a choline-inositol-methionine combination) and other products from Dr. Atkins, contact: Complimentary Formulations, 125 Wilbur Place, Bohemia, NY 11716; tel: 800-628-5467. To contact **Carolyn Dean M.D., N.D.**: 325 East 65th Street, New York, NY 10021; tel: 212-861-9657.

QUICK DEFINITION

Castor oil packs are often used for relief of menstrual cramps, or at joints to relieve pain. To prepare a castor oil pack, lightly heat enough castor oil to thoroughly wet but not soak a 10" x 12" flannel cloth. Immerse the flannel in the hot oil, then fold to make three to four layers and place against the skin. (The oil helps to draw out toxins, release tension, and improve blood circulation, especially in the lower abdomen.) Wrap a heating pad or hot water bottle in a towel and place this over the pack, then cover pack and bottle with another towel to retain heat. Keep in place for one to two hours. Following the treatment, the oil-soaked flannel may be wrapped in plastic and stored in a refrigerator for later use. After the flannel has been used 20 times, discard it.

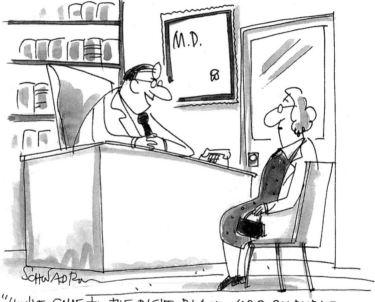

"YOU'VE COME TO THE RIGHT PLACE, MRS. COLBURNE. I SPECIALIZE IN UNNECESSARY SURGERY."

CHAPTER

4

Cysts on the ovaries can be
a painful condition, but not one that need result
in surgery. Natural hormonal therapy,
homeopathy, acupuncture, and herbal medicine
are among the alternative medicine
therapies that can permanently dissolve cysts
and prevent their recurrence.

CHAPTER 4

Ovarian Cysts

A DIAGNOSIS OF OVARIAN CYSTS (fluid-filled sacs that form on or in the ovaries) throws many women into a panic arising from fear that they are on the road to ovarian cancer. This is usually not the case, although ovarian cysts themselves can be painful and a complete medical exam is necessary to rule out cancerous tumors.

Ovarian cysts can develop on or in an ovary at any age between puberty and menopause. Often cysts produce no symptoms, but if they are large, there may be a sensation of pelvic pressure and fullness. Usually the fluid inside the cysts is yellowish, straw-colored, or blood-stained. When there are numerous small cysts (about 1 cm in diameter) in an ovary, the condition is called polycystic ovaries; this condition, in which both ovaries are enlarged, typically occurs in women age 30 and older.

Although ovarian cysts may produce no symptoms, if the growth is large, the ovary is twisted, or there is abnormal hormone production, one or more of the following symptoms may occur:

- Abdominal fullness or heaviness
- Pressure on the rectum or bladder
- Irregularities in the menstrual cycle
- Pelvic pain shortly before the onset or end of menstruation
- Pelvic pain during intercourse
- Nausea, vomiting, breast tenderness

A pelvic exam and ultrasound (SEE QUICK DEFINITION) are used to diagnose ovarian cysts. After a diagnosis, the cysts should be monitored regularly by the physician to check for unusual growth activi-

Causes of Ovarian Cysts

- **Hormonal imbalance**
- **Hypothyroidism**
- **Dietary factors**
- **Genetic predisposition**
- **Cigarette smoking**
- **Psychological/ emotional/sociological influences**

ty or pain. The conventional medical treatment, especially if there is significant pain, is often surgery to remove the cysts (cystectomy). However, in many cases, surgery is not necessary. "An operation need not be a first option unless the findings are suspicious for malignancy or there are other clear indications for surgery," says noted natural health specialist Ralph Golan, M.D., of Seattle, Washington. Often the cysts shrink and disappear by themselves, says Dr. Golan.[1]

Unfortunately, cystectomy can, without prior warning, expand into an operation to remove the ovaries (oophorectomy) and sometimes even the uterus as well (hysterectomy). As you already know, removing the ovaries and uterus will send a woman into premature menopause, with all its attendant physical and emotional trauma.

This chapter presents viable alternatives to such unnecessary surgery—natural therapies that can shrink ovarian cysts and improve your overall health. Another option is to combine conventional and alternative approaches, having the cysts suctioned and drained to relieve the pressure and at the same time implementing alternative medicine therapies to prevent a recurrence of the problem.

What Causes Ovarian Cysts?

As is true of other women's health conditions, hormonal problems (including hypothyroidism which is intimately related to imbalances in hormones) are often central to the formation of ovarian cysts. Other factors include a diet high in sugar, alcohol, and milk products[2] and a genetic predisposition (meaning, ovarian cysts tend to run in families).[3] In addition, a range of lifestyle and emotional/psychological factors have been linked to this disorder. Here, we explore some of these causes in more depth.

Hormonal Imbalance

Ovarian cysts result from a failed or disordered ovulation due

---

Alternative Medicine Therapies for Ovarian Cysts

- Acupuncture
- Castor oil packs
- Dietary recommendations
- Herbal medicine
- Homeopathy
- Natural progesterone therapy
- Nutritional supplements
- Sitz baths

QUICK DEFINITION

Ultrasound, or ultrasonography, is the standard diagnostic tool for determining if a woman has ovarian cysts or a fibroid. The state of deep structures within the body (e.g., the ovaries or uterus) can be visualized by recording the reflections made from pulsing ultrasonic waves directly into the targeted tissues. The ultrasound reflections are then displayed on a computer monitor and are interpreted by a trained medical technician. Generally, the technician is able to accurately identify a cyst or fibroid and assess its approximate size and extent. However, an ultrasound diagnosis is not infallible. Cases have been reported of a prolapsed uterus, prolapsed colon, or ballooned-out, impacted small intestine being misread as a fibroid.

to hormonal imbalances, says John R. Lee, M.D., of Sebastopol, California. For example, the egg follicle sac may fail to ripen and burst, staying in the ovary and forming a cyst. Each month it will continue to enlarge and swell more when it gets a surge of luteinizing hormone (LH, SEE QUICK DEFINITION) at ovulation. LH is the hormone that stimulates ovulation and transforms the egg follicle into the corpus luteum, which produces progesterone. Dr. Lee states that the condition can be treated with natural progesterone cream therapy (see Chapter 3: Fibroids, pp. 113-117).[4]

For more about **hormonal imbalance and hypothyroidism**, see Chapter 1: Menstrual Problems, pp. 24-26, and Chapter 5: Infertility, pp. 163-165.

Ovulation may not occur as a woman nears menopause and, in that case, the pituitary gland does not secrete LH, explains Jennifer Brett, N.D., of Stratford, Connecticut. Without LH, the follicle that grew during the first phase of the menstrual cycle does not rupture and release the egg at ovulation. The woman's body keeps making follicle-stimulating hormone (FSH, SEE QUICK DEFINITION) and the follicle keeps growing and becomes a cyst.

Cigarette Smoking

A study of more than 5,000 women, 21 to 80 years old, found that smoking is linked to the occurrence of ovarian cysts. Women who smoke or who are ex-smokers increase their risk of ovarian cysts by about one-and-a-half times compared to nonsmokers, the researchers report.[5]

The key to smoking's impact on ovarian health lies in the fact that it lowers blood estrogen levels by making the liver more toxic, says nutrition specialist Susan Brown, Ph.D., of Syracuse, New York.[6] Lowered levels of estrogen, in turn, disrupt the menstrual cycle, possibly resulting in abnormal ovulation and the development of cysts. Smoking also depletes vitamin C levels and raises the amount of body toxins such as lead, cadmium, and nicotine, among others.[7] Such deficiencies and toxicities can also affect hormone balance and lead to cyst formation.

Psychological, Emotional, and Sociological Influences

As noted throughout this book, the body-mind link is undeniably integral to health and illness. People who understand this link automatically think of psychological and emotional factors, but women's reproductive systems, being the site in the body of gender identity and sexual issues, are affected by sociological patterns as well. According to W. John Diamond, M.D., of Reno, Nevada, women's health problems often trace back to a precipitating emotional event or preexisting social condition. Along with other alternative medicine physicians, he points to past sexual abuse as a common factor in women with female health problems such as ovarian cysts. Sexual abuse fits all three categories: emotional, psychological, and sociological—the latter because such abuse reflects societal devaluation of women. Changing social roles and delayed childbearing are two other sociological phenomena which Dr. Diamond believes are contributing to an increase in reproductive disorders.

Past History of Sexual Abuse—In Dr. Diamond's experience, a current health problem usually has a link to past trauma. "When I see problems such as ovarian cysts, endometriosis, or fibroids, I am always

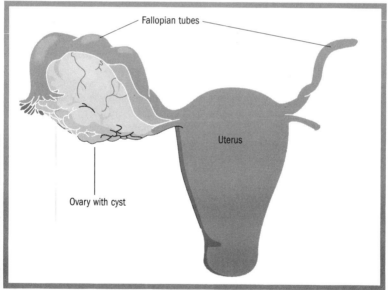

THE OVARIAN CYST. **Cysts can develop on or in an ovary at any age between puberty and menopause. Typically, the cyst fills with a yellowish, straw-colored, or blood-stained fluid; when the cyst becomes large, it can produce a sensation of pelvic pressure and dullness.**

Seven Types of Ovarian Cysts

1) Follicular cysts—These cysts arise from normal ovarian function (as such, they are in the category of "functional" cysts). An egg develops inside a follicle, a cyst-like spherical structure in the ovary. During normal ovulation, the follicle bursts, releasing the egg, then dissolves in two to three weeks. If the follicle fails to burst, it may become a follicular cyst. If it continues to fill with fluid, it can become quite large, produce estrogen, and mimic a tumor.

This kind of cyst may result from hormonal irregularities; however, most follicular cysts regress spontaneously after six to eight weeks. A sign of a follicular cyst can be a sudden onset of pain on one side of the abdomen, occurring mid-cycle and lasting a few hours.

2) Corpus luteum cysts—In some cases, the follicle releases the egg normally, but the remaining hormone-producing structure (corpus luteum) stays intact and eventually becomes a cyst. Although corpus luteum cysts usually dissolve over a period of weeks, they tend to be larger than follicular cysts and may twist the ovary, causing pelvic or abdominal pain. Also called a granulosa-lutein cyst, the corpus luteum cyst can be a signal to check for ectopic or uterine pregnancy. The sign of a corpus luteum cyst can be abnormal or slight bleeding.

3) Dermoid cysts—Among the most common benign tumors of the ovaries, dermoid cysts are rarely cancerous but can become large and twist the ovary causing pain.

4) Cystadenomas—These ovarian tumors are classified as either water-filled or mucus-filled. While both types are benign, they may grow to a large size, causing pelvic or abdominal pain.

5) Polycystic ovarian syndrome (PCO)—This benign condition involves the growth of numerous cysts, usually on both ovaries, and is unrelated to the menstrual cycle. Symptoms of PCO include irregular or absent periods, obesity, increased hair growth, and infertility.

6) Ovarian edema—In this condition, an ovary becomes enlarged by swelling with fluid; in 75% of cases, only one ovary is affected. It typically arises in women in their twenties and produces pain and menstrual irregularities.

7) Endometriomas—If tissue from the uterine lining migrates onto the surface of the ovary, an endometrioma is formed. These blood-filled cysts, regardless of location, often accumulate and shed blood according to the menstrual cycle (a condition called endometriosis). Endometrial implants on the ovaries, though technically a type of endometriosis, will be treated as ovarian cysts in this chapter.

suspicious of previous sexual molestation." Sexual trauma causes an energy disturbance which, in turn, may trigger any one of these conditions, often much later in a woman's life. Dr. Diamond estimates that about 50% of the women he treats for reproductive disorders have a history of sexual abuse.

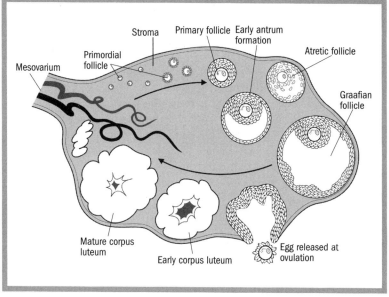

THE ANATOMY OF OVULATION. **Pictured above is a diagram of the ovary showing the stages through which the follicle develops and is released as an egg (the first 14 days of the cycle), and the subsequent changes in the corpus luteum (leading up to menstruation).**

Changing Social Roles—Changes in attitude toward women's social roles open the female psyche to all kinds of disturbances. "Many women are role-distorted, not sure of how they are supposed to be as women," Dr. Diamond notes. "Is a woman a mother or a professional, or both?" The confusing position of women in contemporary American society has an undeniable impact on women's psychological and emotional—and therefore physical—health.

Delayed Childbearing—Women in the U.S. and Canada are having babies much later in life than their mothers and grandmothers did. This resetting of the "biological clock" negatively affects reproductive function, as childbirth clears the energy of the reproductive system better than any therapeutic technique.

During gestation, the entire lower abdomen has a great increase in vascularity, Dr. Diamond explains. More blood vessels form to deliver more blood to this now critical region. Anything that has been deposited there—energy traces, suppressed emotions, "seeds" of physical problems, hormonal imbalances, mentrual pain or irregularity—is removed through the childbirth process.

143

Qi (pronounced *CHEE*) is a Chinese word variously translated to mean "vital energy," "essence of life," and "living force." In Chinese medicine, the proper flow of *qi* along energy channels (meridians) within the body is crucial to a person's health and vitality. There are many types of *qi*, classified according to source, location, and function (such as activation, warming, defense, transformation, and containment). Within the body, *qi* and blood are closely linked, as each is considered to flow along with the other. The manipulation and readjustment of *qi* to treat disease and ensure maximum health benefit is the basic principle of acupuncture, although other remedies and therapies can be used to influence *qi*.

In effect, childbearing cleanses or "energetically recalibrates" years' worth of built-up stagnation in the uterus. "The longer a woman waits to have a child (if she ever does)," Dr. Diamond points out, "the greater the chance that reproductive problems and the psychological issues associated with them may develop or accumulate."

To illustrate his point, Dr. Diamond compares the Western woman's pattern of delayed childbearing to the social norms of other cultures. Among the tribal natives in South Africa, for example, women get pregnant early in life, have babies in quick succession (often over a period of ten years), and breastfeed their children until they reach age five. Interestingly, the tribal women of South Africa have no problems with ovarian cysts, endometriosis, or uterine fibroids.

The South African woman's almost constant pregnancy means that she has barely a half dozen menstrual cycles during her early adult years. In contrast, a Western woman without children has a dozen periods annually. If you bear in mind that with each period there is a loss of vital energy (or *qi*, SEE QUICK DEFINITION), you begin to see the cost to women's physical health from the expansion of women's role in the world.

Given the sociological complications in countries such as the U.S. and Canada, "it's almost as if not having a child before age 30 means a woman will develop endometriosis, fibroids, or an ovarian cyst instead," Dr. Diamond says. The emotional issues associated with a woman's reproductive system must be either cleansed (through childbirth or psychotherapy) or expressed as gynecological disturbances.

The following two cases emphasize the role psychological, emotional, and sociological issues can play in ovarian cysts and the importance of addressing these components as part of treatment; in one case, the limits of not doing so, and in the second, a more successful outcome as a result of being willing to take on the challenge.

Success Story: Ovarian Cyst Pain Eliminated –But What About the Emotions?

W. John Diamond, M.D., recounts how a patient's refusal to examine internal emotional issues limits complete resolution of health problems:

Daisy, 40, came to me with a left-sided ovarian cyst the size of a grapefruit. Even though it had doubled in size in the previous two months, Daisy's gynecologist, after studying an ultrasound of her uterus, decided against surgery and in favor of watchful waiting. Just before menstruation started each month, Daisy had pain and cramping; as the blood flow began, these symptoms eased off. This had been her pattern since adolescence.

When the cyst continued to grow, accompanied by pain in the same region, Daisy's gynecologist recommended either draining the fluid from the cyst or cutting it out in a cystectomy. Daisy decided against both and asked me to give her acupuncture treatments instead. I informed her that hers was not a case for acupuncture, that she would respond better to homeopathic (SEE QUICK DEFINITION) remedies. However, Daisy insisted on acupuncture.

I treated *chong mo* acupuncture points around her uterus (*chong mo* refers to an acupuncture meridian—SEE QUICK DEFINITION—that influences the pelvic area) in three weekly sessions for two weeks, a timetable determined by Daisy. "I want acupuncture, so I'm coming in three times a week until this is better," she told me. This insistence, along with other aspects of her personality, were clues pointing to the appropriate homeopathic remedy. Daisy was self-centered, suspicious, highly talkative, and generally difficult to deal with, qualities which pointed to *Lachesis* (made from American pit viper venom). I gave her one dose of *Lachesis* at high potency (10M).

The next day, Daisy said she had no more pain nor any further pressure sensation in her uterus, as before. As far as she was concerned, she was healed. When I asked her a few weeks later if she wanted any more treatments, Daisy said, "The pain is gone, I think everything is gone." I suggested she see her gynecologist for a follow-up ultrasound, but I don't know if she acted on my advice. I haven't seen Daisy since.

These results illustrate a general principle I find often demonstrated in clinical practice. Once you get the physiology under control, whatever the problem, the pathology usually stops at that stage. The condition, such as a cyst, may or may not regress, but generally it will no longer pose any problems for the individual.

Homeopathy was founded in the early 1800s by German physician Samuel Hahnemann. Today, an estimated 500 million people worldwide receive homeopathic treatment; in Britain, homeopathy enjoys royal patronage. Homeopathy is now practiced according to two differing concepts. In classical homeopathy, only one single-component remedy is prescribed at a time, in a potency specifically adjusted to the patient; the physician waits to see the results before prescribing anything further. In complex homeopathy, typified by *Hepar compositum*, a prescription involves multiple substances given at the same time, usually in low potencies.

Acupuncture meridians are specific pathways in the human body for the flow of life force or subtle energy, known as *qi* (pronounced CHEE). In most cases, these energy pathways run up and down both sides of the body, and correspond to individual organs or organ systems, designated as Lung, Small Intestine, Heart, and others. There are 12 principal meridians and eight secondary channels. Numerous points of heightened energy, or *qi*, exist on the body's surface along the meridians and are called acupoints. There are more than 1,000 acupoints, each of which is potentially a place for acupuncture treatment.

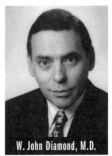

W. John Diamond, M.D.

"In my experience, perhaps 80% of all disease is emotional in origin; the rest is toxicity derived from the environment, including food and water," states Dr. Diamond. **"Women's health problems often trace back to a precipitating emotional event or preexisting social condition."**

W. John Diamond, M.D., is a board certified pathologist; his training in alternative medicine is extensive, including medical acupuncture at the University of California at Los Angeles, classical homeopathy at the Pacific Academy of Homeopathic Medicine in Berkeley, California, and neural therapy at the American Academy of Neural Therapy in Seattle, Washington. Dr. Diamond is coauthor of *An Alternative Medicine Definitive Guide to Cancer* (Future Medicine Publishing, 1997). He may be contacted at: Triad Medical Center, 4600 Kietzke Lane, M-242, Reno, NV 89502; tel: 702-829-2277; fax: 702-829-2365.

However, one of the difficult aspects of Daisy's case was that she was completely resistant to any discussion or probing regarding the possible emotional factors that led to her ovarian cyst. She would talk freely about the physical aspect of her condition, but anything to do with her family life or childhood was out of bounds. This complicated the treatment plan because in my experience, perhaps 80% of all disease is emotional in origin; the rest is toxicity derived from the environment, including food and water. ■

Success Story: Treating the Feelings That Grew the Cyst

"I'd been living to please my dead mother, my husband, and everybody else," says Diana, a 38-year-old woman with a long history of chronic illness, the latest being an ovarian cyst. Like many women who receive the societal message that they should stuff their own needs and put everyone else first, Diana's unresolved emotional issues expressed themselves physically. For treatment of the cyst and other persistent health problems, Diana sought the help of naturopath Kristy Fassler, N.D., of Portsmouth, New Hampshire.

Before exploring the emotional causes behind Diana's ovarian cyst, Dr. Fassler assembled a detailed symptom picture. The cyst was on Diana's right side. Although three ultrasounds over a six-month period showed no change in its shape and size, the cyst had become increasingly painful over the past three to four months. The sensation ranged from chronic aching to "zinging pain." At the same time, Diana began bleeding premenstrually, and the menstrual flow itself was dark and clotted. Diana also experienced chest pain during ovulation, recurrent urinary tract infections, and ezcema, particularly on her nipples and fingers. Bladder irritation added another factor. During the past eight months, Diana started wetting her pants.

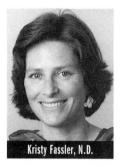

Kristy Fassler, N.D.

The combination of Diana's right-sided ovarian cyst, urinary tract infections, and feelings of shame and worry suggested to Kristy Fassler, N.D., a homeopathic remedy which would address all of these symptoms at once.

While she described her symptoms to Dr. Fassler, Diana became more comfortable talking about her emotional state. She was currently putting her husband through school, and she worried constantly about money. Diana was so concerned about what others think and feel that she had trouble identifying her own emotions. "Her predominant emotion was shame," observes Dr. Fassler. "Diana had a strong need to please other people before she felt entitled to please herself."

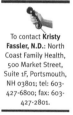

To contact **Kristy Fassler, N.D.**: North Coast Family Health, 500 Market Street, Suite 1F, Portsmouth, NH 03801; tel: 603-427-6800; fax: 603-427-2801.

The combination of Diana's right-sided ovarian cyst, urinary tract infections, and feelings of shame and worry suggested to Dr. Fassler a homeopathic remedy which would address all of these symptoms at once. She prescribed a single dose of *Palladium* 200C, which is commonly given for tumors on the right side of the body.

Seven weeks later, Diana returned for her follow-up visit to report an initial increase in lower abdominal pain, which then gradually lessened until it disappeared completely. Her chest pain had also stopped, although the eczema and bladder irritation continued to bother her. More importantly, Dr. Fassler noted a subtle change in Diana's demeanor. "Her physical complaints aside, Diana was blossoming as a person." By taking charge of her physical health, Diana had developed a more confident attitude toward her life. Her worry and frustruation, previously stuffed down inside of her, was no longer expressing itself as physical pain.

After another single dose of *Palladium*, this time at 30C, Diana's skin and bladder problems improved. Six weeks later, she was strong enough to undergo surgical removal of her cyst, which was benign. Since then, Diana has not experienced any more chest pain, bladder irritation, or lower abdominal pain.[8]

The next case is a powerful illustration of just how much alternative medicine therapies can accomplish, even after conventional medicine has seriously damaged a woman's reproductive system.

Success Story: Acupuncture Reverses Cysts and Enables Pregnancy With Only ¼ Ovary

Maria, 36, was planning to be married in six weeks when she started having pain around the area of her left kidney. On the basis of an ultrasound, her conventional physician diagnosed ovarian cysts and sent her to a gynecologist who immediately scheduled her for a cystectomy.

The surgeon found several dermoid cysts (nonmalignant cysts that grow teeth, skin, and hair) the size of grapefruits which he began to remove, along with both ovaries, when Maria's physician entered the operating room. He informed the surgeon that Maria was getting married and wanted to have children, and that the surgeon needed to leave at least part of the ovaries intact. Maria was left with one-quarter of one ovary.

Following the surgery, Maria, who previously had had regular menstrual periods with little distress, developed erratic menstrual cycles and frequent left-sided pain. The pain was due to cysts continuing to develop on the one-quarter of an ovary that was left.

After Maria got married, she and her husband tried to conceive for six months, with no success. Maria then tried taking Clomid, a fertility drug that stimulates ovulation. When that failed, Maria and her husband tried *in vitro* fertilization a number of times, also with no success. At the last trial, the fertility specialist told Maria she had run out of eggs and would never be able to have children. By the time she finished all the fertility treatments, Maria, who had not been overweight before, had gained 15 pounds and became very unhappy.

At this point, Maria consulted acupuncturist Jane Lyttleton of Sidney, Australia. After reassuring Maria that her one-quarter of an ovary was capable of producing many eggs, Dr. Lyttleton gave her an acupuncture treatment designed to accomplish the following:

■ Improve Energy Circulation—The first goal was to improve the circulation of *qi* (vital energy) and blood to the pelvis in order to relieve pain and prevent more cysts from developing. In Dr. Lyttleton's diagnosis, both the *qi* and the blood were "stagnated" or obstructed in the pelvis. The body fluids were not able to move freely and therefore accumulated, creating a buildup of moisture, phlegm, and "dampness." This accumulation of moisture and phlegm, over time, led to the development of the cysts, as reflected in Maria's tongue coating, which was thick, yellowish, and greasy. Further evidence of the phlegm buildup was the dermoid cysts themselves, which are wet and shiny and encased by thick skin.

■ Strengthen Energy in the Reproductive System—The second goal was to restore and strengthen energy in the channels that circulate around and govern the reproductive system, namely the *chong mo* (see illustration, p. 128) and *ren* channels (see illustration, next page). Dr. Lyttleton determined, through Maria's wrist pulses (SEE QUICK DEFINITION), that the energy in her kidney organ system was low. This system governs the reproductive organs, including the ovaries. With the deficiencies in this system, as well as in the *chong mo* and *ren* energy channels, Maria's remaining bit of ovary tissue did not have enough energy to function properly.

■ Soothe the Emotions—The third goal was to calm and soothe Maria who was quite distraught. For this, treatment focused on freeing energy in the acupuncture meridians that feed the liver and spleen. These organs are important in maintaining emotional balance, according to Chinese medicine. Dr. Lyttleton needled acupuncture points mostly on Maria's abdomen, along with several on her feet and two on her hands.

Following the first session, Maria had what is called a "withdrawal bleed" from discontinuing the fertility drugs. The bleeding, in which the uterus expels drug-stimulated tissue and blood accumulation, lasted two days. Dr. Lyttleton continued acupuncture treatment, adding several points on the abdomen, including a special point, *zigong*, to stimulate ovarian function. After that, Maria experienced three days of abdominal pain, similar to what she had when she had ovulated in the past.

After a total of five treatments (the time elapsed was 34 days from the withdrawal bleed), Maria had still not had a menstrual period. However, Dr. Lyttleton noted that Maria's pulse associated with the kidneys had taken on a new quality which, under some conditions, can indicate pregnancy. Chinese practitioners call this quality a "slippery" pulse, meaning the beat of the pulse has a fluid, wave-like feel to it. A week later, several other of Maria's pulses were "slippery." Dr. Lyttleton gave Maria a pregnancy test which, to everyone's amazement, came out positive.

QUICK DEFINITION

In Chinese medicine, the **pulse** can be felt or "read" at three different positions and three different depths on each wrist. A total of 28 different energy qualities may be discerned from reading a patient's pulse; these include wiry, thready, choppy, tight, knotted, intermittent, rapid, slow, deep, floating, large, slippery, and empty. The quality of the pulse indicates a specific energy state or disharmony of the body and its organs. In conventional Western medicine, the pulse is simply the rhythmic rate of an artery as blood moves through it, pumped by the heart.

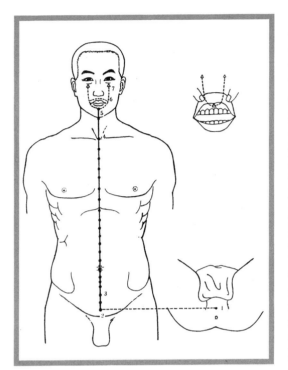

THE *REN* CHANNEL. This acupuncture meridian runs from the bottom of both eyes, through the chin, and down the center of the body to the perineum. It is used to send energy to the reproductive organs.

Maria delivered a healthy baby by Caesarean section, three weeks prematurely. After she stopped breastfeeding two months later, Maria's ovarian pain returned. Dr. Lyttleton continued to treat Maria with acupuncture, noticing some signs that Maria was getting weaker and damper again. However, about five months after the birth of her first child, Maria was pregnant again. Dr. Lyttleton was concerned because she felt Maria was in too weakened a condition to carry a pregnancy to term, but she continued to treat Maria, who delivered another healthy baby.

Unfortunately, after the delivery, Maria bled heavily, developed an infection, and became generally ill. She had constant low back pain, and her pulses and tongue showed increasing weakness and dampness. Maria continued with the acupuncture and became pregnant again, but she miscarried this third child. Six months after the miscarriage, and still under the care of Dr. Lyttleton, Maria had recovered reasonably good health, including a return of her menstrual periods. In all, Maria's treatment program, pregnancies, and return to health spanned four years.[9]

Success Story: Cyst Disappears With Herbs, Homeopathy, and Sitz Baths

In the case of Rita, 32, the solution to her ovarian cyst was in a combination of natural therapies, including homeopathy (as discussed by Dr. Diamond earlier).

Rita came to naturopathic physician Jennifer Brett, N.D., when her daughter had just turned one year old. From the time the baby was about six months old, Rita had experienced frequent pain in the lower left side of her abdomen. The pain, which was intermittent, did not follow Rita's menstrual cycle or any particular pattern, but was so severe that she was doubled over with it. The pain, which felt better with heat application and with pressure, was always worse when Rita was constipated.

Suspecting possible colon problems, Dr. Brett ran a stool culture which revealed no abnormalities. Next, Dr. Brett did an ultrasound which showed a 1cm by 4 cm cyst on Rita's left ovary. Dr. Brett diagnosed the cyst as an endometrioma (blood-filled cyst).

To begin treatment, Dr. Brett gave Rita a homeopathic remedy, *Colocynthis* (from bitter apple), indicated for stabbing stomach pain, violent cramp-like pain, or pain around the ovaries. Rita was to take a 30C dose daily for three weeks, and then as needed for pain. Dr. Brett also gave Rita an herbal tincture called Turska (see sidebar: "Turska Helps to Dissolve Cysts Herbally," p. 152) designed to move blood, tumors, and masses; the dosage was five drops twice a day.

In addition, Dr. Brett had Rita do alternating hot and cold sitz baths, every day for about 15 minutes (see sidebar). The baths would relieve pain and improve blood and lymphatic flow through Rita's pelvis.

To further improve pelvic lymph and blood circulation, Rita was to rest on a slant board (Rita used an old door in her basement) for about 15 minutes. For this, Rita set one end of the board on a chair and the other on the floor, then she lay on the board with her head facing the

How to Take a Sitz Bath

Sitz baths are a traditional European folk remedy in which the pelvis is immersed in hot or cold water. A hot sitz bath is particularly helpful for problems involving the pelvic region, including uterine cramps and painful ovaries. A cold sitz bath, taken for two minutes or less, can be used for inflammation, constipation, and vaginal discharge.

To prepare a sitz bath, find two basins adequate to sit in so that water will reach up to the level of the navel. Fill one of the basins with hot water and fill the other with ice water. Alternate soaks, starting with three to four minutes in the hot, then 30 to 60 seconds in the cold. Repeat three to five times, ending with the cold water. You can also use a cold towel instead of the ice water tub if two basins are not available. Use caution when getting in and out of the basins.

Turska Helps to Dissolve Cysts Herbally

Turska Formula, taken orally and available only by prescription, is a tincture consisting of the extracts of four strong herbs known for moving blood, tumors, and masses. The herbal extracts are mixed with alcohol and water to form the tincture. Turska contains phytolacca or pokeroot

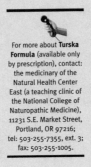

For more about **Turska Formula** (available only by prescription), contact: the medicinary of the Natural Health Center East (a teaching clinic of the National College of Naturopathic Medicine), 11231 S.E. Market Street, Portland, OR 97216; tel: 503-255-7355, ext. 3; fax: 503-255-1005.

(*Phytolacca americana*), aconite or monkshood (*Aconitum napellus*), gelsemium or yellow jasmine (*Gelsemium sempervirens*), and bryony (*Bryonia spp.*). Dosage varies, depending on the patient's sensitivity, and the exact proportions of the extracts, alcohol, and water.

floor and her pelvis higher. This position allows the pelvic congestion caused by accumulation of lymph fluid to drain, leaving room for new blood. "Naturopaths used to call this condition pelvic congestion syndrome and prescribed this simple remedy," explains Dr. Brett. "The goal was to get fresh blood into the pelvis."

Rita followed this regimen for six weeks, when a second ultrasound revealed that her ovarian cyst was completely gone. Also gone was Rita's pain, aside from a recurrence about every six months. At these times, Rita took another dose of *Colocynthis* and the pain went away. "Although we couldn't identify it on ultrasound, my suspicion is that she had another endometrioma somewhere, potentially on her colon, that didn't completely go away," Dr. Brett concludes. "However, it was certainly controllable."

Success Story:
Balancing Hormones Shrinks Large Cyst

In this next case, Dr. Brett again is successful in shrinking an ovarian cyst, this time a much larger one and occurring in a perimenopausal (SEE QUICK DEFINITION) woman.

Marie, 47, went to her gynecologist complaining of heavy bleeding during the previous three menstrual cycles. She had no pain, but was concerned about the heavy bleeding. The gynecologist did an ultrasound and found a large, 4 cm by 8 cm cyst on Marie's right ovary. His solution was to monitor the cyst and if after two months it had not shrunk or disappeared, he would recommend a cystectomy.

Marie wanted to avoid surgery and consulted Dr. Brett. Marie's heavy

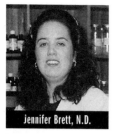

After six weeks of the herbal, vitamin, and homeopathic therapy, Marie's cyst had shrunk to 1 cm by 1 cm, says Dr. Brett. When Marie returned in four weeks, the cyst was completely gone.

bleeding, along with her moodiness and insomnia (both of which are typical symptoms of perimenopause), indicated that she was perimenopausal. Accordingly, Dr. Brett suspected that the cyst was of the follicular variety, common in perimenopausal women.

Dr. Brett explains that such cysts can happen when a woman fails to ovulate. Since there is no ovulation, the pituitary gland does not secrete luteinizing hormone (LH). As explained earlier, without LH, the follicle containing the egg does not rupture as it normally would. The woman's body continues producing follicle-stimulating hormone (FSH) and the follicle grows larger, becoming a cyst.

"It was most important to reduce Marie's FSH levels," Dr. Brett says. To accomplish this, she gave Marie a standardized herbal extract of chastetree berry (*Vitex agnus-castus*) which is a hormone stimulant and has the ability to normalize FSH levels. Marie took two capsules of Vitalex (containing 175 mg of chastetree per capsule) a day, along with vitamin B6 (100 mg, three times daily). Vitamin B6 also lowers FSH levels, according to Dr. Brett.

In addition, Marie took a combination homeopathic-herbal remedy called Estrex (two or three tablets under her tongue every night before bed). Estrex contains homeopathically prepared estradiol, estrone, and testosterone hormones, *Sepia*, *Lachesis*, black cohosh (*Cimicifuga racemosa*), wild yam (*Dioscorea villosa*), and homeopathic Ovary and Adrenal.

All of the homeopathic substances in the remedy were to address underlying hormonal imbalances, says Dr. Brett. "If there's not enough testosterone, for example, the remedy will stimulate the body to produce more, and if there's too much testosterone—as is more common with ovarian cysts—it will slow down testosterone production." The *Estradiolosum* and Estrone are derived from and affect those

Perimenopause is a newly-described condition characterized by the early onset of selected menopausal symptoms. The average American woman enters menopause around age 52; since perimenopause can begin as early as age 35, a woman may be vulnerable to the effects of menopause-related hormonal changes for as long as 17 years. Symptoms of perimenopause include moodiness, anxiety, weight gain, food cravings, irritability, headaches, bloating, "fuzzy" thinking, and depression. As with menopause, perimenopause (peri meaning "before," and menopause meaning "the end of the menses") is associated with a drop in progesterone relative to estrogen (two key female hormones). Increases in environmental estrogens, or substances (such as certain pesticides and other men-made chemicals) which function as estrogens once in the body, can exacerbate the effects of perimenopause.

To contact **Jennifer Brett, N.D.**: 998 Nichols Avenue, Stratford, CT 06497; tel: 203-377-1525; fax: 203-380-2831. For **Estrex**, contact: NF Formulas, 9775 S.W. Commerce Circle C-5, Wilsonville, OR 97070; tel: 800-547-4891 or 503-682-9755; fax: 503-682-9529. For **Vitalex**, contact: Nature's Way, 10 Mountain Spring Parkway, Springville, UT 84663; tel: 801-489-1500; fax: 801-489-1700. PhytoPharmica also makes a *Vitex* extract with 225 mg *Vitex* per capsule; contact: PhytoPharmica, P.O. Box 1745, Green Bay, WI 54305; tel: 800-553-2370 or 800-376-1525; fax: 414-469-4418.

specific estrogens, estradiol and estrone, while the Ovary and Adrenal homeopathic remedies are made from potentized dilutions of the glands' energetic essences and thus can affect the functions of those two glands. Black cohosh and wild yam are known for their hormone-balancing properties, as are *Sepia* and *Lachesis*.

After six weeks of the herbal, vitamin, and homepathic therapy, Marie went for a follow-up visit to her gynecologist. He found the cyst had shrunk to 1 cm by 1 cm. The gynecologist said he would wait one more menstrual cycle before proceeding with surgery. When Marie returned in four weeks, the cyst was completely gone.

For long-term preventive maintenance, Dr. Brett took Marie off the Estrex and B6, but kept her on the Vitalex, reducing the dose to one capsule a day. Marie has been fine ever since.

Self-Care for Ovarian Cysts

The following are steps you can take to start shrinking your ovarian cysts. As always, however, before embarking on any self-care program, you need to first determine if other pathology is involved. In addition, serious health conditions such as ovarian cysts are best treated under the guidance of a qualified medical practitioner.

Natural Progesterone Therapy

As Dr. John Lee mentioned previously, natural progesterone can bring relief to ovarian cysts by helping to restore proper hormonal balance. Natural progesterone, delivered topically before ovulation, can inhibit the levels of LH (luteinizing hormone), says Dr. Lee. Within one to two cycles, as the cyst is no longer stimulated, it will "very likely shrink and disappear without further treatment."

Dr. Lee prefers natural progesterone in cream or oil formulation because transdermal (through the skin) absorption is more efficient than taking it orally, and the effect lasts longer without the emotional highs and lows associated with the oral drops. For ovarian cysts, Dr. Lee typically recommends 1/8 to 1/2 teaspoon of cream per day or three to ten drops of oil. The cream should be applied to the palms, face, neck, upper chest, breasts, inside of the arms, or behind the knees from day ten to 26 of the menstrual cycle, says Dr. Lee.

The key criterion for the type of cream or oil to use is the amount of progesterone it contains. Under healthy conditions, a premenopausal woman's system produces about 20 mg daily of progesterone between days 15 and 26 of the cycle. When using the cream, amounts in the range of 20-30 mg daily are often sufficient; relief from the primary symptoms will indicate a woman is taking the appropriate dosage.[10]

Diet and Nutritional Supplements

In cases of ovarian cysts, women's health specialist Tori Hudson, N.D., of Portland, Oregon, focuses on possible toxemia of the liver and designs treatments to maintain healthy liver function. (As noted in previous chapters, the liver, as the body's filter for toxins and excess estrogen, is essential to maintaining proper hormonal balance.) Dr. Hudson's program includes dietary changes and supplements. She recommends a vegetarian diet of organic foods with an emphasis on liver-nourishing foods such as beets, carrots, and lemons. She also strongly advises eliminating fried foods, sugar, coffee, cigarettes, and alcohol.

Helpful supplements include vitamins A, E, and C, beta carotene, and zinc, as well as black currant and evening primrose oils, says Dr. Hudson. Studies have shown that supplementing with vitamin E (800-1,200 IU daily) may relieve some of the symptoms associated with ovarian cysts.[11] As support for the liver, Dr. Hudson frequently prescribes a lipotropic supplement called SLF Forte. Lipotropics metabolize fatty deposits in the liver and thus help restore this organ's toxin-processing function, which in turn is helpful in eliminating ovarian cysts. SLF Forte contains vitamins B6 and B12, choline and inositol (also in the B-complex family), the amino acid methionine, beet powder, and dandelion.[12]

Ralph Golan, M.D., encourages women who suffer from ovarian cysts to adopt a diet emphasizing whole foods over refined or processed foods. Since eating too many fatty or mucus-stimulating foods can contribute to the formation and growth of ovarian cysts, Dr. Golan suggests limiting intake of fruit and fruit juices, buttery or oily foods, animal fats, dairy products, and sugar. He also recommends avoiding alcohol and caffeine (coffee, tea, chocolate, soft drinks, and even caffeine-containing medications).

Self-Care Homeopathic Remedies

In addition to the constitutional or combination formulas employed by

For a list of brand names of **natural progesterone creams**, along with their progesterone content, see Chapter 3: Fibroids, pp. 114-115. For more about **the use of progesterone creams**, see Chapter 1: Menstrual Problems, pp. 31-34.

While Dr. Lee's recommendations represent a self-care option, women are advised to consult a qualified health-care professional for supervision of treatment because ovarian cysts can be a serious health problem.

Natural progesterone cream is available at health food stores. The brand *ProGest* is also available from: Transitions for Health, Inc., 621 S.W. Alder Street, Suite 900, Portland, OR 97205-3627; tel: 800-888-6814.

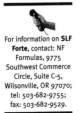

For information on **SLF Forte**, contact: NF Formulas, 9775 Southwest Commerce Circle, Suite C-5, Wilsonville, OR 97070; tel: 503-682-9755; fax: 503-682-9529.

Drs. Diamond and Brett, the field of homeopathy also includes remedies which can be used for symptom relief. The following is a general guide to homeopathic remedies for ovarian cysts, according to the cyst's location and the type of pain involved.[13] Remedies should be taken every three to four hours as needed. For severe or persistent symptoms, seek proper consultation with a qualified healthcare practitioner. These protocols are indicated for first aid, not deep treatment.

■ Left ovary—localized pain which is sharpest in the morning and less severe as the day progresses; *Lachesis* 12C

■ Right ovary—stinging pains, associated with pain during menstruation and tenderness in the pelvic area; *Apis* 6C

■ Lower abdomen—wedge-like pain between the ovary and the uterus; *Iodum* 6C

■ Lower abdomen—shooting pain so intense that the sufferer must bend over for relief; *Colocynthis* 6C

Castor Oil Packs

Castor oil packs, as mentioned previously in this book, can provide pain relief, draw out impurities, and help dissolve tumors and cysts. Dr. Golan recommends using a castor oil pack over the lower abdomen for one hour daily, for up to one month or sometimes longer.[14]

To prepare a castor oil pack, lightly heat enough castor oil to thoroughly wet (but not soak) a 10" x 12" flannel cloth. Immerse the flannel in the hot oil, then fold to make three to four layers and place against the skin. The oil will help to draw out toxins, release tension, and improve blood circulation. Place a heating pad or hot water bottle (wrapped in a towel) over the pack, then cover pack and bottle with another towel to retain heat. Keep in place for one to two hours. You can store the flannel cloth wrapped in plastic in a refrigerator for later use; discard after 20 uses.

CHAPTER

5

There are alternative medicine
therapies which are far more effective than
the costly and invasive surgeries
and fertility drugs commonly offered to women who
suffer from infertility. So-called infertility
is often quickly resolved when underlying conditions
contributing to it are treated.
Traditional Chinese medicine is one of the more
powerful treatment methods available
and has restored many women to fertility.

Infertility

I N F E R T I L I T Y, or the inability to conceive children, can be heartbreaking and frustrating. In the U.S. alone, there are an estimated 5.3 million people who suffer from infertility[1] and the numbers seem to be on the rise. Most doctors diagnose infertility after the people involved have been trying to conceive for a year without success. However, if the woman is 35 or older, she is often advised to seek medical help after six months because of her naturally declining fertility. Conventional fertility specialists are doing a booming business plying drugs and expensive procedures to people who desperately want a child.[2] The complex, invasive medical treatments used to reverse the problem command a yearly price tag of *at least* $1 billion.[3]

Alternative medicine has proven successful in helping women conceive, even after these expensive procedures—such as fertility drugs or *in vitro* fertilization—have failed. The reason, as found throughout this book and as you will see in the case studies in this chapter, is that the alternative medicine physician treats the underlying problems causing the infertility in the woman or man or both. With this approach, the woman can avoid the side effects of fertility drugs and, not only become a parent, but end up healthier.

The Many Causes of Infertility

As conception is a joint proposition, so, at least in terms of medical investigation, is infertility. Alternative medicine practitioners will not stop with checking reproductive hormone levels in each partner (although those certainly will be taken into account). They will also address the full range of health issues, from nutritional deficiencies, stress levels, and digestion and elimination, to dietary and lifestyle habits, thyroid function, and toxic exposures or accumulations. Disturbances in any of those areas can become causal factors in infertility.

Medical researchers estimate that 60% of the cases of infertility are due to problems with the woman. These range from malnutrition to structural abnormalities in the female reproductive system. For example, 20% to 30% of infertility cases are due to pathologies in the fallopian tubes: scarred fallopian tubes from pelvic inflammatory disease, sexually transmitted diseases, or an infection related to an IUD (intrauterine device), can produce infertility.

A fibroid, cancerous tumor, or endometriosis can also block the egg from moving through the fallopian tubes or even prevent its production. About 10% of infertility cases are caused by fibroids, cysts, or other uterine disturbances while about 15% are due to abnormalities in ovulation or the menstrual cycle, or a failure to ovulate or bleed.[4] Other causes for the woman include hormonal imbalances, inability to ovulate, excessive radiation or X-ray exposure, advanced age, and emotional factors.[5] Long-term use of birth control pills can also result in infertility.

Approximately 40% of the factors contributing to infertility derive from the male.[6] These include immunologic factors (such as antibodies that work against semen); semen that is infected or has an abnormal stickiness (viscosity); ejaculatory disturbances preventing sperm from being delivered to the uterus; abnormally low sperm count, motility (ability of the sperm to move about), and penetration; abnormally shaped sperm; insufficient seminal fluid; undescended or injured testicles; childhood diseases such as mumps; viral infections; varicocele (varicose vein in the scrotum); excessive radiation and X-ray exposure; and prostate disorders.[7]

Given that this book is devoted to women's health, this chapter focuses on the woman's infertility, although some of the case studies touch upon the infertility of the male partner. The following detailed

Causes of Female Infertility

- Preexisting endometriosis
- Underactive thyroid gland
- Nutritional deficiencies
- Inappropriate body fat ratio
- Environmental estrogens
- Fluoride toxicity
- Birth control pills
- Douching
- Use of addictive substances
- Depression and stress

Alternative Medicine Therapies for Infertility

- Acupuncture
- Aromatherapy
- Detoxification
- Herbal medicine
- Homeopathy
- Nutritional supplements

For more about **fibroids,** see Chapter 3: Fibroids, pp. 100-137.

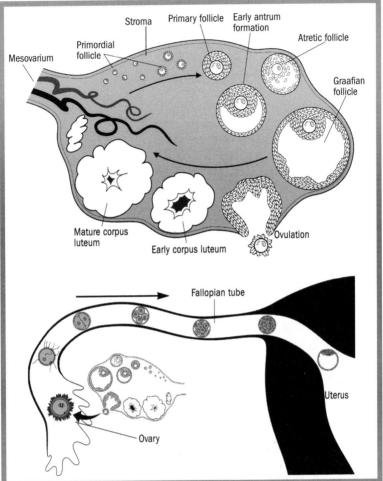

THE MOMENT OF FERTILITY. **The stages leading from follicle to ovulation and the release of the egg (ovum) are shown in the top illustration. The egg moves from the ovary through the fallopian tube to be deposited in the uterus where it awaits fertilization (bottom).**

causal factors of infertility include many which may not be considered by a conventional physician.

Preexisting Endometriosis

Physicians and researchers have long known that moderate to severe endometriosis causes infertility by blocking the fallopian tubes or ovaries

The Fertile Period of Each Sexual Cycle

Once the egg (ovum) has been released from the ovary, it remains viable (capable of being fertilized) for about 24 hours. Sperm can remain viable within the uterus for up to 72 hours, although a 24-hour life span is more typical. Generally, for pregnancy to take place, sperm must be introduced within one to two days before ovulation and up to one day after ovulation. Some women have brief pelvic pain lasting a few minutes to a few hours near the time of ovulation or immediately afterward; this is called "mittelschmerz."

Ovulation is triggered at mid-cycle (approximately day 14 of a normal 28-day menstrual cycle) when the egg made in the ovary and enclosed in what is called a follicular cyst is almost ripened. At that point, the follicular cyst receives a surge of luteinizing hormone (LH, SEE QUICK DEFINITION) from the pituitary gland in the brain. The luteinizing hormone causes the follicular cyst to burst open and spill the egg into the abdominal cavity. After that, the egg finds its way to the fallopian tubes (one on either side of the uterus) which convey the egg to the uterus where it may be fertilized.

QUICK DEFINITION

Luteinizing hormone (LH), produced by the pituitary gland in hte brain, is primarily responsible for ovulation in women. Its name comes from lutein, the yellowish fluid which fills the corpus luteum. This is a hormone-secreting body of endocrine tissues which forms the follicle or sac containing a developing egg. The corpus luteum controls the production of the key female hormones estrogen and progesterone during the second half of the menstrual cycle (called the luteal phase). At mid-cycle, the body secretes increasing amounts of estrogen, which triggers a dramatic surge of LH and another hormone, called follicle-stimulating hormone (FSH). This usually occurs between days 12 and 16 of the cycle, with ovulation (the release of the egg) at day 14. The sudden increase in LH/FSH causes the corpus luteum (also called the follicular cyst) to burst, allowing the mature egg to travel down into the fallopian tubes. Following ovulation, the corpus luteum gradually shrinks, producing less estrogen and progesterone. The steady decline of these hormones ends in the shedding of the uterine lining (menstruation) and the beginning of a new cycle.

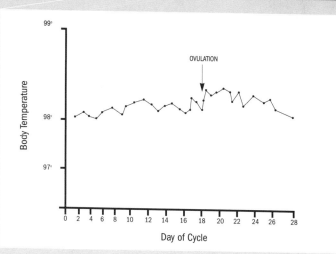

BODY TEMPERATURE RISES AT OVULATION. Shortly after ovulation, there is a distinct peak in body temperature, which does not return to its starting point until just before menstruation.

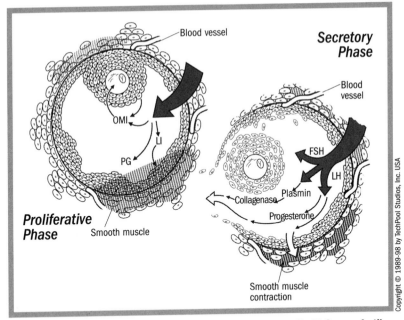

Proliferative Phase

Secretory Phase

Blood vessel

OMI

LI

PG

Smooth muscle

Blood vessel

FSH

LH

Collagenase

Plasmin

Progesterone

Smooth muscle contraction

Copyright © 1989-98 by TechPool Studios, Inc. USA

INSIDER'S VIEW OF A FERTILIZED EGG (OVUM) IMPLANTING IN THE UTERUS. **(Left) Once a fertilized egg attaches to the uterine wall, hormones are released to prevent further ovulation and the shedding of the uterine lining, i.e. menstruation. (Right) If a fertilized egg fails to implant in the uterus, menstruation follows—including the ejection of the egg itself.**

For more about **endometriosis**, see Chapter 2: Endometriosis, pp. 68-99.

with scar tissue. A recent study, however, provides strong evidence that even minimal or mild cases of endometriosis can cause not only infertility but sterility, even when ovulation is normal and there are no blockages.

The study involved 717 women who had been unable to get pregnant for one to four years. All were examined by laparoscope, a slender optical instrument inserted into the abdominal cavity. Of the 717 women, 341 were diagnosed with minimal or mild endometriosis, with no other complicating factors. The study did not offer an explanation as to how the infertility was caused by the mild endometriosis, but said many of the women got pregnant after their endometriosis was treated surgically.[8]

Some insight into the linkage between endometriosis and infertility may be forthcoming. Research under way at the University of North Carolina, in Chapel Hill, could lead to a special test for endometriosis and help explain why even the mildest cases of endometriosis can cause infertility. The research involves a protein called alpha-v/beta-3, which appears on the surface of normal endometrial cells six or seven days after ovulation.

The protein appears to help embryos attach to the uterus and so may be crucial for fertility, but it's missing in up to 50% of women with endometriosis. If the test is approved, women suspected of having endometriosis could have a few endometrial cells biopsied at the critical time to check for the presence of alpha-v/beta-3. In the research in progress, of 33 women who were missing the protein, 30 were found upon laparoscopic examination to have endometriosis.[9]

Underactive Thyroid Gland

As explained in previous chapters, hypothyroidism contributes to a relative excess of estrogen. Specific to fertility issues, the unhealthy side

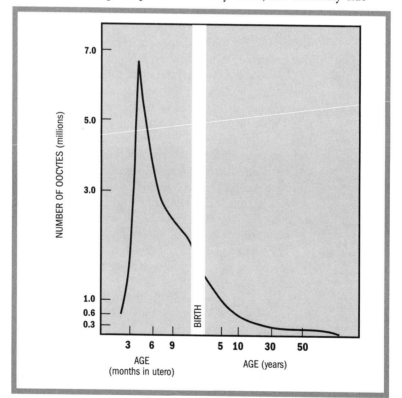

THE MOST FERTILE TIMES IN LIFE. Ironically, the female body has the highest number of potential eggs (oocytes) as a six-month-old fetus. After birth, the number drops dramatically and continues to decline until menopause.

For more about **hypothyroidism and thyroid testing**, see Chapter 1: Menstrual Problems, pp. 24-26.

For more about the **thyroid and health**, see "Reviving the Thyroid," *Alternative Medicine* #23, pp. 54-59.

QUICK DEFINITION

An **antibody** is a protein molecule containing about 20,000 atoms, made from amino acids by B lymphocyte cells in the lymph tissue and set in motion by the immune system against a specific foreign protein, or antigen. An antibody is also referred to as an immunoglobulin and may be found in the blood, lymph, colostrum, saliva, and the gastrointestinal and urinary tracts, usually within three days after the first encounter with an antigen. The antibody binds tightly with the antigen as a preliminary for removing it from the system or destroying it.

effects of excess estrogen which could be discouraging to conception include stimulation of cell growth into tumors in the female reproductive organs, an increase in cardiovascular problems, and tissue damage.[10]

Hypothyroidism can actually cause the body to reject a fetus. Broda O. Barnes, M.D., a pioneer in hypothyroidism research, found a link between hypothyroidism and miscarriage. Of 301 female hypothyroid patients in his practice, 164 had miscarriages. In treating the women, he found that successful conception and pregnancies often were correlated with times when the women were taking thyroid supplements.[11]

"Thyroid secretions in adequate amounts appear to be essential for the development of the egg and for proper ovarian secretions," said Dr. Barnes. "If thyroid function is low, an egg may be discharged from an ovary, but it may not be fertilizable or, if fertilized, may not be capable of nesting, so that pregnancy is quickly aborted."[12]

As noted in Chapter 1, standard thyroid tests often fail to detect an underactive thyroid. Even if the tests are normal, a failure to ovulate or an ovarian hormone imbalance could indicate low thyroid function, states natural health specialist Ralph Golan, M.D., of Seattle, Washington. If more accurate testing uncovers hypothyroidism, Dr. Golan advises taking thyroid hormone supplements while trying to conceive, and then continuing them during pregnancy and post-partum. Consult with your practitioner on the dosages, which must be based on the results of testing your thyroid hormone levels, Dr. Golan says.[13]

The thyroid gland, in addition to causing infertility if it is underactive, can also influence reproduction through its antibodies (SEE QUICK DEFINITION). In a recent study, the presence of a thyroid antibody (thyroglobulin or TG, an iodine-bearing secretion) was shown to have an association with a risk of early miscarriage.

In the study, performed at the University of California at Irvine, researchers tested 487 women for TG antibodies, finding that 106 or 22% of participants carried the antibodies, meaning their bodies were reacting against their own thyroid hormones. Women who tested positive for TG antibodies were found to experience a 32% miscarriage rate, compared with a 16% miscarriage rate in women who tested negative. According to the study, the presence of these antibodies can serve as a useful marker for identifying women at risk for clinical miscarriage.[14]

The results of this study suggest that there may be an autoimmune process involved in infertility, certainly an observation not yet widely discussed. For some reason, the body regards its own thyroid secretions as "foreign" and stages an immune response against them. Meanwhile, given the expensive and often invasive nature of modern reproductive technology, the possibility of a connection between the body's internal environment and infertility calls for further research into viable alternatives to hormone therapy and surgery.

Nutritional Deficiencies

Nutritional deficiencies can adversely affect the functioning of the female reproductive system and cause infertility. In particular, deficiencies in folic acid, vitamins B6 and B12, and iron have been studied for their ability to help reverse infertility, says Melvyn Werbach, M.D., of Tarzana, California.[15] In addition to these nutrients, other deficiencies seen as causal in women's infertility are vitamins B1, B2, C, and E, zinc, and magnesium.[16]

Here is a sampling of the supporting research on some of these nutrients:

■ Folic Acid—According to case reports published in the *British Journal of Obstetrics and Gynaecology*, three women (29 to 32 years old) who had been experiencing fertility problems for several years were given 5 mg of folic acid three times daily. All became pregnant within three to 15 months after they began the protocol.[17]

■ Vitamin B6 (pyridoxine)—In a study reported in *Medical World News*, 12 infertile women, 23 to 31 years old, all sufferers of premenstrual syndrome (PMS), were able to become pregnant after taking a dietary supplement of pyridoxine (100-800 mg) once daily over a period of months. Dosages depended on the amount of pyridoxine necessary to relieve PMS symptoms for at least six months. Eleven of the pregnancies occurred within the first six months of therapy.[18]

■ Vitamin C—In England, 113 infertile women between the ages of 18 and 54 were treated with dietary supplements after experiencing an increase in hair loss; specifically, a daily dose of oral iron (35 mg) and vitamin C (200 mg). Seven of the women became pregnant within 28 weeks. Three of those seven had been pursuing fertility treatment for as long as nine years prior to the supplement program, and the remaining four had not become pregnant in the previous 30 months, despite having normal periods and unprotected intercourse.[19]

One study showed that women who were 85% of their "ideal" weight or less experienced a nearly fivefold increase in the risk of infertility, while women who were 120% of their "ideal" weight or more experienced a similar increase in risk.

Inappropriate Body Fat Ratio

For more about **amenorrhea**, see Chapter 1: Menstrual Problems, pp. 63-66.

While it seems quite logical that nutritional deficiencies could affect fertility, it is surprising, on the other hand, to find that the amount of body fat on a woman is also a causal factor in her ability to become pregnant. Clinical research has shown that body fat—both too much and too little—has a significant effect on a woman's chances of conception. A study performed at the University of Washington documented 376 infertile women who experienced difficulties in ovulation and compared them to fertile women of similar age and health status.

According to study results, women who were 85% of their "ideal" weight or less experienced a nearly fivefold increase in the risk of infertility, while women who were 120% of their "ideal" weight or more experienced a similar increase in risk. The authors of the study estimated that 6% of infertility in which ovulatory dysfunction is present results from being excessively underweight, and another 6% results from being excessively overweight.[20]

In addition to how much or how little extra weight a woman is carrying, research points to how that weight is distributed as an important factor in fertility. A large fertility clinic in the Netherlands reports that of 500 women participating in their donor insemination program, those women with a higher waist-hip ratio experienced a 30% decrease in the probability of conception during each menstrual cycle. After taking into account the added factors of age and body weight, researchers concluded that body fat distribution in women attempting pregnancy seems to have more of an impact on fertility than either age or body weight.[21]

The connection between body fat and fertility has been well-documented. In particular, women who have experienced a rapid weight loss are at a greater risk of temporary infertility due to amenorrhea (a break in the menstrual cycle during which a woman ceases to ovulate).[22] This condition may be reversed over a period of weeks, however, with improved diet and nutrition.

Environmental Estrogens

As they are with many of the health conditions included in this book, environmental estrogens (SEE QUICK DEFINI-TION) or xenoestrogens can be behind infertility. The mechanism by which they reduce fertility can be found in their effect on the endocrine glands (SEE QUICK DEFINITION).

Environmental estrogens are increasingly prevalent in Western societies; once in the body, they accumulate and persist for decades, contributing to a range of reproductive disorders. In fact, there is no doubt that something is seriously interfering with normal human hormonal and endocrinal functioning, states Theo Colborn, Ph.D., a senior scientist with the World Wildlife Fund and an environmental author.[23] Since 1945, synthetic chemicals (such as DDT, DES, PCBs, dioxins, among many others) have been released into our air, water, soil, food, and body. At least 51 of these have been conclusively shown to disrupt the human endocrine system.

Each year, an estimated 1,000 new synthetic chemicals enter the world market, swelling the planetary total to well over 100,000. All of these are completely foreign and potentially harmful to endocrine function; almost none have been thoroughly tested for long-term, transgenerational health effects.

Evidence is accumulating that these chemicals, even at very low concentrations and exposures, can, by disrupting the endocrine system, cause "hormone havoc:" autoimmune diseases, clinical depression, genital and reproductive system defects (such as infertility), and long-term, delayed developmental effects across the generations. The result is that it is no longer possible to "define a normal, unaltered human physiology," says Dr. Colborn.

Obviously it is prudent for everyone—but particularly women suffering from infertility—to lower their exposure to environmental estrogens as much as possible. Eating organically raised food is one step you can take immediately to cut out the xenoestrogen-laden pesticides you are ingesting with your meals. Given that none can fully protect themselves from these damaging estrogen-mimicking substances, undergoing detoxification protocols can help eliminate the toxins stored in the body and prevent further buildup.

Environmental estrogens are foreign compounds and/or chemical toxins that mimic the effects of estrogen. Environmental estrogens, also called xenoestrogens, are present primarily in man-made chemicals ("greenhouse gases," herbicides, and pesticides such as DDT) and industrial by-products (from manufacture of plastics and paper, as well as from the incineration of hazardous wastes). Environmental estrogens often cause an imbalance of estrogen relative to progesterone, another key hormone. When a woman's body has too much estrogen (a condition called estrogen dominance), a variety of health problems can result, including breast cancer, fibroids, and endometriosis, among others. According to some researchers, environmental estrogens also affect men, and may contribute to testicular cancer, urinary tract disorders, and low sperm count. Dioxins are one kind of xenoestrogen. The World Health Organization puts the "tolerable" intake of dioxins for a human being at 10 picograms a day; at that rate, one gram of dioxins would provide every person in the United States with their "safe" daily intake for 100 years.

Endocrine glands, including the testicles, ovaries, pancreas, adrenals, thyroid, parathyroid, and pituitary, are central to the regulation and normalization of all the body's complex, interconnected systems, from metabolism and heat production to spermatogenesis and uterine preparations for pregnancy.

"The chemicals in the birth control pill may suppress the natural production of hormones, increase the risk of sexually transmitted diseases, and upset the assimilation of nutrients—all of which can affect fertility and pregnancy," states Barbara Seaman.

Fluoride Toxicity

If the water you drink contains fluoride, a frequent additive in public water systems, it could be affecting your ability to conceive. Although clinical research has long documented the effects of fluoride toxicity on reproduction in various animal species, a study performed at the National Center for Toxicological Research in Jefferson, Arkansas, has finally established a link between human infertility and fluoride levels in local water supplies.

The study, which used a U.S. database of drinking water systems to track fluoride levels across the country, showed that in every region which had greater fluoride concentrations in their water supplies, there was a corresponding decrease in the annual total fertility rate (among women between the ages of 10 and 49).[24] Finding a source of flouride-free drinking water can thus be an important step in becoming more fertile.

Birth Control Pills

Another potential toxin which decreases fertility is the birth control pill. Even though the doses of estrogen and progesterone in the pill have been lowered since it was first introduced in the late 1950s, long-term use of birth control pills can still contribute to infertility, says women's health advocate Barbara Seaman, co-founder of the National Women's Health Network, based in New York City.

"The chemicals in the pill suppress the natural production of hormones, increase the risk of sexually transmitted diseases, and upset the assimilation of nutrients—all of which can affect fertility and pregnancy," states Seaman.[25] Deficiencies in B vitamins, including thiamine (B1), riboflavin (B2), pyridoxine (B6), and B12, folic acid, vitamins C and E, zinc, and magnesium are all associated with birth control use and are the same nutrient deficiencies that can cause infertility, Seaman observes.[26]

She also cautions that the pill may raise levels of vitamin A and copper which, in excess, could contribute to infertility and birth defects (as well as emotional disturbances and hair loss). Moreover, women going off the pill can experience "post-pill amenorrhea," or the failure to menstruate or ovulate after they stop using the pill. This happens because the pill disrupts the normal flow of hormones from the hypothalamus in the brain to the pituitary gland and from there to the ovaries.[27]

Post-pill amenorrhea is often resolved after a waiting period of a few weeks to many months, Seaman says, and especially if the woman takes nutritional supplements. However, she notes that not all women are knowledgeable on this issue and may immediately turn to fertility drugs instead of waiting for their natural hormonal rhythms to return.[28]

Similarly, women who have been on birth control pills sometimes develop pituitary gland insufficiency, says natural medicine authority Joseph Pizzorno, Jr., N.D., president of Bastyr University in Seattle, Washington. The pituitary gland secretes hormones that stimulate the ovaries to mature and produce a viable egg. Birth control pills may adversely affect that function.[29]

Douching

Vaginal douching, touted by advertisers as a healthy feminine hygiene practice, can be detrimental when it comes to reproductive potential. A study involving 840 married women of childbearing age found that women who douched were 30% less likely to conceive for each month they attempted pregnancy. The data also revealed that For more about the **negative effects of douching**, see Chapter 6: Cystitis, p. 206. women 18 to 24 years old experienced a 29% reduction in fertility, compared with only a 6% reduction in women between the ages of 30 and 39. Although the study associated douching with reduced fertility, it is not known whether douching contributes directly to infertility.[30]

Use of Addictive Substances (Caffeine, Alcohol, Cigarettes)

Certain lifestyle choices such as smoking cigarettes or drinking alcohol or coffee may affect your fertility. A 1995 study at the University of California at Berkeley found that women who smoked cigarettes took about twice as long to conceive than women who did not. The study added to a growing body of evidence for a connection between smoking and infertility.[31]

Researchers have offered various explanations for the negative effect of smoking on fertility. One study presented evidence that when cotinine (a product of the body's attempt to metabolize nicotine) is present in bodily fluids, the possibility of successful conception is sig-

In one study, women who had a history of depression in the months or years before trying to conceive had a substantially greater chance of encountering infertility.

nificantly reduced. The study showed that while an average nonsmoking woman had a 37% chance of pregnancy per cycle, the chances went down to 27% if the woman smoked.[32]

Research has also established a connection between excessive caffeine intake and difficulty in conception. In a two-year study involving 1,430 women, researchers found that coffee drinkers who consumed more that 300 mg of caffeine daily (about three cups of strong coffee) had a greater risk of delayed conception. The study noted, however, that a daily intake of less than 300 mg of caffeine had no noticeable effect on fertility.[33]

Excess caffeine produces its effect on reproductive ability by decreasing the concentration of serum prolactin, a pituitary gland hormone that stimulates milk production; too little prolactin (hypoprolactinemia) is associated with inferility, according to Melvyn Werbach, M.D. Excess alcohol consumption also results in hypoprolactinemia. Caffeinated soft drinks can be even more harmful to fertility than coffee, cautions Dr. Werbach. Drinking even one caffeinated soft drink a day can reduce the monthly chances of conception by 50%, according to a published study, Dr. Werbach notes.[34]

Depression and Stress

While it is important for fertility to avoid eating, drinking, or inhaling toxic substances, toxic thoughts and feelings can also hamper your ability to conceive. Volumes of research have firmly established the contribution of the mind and emotions to physical health. While any psychological or emotional issues can be involved in an individual's inability to conceive, the following studies pinpointed depression and stress as particular factors in infertility.

In one study, women who had a history of depression in the months or years before trying to conceive had a substantially greater chance of encountering infertility. The researchers, from the Memorial Hospital of Rhode Island in Pawtucket, questioned 339 women, 22 to 47 years old, in the Pawtucket area. Of 58 women who said they had a history of depressive symptoms, 24% reported infertility. Of 281 women who said they had no prior depression, only 13.5% reported infertility.[35]

Stress also has a negative impact on fertility. In a study of 38 patients at the University Medical Center in Front Royal, Virginia, women were grouped according to whether their infertility was anatomical or non-anatomical. The non-anatomical group reported more psychosocial stress.[36]

More Reasons for Infertility: The Chinese Medicine Perspective

A traditional Chinese medicine physician looks at infertility with a slightly different view than the Western eye (see sidebar: "A Glossary of Traditional Chinese Medicine Terms," p. 172). Master acupuncturist **Y.C. Chiang, O.M.D., Ph.D.**, of El Cerrito, California, explains the numerous reasons, according to the Chinese medical model, why women cannot get pregnant and illustrates the TCM treatment approach with a case history from his patient files:

In Chinese medicine, energy is very important. I will explain the energy of fertility in terms of an analogy common to Chinese medical thinking. Before birth, while you are a fetus in your mother's womb—we call this "Before Heaven"—you are dependent on what you can receive through the umbilical cord and the energy of your kidneys. There is a circuit of energy from your kidneys, up your spine, through your mouth, down to the genitals, and back to the kidneys again. This is the route of the "Before Heaven" energy that comes from the kidneys.

When you are born, you cry and urinate. This breaks the circuit of "Before Heaven" power. Now you must breathe and eat on your own—this is called "After Heaven"—and its energy comes from the spleen. This is the second basic life power. It is like an engine with the kidney energy being the spark plugs and the spleen energy the motor.

However, the kidneys are also involved in "After Heaven" energy. "Before Heaven" is a finite amount, an irreplaceable store of energy. If you damage "Before Heaven" power, you shorten your life, unless you make up for it by replenishing the "After Heaven" power. Your "Before Heaven" power may also be low because of what you received from your mother's body while in the womb or by inheritance. You can make up for this by building your "After Heaven" energy through proper diet, exercise, and energy practices such as *qigong* or *tai chi*.

With these concepts made clear, I can now explain the specific causes of infertility which include the following:

A Glossary of Traditional Chinese Medicine Terms

Traditional Chinese medicine (TCM) originated in China over 5,000 years ago and is a comprehensive system of medical practice that heals the body according to the principles of nature and balance. A Chinese medicine physician considers the flow of vital energy (*qi*—pronounced CHEE) in a patient through close examination of the patient's pulse, tongue, body odor, voice tone and strength, and general demeanor, among other elements. Underlying imbalances and disharmony in the body are described in terminology analogous to the natural world (heat, cold, dryness, or dampness). The concept of balance, or the interrelationship of organs, is central to TCM. In TCM, imbalances are corrected through the use of acupuncture, moxibustion, herbal medicine, dietary therapy, massage, and therapeutic exercise.

Acupuncture is an integrated healing system developed by the Chinese over 5,000 years ago and introduced in the United States in the mid-1800s. The treatment is administered by an acupuncturist using hair-thin, stainless-steel needles, generally presterilized and disposable; these are lightly inserted into the skin at any of over 1,000 locations on the body's surface, known as acupoints. Acupoints are places where *qi* can be accessed by acupuncturists to reduce, enhance, or redirect its flow. Acupuncture is employed for a wide variety of conditions (the World Health Organization counts 104), including pain relief, asthma, migraines, and arthritis.

Acupuncture meridians are specific pathways in the human body for the flow of *qi*. In most cases, these energy pathways run up and down both sides of the body, and correspond to individual organs or organ systems, designated as Lung, Small Intestine, Heart, and others. There are 12 principal meridians and eight secondary channels. Numerous points of heightened energy, or *qi*, exist on the body's surface along the meridians and are called acupoints. There are more than 1,000 acupoints, each of which is potentially a place for acupuncture treatment.

The Fallopian Tube is Narrow—The egg cannot get to the uterus because the "Before Heaven" power in the kidney is low. When the kidney is low in energy, it cannot provide power to the uterus, ovaries, and vagina. If no power services the ovaries, the fallopian tubes will be very narrow so the egg cannot go down.

Women with low energy in the kidneys often have cold hands and feet and don't like making love. There is no "fire" in the kidneys to get the "heat" out to the extremities, such as the hands. If they make love, the kidneys lose even more energy. Also if the kidneys are low in energy, the bladder will be low in energy—just as if the parents are poor, the child will be poor. When we treat the kidneys to restore the balance, the fallopian tubes open.

The main problem in infertility is low energy in the kidneys, uterus, and ovaries. When there is no energy in the body, there is no "heat" or basic life force, so no eggs go down the fallopian tubes and women do not get pregnant, says Dr. Y.C. Chiang.

"After Heaven" Energy is Low in the Kidneys and Spleen—Perhaps you have expended too much of this energy or have damaged your kidneys. As a result, you aren't building up your "After Heaven" energy through diet, exercise, or physical practice, so you keep draining the kidneys and therefore the spleen. Consequently, no energy gets to the uterus and the ovaries. In this case, we treat the kidneys and the spleen to restore the energy balance.

The main problem in infertility is low energy in the kidneys, uterus, and ovaries. When there is no energy in the body, there is no "heat" or basic life force, so no eggs go down the fallopian tubes and women do not get pregnant. The next most common factor is a fibroid tumor or endometriosis, followed by an energy or fertility problem in the husband.

Low Reserves of Body Energy—The body is low in energy and cannot produce viable eggs every month. This may be because the woman has inherited a condition of low energy in the blood or bones or because she is depleting her reserves with no exercise, a bad diet, or emotional stress.

According to Chinese medicine, the mother gives the child its blood and muscle energy and the father gives the energy for the bones. If you inherit low energy in one or both of these categories, it will affect your energy as an adult. Your "After Heaven" power will be low in energy. Since the kidneys "control" the growth of the bones, and the heart "controls" the transportation of blood, and the kidneys help maintain balance in the heart, once again, we treat the kidneys to correct the imbalance.

Vaginal Discharge or "Cold" Uterus—Vaginal discharge is a poison that drains energy from a woman's body. "Cold" does not mean chilled or deficient in temperature; rather it means a state of slow, sluggish, damp energy. From the color of the discharge, we can know which organ has the problem.

Sometimes the vaginal discharge has a strong smell like fish. This means the body has too much water. Fish is a "water smell" that indi-

Women in the U.S. often have too many stresses and worries that affect their emotions. Their nerves can never relax, so their periods become irregular and the eggs don't go down the fallopian tubes, Dr. Chiang explains.

To contact **Y.C. Chiang, O.M.D., Ph.D.:** Wen Wu School of Martial Arts, Inc. and Chung Hua Clinic of Acupuncture and Chinese Herbal Medicine, 10124 San Pablo Avenue, El Cerrito, CA 94530; tel: 510-524-1057. Chinese fertility herbs similar to those used by Dr. Chiang in his preparations are available from: Mayway Corp., 1338 Mandela Parkway, Oakland, CA 94607; tel: 510-208-3113; fax: 510-208-3069.

cates the bladder and kidneys are out of balance. If the discharge is yellow or brown, that points to low energy in the spleen. If the discharge is white, the imbalance is in the large intestine or the lungs. If the discharge is blue or green, it's liver or gallbladder trouble; anger often goes with this symptom. Sometimes the discharge is black, which indicates low energy in the kidneys.

A discharge also means the woman's pelvic area is "cold" or low in energy. The organs which are out of balance are not providing the power the uterus needs. The imbalance produces the discharge, which can kill the eggs and the man's sperm. For a woman with a "cold" uterus, we have to build up the blood with herbs to give the patient more energy and better circulation so she can become pregnant.

Irregular Menstruation—Irregular periods from internal causes can disturb fertility. Sometimes menstruation is late, sometimes early, sometimes it lasts a short time, sometimes too long. This inconsistency makes it difficult to get pregnant.

Month to month, the eggs go down the fallopian tubes at different times, or can't get through at all. If the blood is not strong, the eggs are not strong either. They go down like a bubble and then break. It's mainly the spleen and the liver that make the period irregular. Here, we help regularize the woman's periods, mostly with acupuncture treatments (see sidebar: "A Glossary of Traditional Chinese Medicine Terms," p. 172). Women in the U.S. often have too many stresses and worries that affect their emotions. Their nerves can never relax, so their periods become irregular and the eggs don't go down the fallopian tubes. Being emotionally high-strung or having obsessive thoughts works through the spleen, while the energy of anger goes through the liver.

Weakened Male Energy—The man's sperm is weak. It might be low in energy, not strong; it moves too slowly or is weak because he has been exposed to toxic chemicals. The man's whole body, including his kidneys, is low in energy, so the sperm is not strong either. This can be due to excessive sex or excessive ejaculation during adolescence, which exhausts the kidneys and therefore affects sperm production. Underdeveloped testes or a blockage in the sperm duct are also due to insufficient kidney energy.

Success Story: Reversing a Dismal Prognosis

While conventional medicine could offer only a poor outlook for the following patient, **Dr. Y.C. Chiang** explains how he used acupuncture and herbs to reverse her endometriosis and enable her to successfully carry a child to term:

Jan had consulted many different conventional doctors over five years, trying to find the source of her persistent abdominal pain. Finally, one doctor diagnosed it as endometriosis; he confirmed his diagnosis by conducting minor exploratory surgery. Endometriosis is a common cause of infertility and Jan wanted to have a child.

Jan's doctor told her she had four choices regarding the endometriosis. The first choice he gave her was a Catch-22: she could have a child, as pregnancy sometimes clears up endometriosis, but it was unlikely because of the endometriosis that she could carry a baby to term if she could get pregnant at all. The other three choices he offered her were to take birth control pills, have surgery to remove the endometrial adhesions, or learn to live with the pain for the rest of her life.

> In general, if you can't remove the endometriosis, you can't get pregnant, says Dr. Chiang. In Jan's case, it took about four months to clear up her endometriosis, then another two months for her to get pregnant.

When I met Jan, I told her she had a fifth option: Chinese medicine. I treated her with acupuncture and herbs; specifically, an herbal formula containing perilla leaf, *angelica dan gui* root, schizandra fruit, raspberry, cnidium seed, citrus peel, wild ginger, lycil berry, and honey-fried licorice root.

In general, if you can't remove the endometriosis, you can't get pregnant. It took about four months to clear up Jan's endometriosis, during which her abdominal pain gradually disappeared. Then after another two months, she became pregnant; when I saw her recently, she had a strong 15-month-old son.

The herbal formula I prescribed for Jan was specifically designed for her; it is not necessarily effective or appropriate for all women, and each woman will require a specially adapted formula. Choosing the right formula can come only after a long and thorough examination of the patient. You can't always see the problem on an X ray, although Western medicine depends on tests like these for information about baffling conditions.

That's why in Chinese medicine, we collect valuable information about the patient's condition by listening to the pulse, examining the tongue, and noting the color of the skin (and in the case of infertility, the color of the vaginal discharge, see pp. 173-174). The pulse, tongue, and skin color are like the stalk, leaf, and flower of a plant. If you see something wrong in the plant, the problem is in the roots. Then you need to treat the foundation of the problem. If the foundation is damaged, we correct the foundation, then there is no more problem.

If you don't treat the problem in the foundation, the symptoms will go away only temporarily. It's not a complete treatment. If you try to treat the leaves—such as giving Jan birth control pills or performing surgery—the problem will return. You have to treat the roots and the soil.

Acupuncture and herbs can correct energy imbalances and normalize a woman's body systems. Once a woman is balanced, she is much more likely to conceive, to have a healthy pregnancy, and to give birth to a healthy child. ■

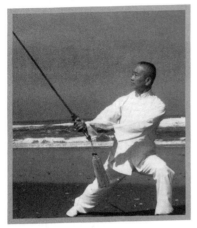

With perfectly smooth skin and a lean body, Dr. Y. C. Chiang could pass as forty-something. He's 76. He credits his youthfulness to good diet and *Ru He Chuan*, a martial arts form of which he is the Eighth Generation master. From *Ru* ("scholar") and *Hee* ("white crane"), it's a kind of intellectual boxing, emphasizing morality, spirit, and physical prowess. As for Chinese medicine, Dr. Chiang has been practicing it for 60 years. He emphasizes the need to treat everyone as an individual and prepares Chinese medicines for his patients accordingly. "Everyone needs something different," he says.

Success Story: Actress Annie Potts Overcomes Infertility With Chinese Medicine

Jan's experience with Dr. Chiang is not unusual. He has successfully treated many women for fertility problems, among them actress Annie

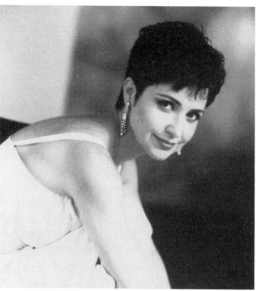

©1993 Jon Ragel-Onyx

"In my heart I felt that *surely* there must be another way to achieve the same end as taking Pergonal for fertility," says actress Annie Potts. There was, but she wouldn't find it until she gave up on conventional medicine and went in search of an alternative. Then, she finally got the baby she wanted.

Potts. Here is the story of how, with Dr. Chiang's acupuncture and herbal treatments, she was able to reverse her seeming infertility and give birth to not just one, but two children.

When she was almost 40, *Designing Women* star Annie Potts—known to fans over the show's seven-year run as the pragmatic Mary Jo Shively—wanted to have another baby but discovered she couldn't get pregnant. She worried that she might be infertile. No problem. After a few false starts with conventional doctors, she'd find that alternative medicine could help her out again as it had so many times before.

Ever since she broke nearly every bone below her waist in a dramatic car accident when she was 21, Annie Potts had been designing her health using the best that alternative medicine had to offer, from reflexology to chiropractic, yoga to Pilates Method physical therapy, herbs to Chinese medicine. Annie's faith was well-placed because four months after consulting Dr. Chiang, she was pregnant. That baby was Jake; when Annie was 43, she gave birth to another child, again with the aid of Chinese herbs from Dr. Chiang.

"In this last pregnancy, I used Chinese medicine the whole time," says Annie, in her trademark Kentucky twang. "I bounced back so quickly. I was back at the gym only three weeks after my baby was born. I'm only five pounds over my weight before I got pregnant, and I feel great."

Even though she had given birth to a son named Clay 15 years earlier, somehow, in the intervening years, Annie had become seemingly infertile. At 39, she wanted another child. She spent a year trying to conceive, but was unsuccessful. When she consulted conventional physicians, they put her on Clomid. They assured her that only 2% of women experience the negative side effects, such as abdominal discomfort, uterine bleeding, breast tenderness, depression, dizziness, and about 14 others. Annie soon found that she was one of the unlucky 2%.

"I nearly went insane," she recalls. "I never had PMS in my life before this. Suddenly I became somebody I didn't recognize. I had terrible mood swings, weeping, and hot flashes in the middle of the night. I'd wake up and the sheets would be soaked from my sweating. It was awful." Annie wanted a baby so much that she endured this state of nonstop PMS for six months. But still she wasn't pregnant. Her doctors had an even more upsetting drug for her to try—Pergonal. In effect, it would be a bizarre form of urine therapy.

Pergonal is an injectable drug containing gonadotropins (hormones for the gonads, in this case, ovaries) purified from the urine of postmenopausal women. Annie's doctors believed this drug would stimulate her system to make eggs which could then be fertilized in a test tube. They told her that of the seven or eight eggs that would be incubated, usually only two would take; if three or more took, then they would eliminate the surplus by "selective reduction."

"That phrase chilled me," Annie says. "In my heart I felt that *surely* there must be another way to achieve the same end as taking Pergonal for fertility." There was, but she wouldn't find it until she gave up on conventional medicine and went in search of an alternative. Then, she finally got the baby she wanted.

Dr. Chiang had a reputation for solving health problems against which others had failed. During their first consultation, as he sat with his fingers on her wrist reading her pulse, Annie waited anxiously for his analysis. Finally she asked him, "Do you think I can have another baby?" Dr. Chiang calmly answered in the affirmative, and said it should take only about a month to get pregnant.

It actually took four months because Dr. Chiang first had to balance and strengthen Annie's organs and energy pathways with acupuncture. Then he gave her a combination of herbs in pill and powder form including, among others, white peony root, plantain seed, wolfberry fruit, licorice root, raspberry fruit, and glossy privet fruit. When she didn't get pregnant in the first few months, Dr. Chiang put Annie's husband, TV director Jim Hayman, on herbs as well. Then, Annie was pregnant in a month.

After Jake's birth, Dr. Chiang gave Annie another herbal preparation to strengthen both her and the nursing baby. This formula contained white peony root, licorice root, and glossy privet fruit, along with lily bulb, codonopsis root, pinellia rhizome, ginger, citrus peel, and black jujube date. With Dr. Chiang's herbs, Annie recovered quickly.[37]

Traditional Chinese Medicine Says Look to the Liver

Another traditional Chinese medicine physician Roger C. Hirsh, L.Ac., O.M.D., of Beverly Hills, California, observes that infertility is often a matter of stagnant energy in the liver or "liver qi stagnation or congestion."

The easiest way to understand the concept of "qi stagnation" is to look at a human being the way an acupuncturist or Chinese practitioner does: as a network of energy channels or meridians that circulate all over the body like highways, with special roads branching into each internal organ. The channels not only circulate the energy traffic (qi—SEE QUICK DEFINITION) and keep it flowing, but they also nourish the internal organs with energy.

If the person is stressed, has a poor diet of junk food, suffers a physical trauma, has bad habits such as cigarette smoking or lack of sleep, has nutrient deficiencies, or takes prescription drugs—to name just a few examples— there could be a blockage or obstruction (traffic jam) on one or more of the energy channels. The blockage will slow the flow of energy in that channel and make it sluggish or "stagnated." Since the activity in each channel affects the organs where it circulates, the energy in those organs will also become "stagnated," meaning that their natural rhythms will be disrupted or even shut down.

Since the liver channel flows through the reproductive organs, and the liver's job is to ensure a smooth flow of blood and energy through those organs, a "stagnated" liver can give rise to any or all of the female and male reproductive health problems, including infertility. Unexplained infertility, for which a clear-cut physiologi-

Qi (pronounced *CHEE*) is a Chinese word variously translated to mean "vital energy," "essence of life," and "living force." In Chinese medicine, the proper flow of *qi* along energy channels (meridians) within the body is crucial to a person's health and vitality. There are many types of *qi*, classified according to source, location, and function (such as activation, warming, defense, transformation, and containment). Within the body, *qi* and blood are closely linked, as each is considered to flow along with the other. The manipulation and readjustment of *qi* to treat disease and ensure maximum health benefit is the basic principle of acupuncture, although other remedies and therapies can be used to influence *qi*.

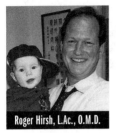

Roger Hirsh, L.Ac., O.M.D.

Unexplained infertility, for which a clear-cut physiological or structural problem is not at fault, represents an estimated 15% of all infertility cases, notes Dr. Hirsh. "Liver *qi* congestion" may be the explanation, he says.

cal or structural problem is not at fault, represents an estimated 15% of all infertility cases, notes Dr. Hirsh. "Liver *qi* congestion" may be the explanation, he says.

One of the principal means by which a stagnated liver (and its energy channel or meridian) affects infertility is through reduced blood flow to the uterus and pelvic area. "Acupuncture given at the right time in the menstrual cycle, in conjunction with an herbal formula and some counseling, very likely can clear the liver congestion in several months," notes Dr. Hirsh. "Couples must realize, however, that the prevalence of liver *qi* stagnation in modern society is not something simple that can be relieved overnight. It may take nine months or more to release the stress, trauma, and toxins in the system, although there are cases that have resolved in a month's time."

The treatment goal, says Dr. Hirsh, is to "make the abdomen happy." This is a metaphor for correcting the digestion, menstruation, and hormones, so that women can conceive, he says. "Of course, raising the man's sperm count and sperm motility is important as well, because it is not just the woman who is infertile in an infertility situation. A key to this is the way the blood flows in the pelvic cavity."[38]

In treating infertility, Dr. Hirsh frequently works in conjunction with conventional doctors and designs acupuncture treatments that complement and support their medical procedures. For example, he often gives acupuncture treatment to women who have just been artificially inseminated and works with patients who are taking Clomid to help regulate their fertility cycle. As Dr. Hirsh states, "Traditional Chinese medicine can increase the success rate of Western medicine, and at the same time slow down the clock on a woman's aging endocrine system."

The following case demonstrates how cooperation between the different modes of medicine can work and the importance of correcting the liver energy imbalance, in this instance, in both partners in the couple trying to conceive. The case firmly establishes how treating both the man and the woman may be necessary to reverse infertility.

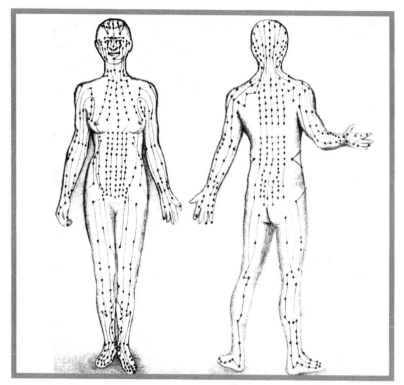

ACUPUNCTURE MERIDIANS IN THE BODY. Acupuncture meridians are specific pathways in the human body for the flow of life force or subtle energy, known as *qi* (pronounced *CHEE*). In most cases, these energy pathways run up and down both sides of the body, and correspond to individual organs or organ systems, designated as Lung, Small Intestine, Heart, and others. There are 12 principal meridians and eight secondary channels. Numerous points of heightened energy or *qi* exist on the body's surface along the meridians and are called acupoints. There are more than 1,000 acupoints, each of which is potentially a place for acupuncture treatment.

Success Story: Acupuncture Helps a Couple Conceive

Buddy and Sally wanted to conceive, but couldn't. After being given a poor prognosis by conventional fertility specialists, they consulted Dr. Hirsh. Buddy, 37, had been diagnosed with primary infertility due to low semen count, specifically 3 million per ml (more than 20 million is normal), and low motility at 21%.

Buddy also complained of lethargy and exhaustion; his short-term memory was poor; his sexual drive was reduced; and he had muscle tension due to stress. His past medical history included allergies, sinusitis, and chest and lower back pain, reports Dr. Hirsh. His diag-

To contact **Roger Hirsh, L.Ac., O.M.D.:** 9730 Wilshire Blvd., Suite 105, Beverly Hills, CA 90212; tel: 800-967-3898 or 310-550-8186; fax: 310-550-1014. Infertility herbs such as those used by Dr. Hirsh are available from: Mayway Corp., 1338 Mandela Parkway, Oakland, CA 94607; tel: 800-2-MAYWAY or 510-208-3113; fax: 510-208-3069. Their name for "Restore the Right Kidney" is "Right Side Replenishing."

nosis, according to Chinese medicine, was that Buddy's liver energy was stagnant and that his kidney energy was deficient, meaning that the vital energy in the channels that normally nourish his kidneys had been depleted by some type of emotional or physical stress to the body.

Dr. Hirsh's treatment included once-weekly acupuncture for liver, bladder, kidney, and spleen points on his body, accompanied by a variation of an herbal formula called You Gui Wan ("Restore the Right Kidney"). Taken daily, it contained the Chinese herbs *Rx. Rehmanniae, Rhizoma Dioscoreae, Fr. Corni, Fr. Lycii, Cortex Eucommiae, Rx. Angelica Sinensis, Cortex* and *Ramulus Cinnamomi, Semen Cuscutae, Cornu Cervi Pantotrichum, Rx. Glycyrrhizae* (honey-baked licorice), *Rx. Ginseng,* and *Rhizoma Anemarrhenae.*

Positive results for Buddy were achieved after two months of treatment. Remarkably, his semen count had climbed to 18 million/ml with 89% sperm motility; he felt less exhausted and felt heightened libido; and he experienced less psychological stress over the infertility issue and his own contribution (or perceived shortcomings) to the problem.

At the same time as he worked with Buddy, Dr. Hirsh also treated 35-year-old Sally. Her presenting symptoms included PMS, headaches, back pain, abdominal distention, and a light menstrual flow (without clots) in a cycle lasting 24 to 28 days. Her past medical history included occasional migraines with dizziness, and nausea and vomiting following cheese consumption. Most of Sally's symptoms, Dr. Hirsh notes, are typical of a woman with liver *qi* congestion.

As with Buddy, Dr. Hirsh gave Sally a series of once-weekly acupuncture treatments, working on points on her spleen, stomach, gallbladder, and liver meridians. Then he prescribed a series of 13 Chinese herbs: *Rx. Angelica sinensis, Rx. Ligustici wallichii, Rx. Rehmanniae, Rx. Paeoniae alba, Rhizoma Gastrodiae, Hb. Loranthi, Fr. Viticis, Fr. Tribuli, Fr. Lycii, Poria cocos, Semen Cuscutae, Flos Chrysanthemi,* and *Rx. Glycyrrhizae* (honey-baked licorice). After about two months on this treatment program, Sally's symptoms were much improved and she was ready to try an artificial insemination procedure using Buddy's sperm. Soon after, she was pregnant, says Dr. Hirsh.

Dr. Hirsh notes that according to conventional medicine, Sally did not require treatment as her hormone levels were sufficient. "However, traditional Chinese medicine points out that the flow of blood to the pelvic cavity is extremely important and is governed by the liver," comments Dr. Hirsh. "Therefore, treatment of her liver stagnation and blood (nutrition) deficiency was most important."[39]

As should be clear by now, traditional Chinese medicine is a powerful therapy for the treatment of infertility. The next case demonstrates the use of TCM in combination with other alternative medicine therapies (including Western herbal remedies, nutritional supplements, thyroid glandular extracts, essential plant oils, and special fertility testing methods) and highlights a number of the causal factors discussed earlier in the chapter.

Success Story: Fertility Testing Pinpoints the Moment of Ovulation

Jane, 34, had been trying, without success, to get pregnant for six years. Conventional physicians had been unable to determine why Jane was infertile. A laparoscopy hadn't detected anything abnormal. Jane's reproductive history included an operation to remove ovarian cysts when she was in her early twenties and irregular and infrequent periods (border-line amenorrhea or failure to menstruate) ever since she started menstruating—sometimes she had only three periods a year.

Discouraged with conventional approaches, Jane went to see acupuncturist and herbalist Rachel Koenig, L.Ac., N.C.C.A.H., of Brooklyn, New York. In the course of taking Jane's medical history, Dr. Koenig learned that Jane had symptoms typical of hypothyroidism, including coldness in her hands and feet, moodiness, a tendency to take on weight, and her infrequent menstruation.

Dr. Koenig also drew a connection between Jane's ovarian cysts and an underactive thyroid. She speculated that Jane's ovaries might be overworking (which would produce the cysts) in an attempt to balance an under-production of hormones in the thyroid and the adrenal glands, which Dr. Koenig suspected were also underactive. Her suspicion regarding the adrenals was based on the fact that these glands control the body's reaction to stress; Jane had been under extreme stress in connection with the fertility problem and its effect on her marriage, as well as coping with a high-profile, full-time professional career.

Dr. Koenig had Jane do a basal temperature test (taking body temperature with a thermometer under the armpit first thing in the morning) in order to determine thyroid activity. While the normal basal body temperature range is 97.8° F to 98.2° F, Jane's basal temperature was around 96° F, another sign of hypothyroidism.

183

The first causal dynamic in Jane's infertility was overall depletion of her *qi*, probably due to stress and poor nutrition, says Dr. Rachel Koenig, and some of her meridians were blocked or "stagnated," also due to stress and nutrient deficiencies.

A further factor in Jane's fertility problem was that she was having trouble identifying her fertile times because her menstrual cycles were so irregular. She had tried a urine "stick" test called the "VU Quick" (available over-the-counter) which measures when a surge in the luteinizing hormone level takes place, indicating that ovulation is about to happen (see sidebar: "The Fertile Period of Each Sexual Cycle," p. 161). Having no way to identify mid-cycle, she repeated the test in a hit-or-miss fashion all month long, an expensive and fruitless practice.

Dr. Koenig had Jane do the Barnes basal temperature test every morning, keeping charts of the results so she could see when the temperatures were rising, signaling she would be ovulating.

Based on the traditional Chinese medicine methods of diagnosis (explained by Dr. Chiang, pp. 171-175), Dr. Koenig had determined that the first causal dynamic in Jane's infertility was overall depletion of her *qi*, probably due to stress and poor nutrition. In addition, some of her meridians were blocked or "stagnated," also due to stress and nutrient deficiencies. This combination of "*qi* deficiency" and a "*qi* stagnation" was affecting Jane's adrenal and thyroid gland function and slowing down her menstrual cycle.

The "*qi* stagnation" was also hampering the ability of the body's organs (primarily the spleen and kidneys) to circulate and distribute moisture properly. This was causing buildup of phlegm, mucus, and moisture—or what the Chinese call a condition of "dampness"—in Jane's throat (thyroid area). The "dampness" was further contributing to her hypothyroidism.

Jane's weak and irregular menstrual activity was evidence that her kidneys, which control the vital "essence" known as *jing qi*, or reproductive organ energy of the body, were depleted, probably also due to stress, poor diet, overwork, and other lifestyle habits.

Dr. Koenig designed a supplement and herbal program to strengthen and boost the circulation of energy in Jane's body, to move moisture and dry the "dampness," and also to nourish her thyroid, adrenals, and kidney organ energy. This individually tailored protocol included:

Take Your Own Basal Temperature

You can do the Barnes basal temperature test (developed by Broda O. Barnes, M.D., Ph.D.) with a standard oral thermometer, but it's easier and faster to do it with a digital thermometer which gives an electronic readout in about five seconds versus the ten minutes of its oral counterpart. Also, a built-in memory saves the last temperature reading, so you can record it later.

Take the reading under your armpit while still lying in bed in the morning, before getting up or doing anything else. Wait until the thermometer beeps, signaling the temperature has registered. (If you're using an oral thermometer, wait ten minutes. Make sure you shake it down before using). Keep a record of the temperatures. If you are still menstruating, start test-

For more about **thyroid health**, contact: Broda O. Barnes Research Foundation, P.O. Box 98, Trumbull, CT 06611; tel: 203-261-2101. The Broda O. Barnes Research Foundation is a non-profit information and education organization that disseminates the work of Dr. Barnes and other experts in the field of endocrine function. They offer information packets, audios and videos, physician referrals, a 24-hour urine test, and consultation services for doctors.

ing on the first day of your period, when temperatures are lowest. If you are testing for possible hypothyroidism, take the temperature for three or four days. Temperatures averaging below 97.8° F may reflect hypothyroidism.

If you are trying to determine your fertile times to see when you are ovulating, you will need to take the temperature for at least two weeks. You should notice a rise (between 0.3° F and 1° F) in temperature shortly before, during, or after ovulation.

Another way to take your basal body temperature is by urinating into a styrofoam cup first thing in the morning and putting the oral thermometer in the cup for five minutes, according to Serafino Corsello, M.D., of New York City and Huntington, New York.[40]

- Thyroplex (to support the thyroid, containing thyroid, pituitary, and hypothalamus glandular extracts, the amino acid L-tyrosine, zinc, manganese, copper, and iodine): two tablets daily
- Cinnamon and Rehmannia Formula by Seven Forests (to nourish the kidneys and, with the inclusion of the herb frittilaria, to help move phlegm from the throat): six tablets daily
- Adrenal Complex (contains adrenal glandular extracts and minerals to support the adrenal function): four daily
- Nutritional Elixir (contains herbs for strengthening estrogen production and the reproductive system, including red clover, nettles, dandelion, and yellowdock in a syrup of marine algae): two teaspoons daily

Jane's acupuncture treatments focused on points designed to release blocked energy in the spleen channel, which oversees the transport of blood, as in menstruation. During treatment, Dr. Koenig

With the personal fertility tester, Jane could tell when she was ready to ovulate because the fern-like patterns derived from a saliva sample become bold and intricate as ovulation nears.

Aromatherapy uses the essential oils extracted from plants and herbs to treat conditions ranging from infections and skin disorders to immune deficiencies and stress. The volatile constituents of the plant oils (its essence) are extracted through a process of steam distillation or cold-pressing. Although the term "aromatherapy" would seem to suggest an exclusive role for the aroma in the healing process, the oils also exert much of their therapeutic effect through their pharmacological properties and their small molecular size, making them one of the few therapeutic agents to easily penetrate bodily tissues. The benefits of essential oils can be obtained through inhalation, external application, or ingestion. The term aromatherapy was coined in 1937 by the French chemist Rene-Maurice Gattefosse, who observed the healing effect of lavender oil on burns.

A **micellized vitamin** (from micelle, which means "a colloid particle") is formulated to resemble a small, fat droplet, which is easily absorbed by the mucosa under the tongue. The result of this high absorbability is that you need less of a micellized vitamin to get the same nutritional benefit. For example, you need only one drop of micellized vitamin A per day to meet recommended daily requirements.

daubed organic aromatherapy (SEE QUICK DEFINITION) essential oils on Jane's abdomen; specifically, a formula of 30 drops of ginger oil (to warm the abdomen and stimulate the energy and blood to move more freely) and a small amount of micellized (SEE QUICK DEFINITION) vitamin E in one ounce of organic hazelnut oil. Dr. Koenig left the needles in for 40 minutes. The results were immediate—Jane began menstruating the next day.

With Jane's new menstrual period to use as a measure for establishing a regular cycle, Dr. Koenig immediately had Jane start counting two weeks from the first day of her period. Then, at day 14, she added Vitex Elixir (two teaspoons a day) to Jane's supplement program. Vitex (*Vitex agnus-castus*), or chastetree berry, has a strong hormone-stimulating action, particularly on progesterone. In the second half of the menstrual cycle, progesterone is dominant because it prepares the uterus for a fertilized egg. The Vitex would help restore the natural balance and rhythm of Jane's hormones and menstrual cycle, says Dr. Koenig.

If Jane didn't get a period about 16 days after she started the Vitex Elixir, which would put her at about day 31, she would stop taking it and wait and see what happened. Jane's first cycle lasted about 40 days. The next cycle went 35 days. Dr. Koenig continued to give Jane acupuncture every five weeks, as close to ovulation as they could approximate.

Next, Dr. Koenig had Jane purchase a personal fertility tester, a palm-sized portable device which allowed Jane to see a magnified view of her saliva. At various times in her cycle, Jane licked the tip of the tester and then examined the result. The saliva shows different fern-like patterns when the body is circulating the hormones in the first half, or estrogen phase, of the cycle. When the "ferns" disappear, a woman can tell she is in the second half, or progesterone phase of the cyle. In this way, Jane could better understand the rhythms of her own cycle, Dr. Koenig explains.

Finally, Dr. Koenig instructed Jane in correlating the "fern" readings with the basal temperature that she was continuing to take every morning. When the basal temperature readings were starting to rise and the "ferns" on the fertility tester were becoming bolder and more intricate, ovulation was near.

As a third and final cross-reference, Dr. Koenig taught Jane how to read her cervical mucus secretions to determine ovulation. These secretions, which are released through the vagina, change in consistency starting about six days prior to ovulation. They become increasingly more wet, profuse, stringy, and slippery, like raw egg white. (They are actually called "spin," for *spinnbarkeit*, which means "string-like" in German.) Jane checked for when the mucus was most egg white–like and stringy.

When all three variables—the secretions, the "ferns" and the temperatures—were in line, she knew she was ovulating and thus could schedule the optimum fertile time for sexual relations with her partner. Five months into the treatment, Jane became pregnant and successfully delivered a beautiful, healthy baby.

What follows is more information on the types of fertility testers available, and the benefits of learning to read your body's cycles.

Self-Testing: When are You Most Fertile?

Women in Europe and South America have been testing their saliva to determine fertility for years. In primarily Catholic countries such as Spain and Argentina, women use saliva testing as a form of natural birth control akin to the rhythm method. In the U.S., small manufacturers are marketing the testing kits as a home fertility aid.

Since the 1940s, researchers have known that hormonal changes during a woman's cycle significantly alter the chemistry of her saliva and cervical fluid. Monthly changes in crystallized saliva and cervical mucus were first discovered in 1948. Since then, numerous independent studies have made the connection between the hormonal changes of the menstrual cycle and the crystallized arrangement of saliva and cervical fluid during ovulation.

When saliva and cervical fluid evaporate, they form distinctive crys-

For more about **Thyroplex,** contact: Karuna Corporation, 42 Digital Drive, Novato, CA 94949, tel: 800-826-7225 or 415-382-0147. For **Seven Forests Cinnamon and Rehmannia Formula,** contact: Institute for Traditional Medicine, 2017 S.E. Hawthorne Blvd., Portland, OR 97214; tel: 800-544-7504 or 503-233-4907; fax: 503-233-4907. For **Adrenal Complex,** contact: Tyler Encapsulations, 2204 N.W. Birdsdale, Gresham, OR 97030; tel: 800-869-9705 or 503-661-5401; fax: 503-666-4913. For **Nutritional Elixir** or **Vitex Elixir,** contact: Gaia, Lancaster Country Road, Harvard, MA 01451; tel: 800-831-7780 or 508-772-5400; fax: 508-772-5764. For **organic essential oils,** contact: Phyto Medicine Company, 6701 Sunset Drive, Suite 100, Miami, FL 33143; tel: 305-662-6396; fax: 305-667-5619. Acupuncturist and herbalist **Rachel Koenig, L.Ac., N.C.C.A.H.,** is not taking any new patients at this writing. For a list of referrals of practitioners with a similar mind, contact: 53 Prospect Park West, Brooklyn, NY 11215; tel: 718-390-8898.

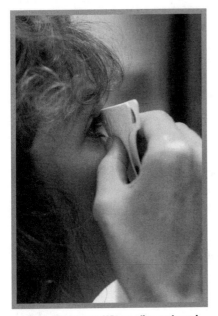

A WINDOW ON FERTILITY. **When saliva and cervical fluid evaporate, they form distinctive crystalline patterns which apparently correspond to the physiological changes occurring during the fertility cycle. Using a home fertility test (pictured above), a woman is able to view these patterns through a miniature microscope.**

talline patterns which correspond to the physiological changes occurring during the fertility cycle. Cell patterns (dots) form before the egg has matured, indicating a period of infertility; canal patterns (straight lines) form just before and during ovulation, when a women has the best chance of becoming pregnant; fern patterns (branching) occur just after ovulation, when conception is still possible, but not likely. The makers of the home fertility testing kits caution that during a "transition phase," when two of these patterns occur at the same time, a woman should assume she is fertile.

Most home fertility tests include a slide for saliva and cervical mucus samples and some form of microscopic lens through which to view the slide. The testing kits are accurate, portable, and reusable, according to their manufacturers. They are also far cheaper than laboratory urine tests, which typically cost $50 to $100 per month. The PFT 1-2-3™ model from Chain Reactions, Inc., provides colored slides to help you see your sample more clearly. The colored slides improve the accuracy of the test by providing you with more than one sample to view, and the different colors of light make the patterns more clearly visible. The PFT 1-2-3 works well with many different light sources.

Another fertility tester, called Ovu-tec, provides its own source of light. The test is shaped like a small lipstick container with an eyepiece on one end and the sample slide and microscopic lens fitted inside. A small lightbulb behind the slide acts as a miniature flashlight, illuminating the sample for better viewing. When you look inside, the sample appears like the patterns of a tiny kaleidoscope pointed toward a light source.

Most manufacturers of home fertility tests recommend testing your saliva immediately after waking up in the morning, before eating or drinking. While saliva tests are still fairly accurate at other times of day, any food or liquids present in the sample may interfere with test results. If you drank liquids or ate food just before doing a test, or if you have any inflammation or infection in your mouth, the manufacturers suggest confirming your results with a cervical fluid sample.

For more about the **PFT 1-2-3™**, contact: Chain Reactions, Inc., 11230 Gold Express Drive, Building 310 #272, Gold River, CA 95672; tel: 916-944-4009; fax: 916-944-4035. For **Ovu-tec**, contact: Ovu-tec, 911 N.W. 30th Avenue, Ocala, FL 34475; tel: 888-337-6464 or 352-629-2110; fax: 352-629-7332.

In the same way, saliva testing can be used as a back-up for cervical fluid testing. If you suspect you have a vaginal yeast infection or experience any itching or inflammation, use the saliva method for best results (make sure to consult your doctor if these vaginal symptoms persist). Swimming, bathing, or douching can also interfere with accurate testing of cervical fluid.

Despite these potential problems, saliva and cervical mucus tests are still the most accurate forms of fertility testing commercially available, according to Dr. Koenig. The fertile phase of a woman's cycle lasts about six days, from three to four days before ovulation to two to three days after. Yet many in-home and laboratory *urine* tests measure the hormone which triggers ovulation, even though that hormone reaches its highest level at the time of ovulation, just *after* the most fertile time has passed. "By then, it's too late," explains Dr. Koenig. "You have to get the sperm in place to wait for the egg to mature."

As demonstrated by the case of Jane and the earlier medical histories, an alternative medicine physician who understands the causal factors in infertility can address each in turn and help a woman achieve a healthy pregnancy and delivery, even in the most discouraging cases. The woman in the next case had tried everything a multitude of conventional fertility specialists had to offer before she sought alternative medicine treatment and learned what was really causing her infertility.

Success Story: Pregnancy After 20 Years of Infertility

Annette, a 41-year-old attorney, first came to see Serafina Corsello, M.D., director of the Corsello Centers for Nutritional Complementary Medicine in New York City and Huntington, New York, not because she was infertile but because her conventional physician thought she had an infection or some other imbalance since her white blood cell count was abnormally low.

During her intake interview with Dr. Corsello, however, Annette

Sexual Practices to Promote Conception

Certain positions in sexual intercourse can be more conducive to conception than others. The best is the missionary position: woman on her back, knees raised, and partner on top, penetrating as deeply as possible. Afterward, the woman should remain lying on her back, with her legs raised, for about a half-hour. A pillow placed under the woman's hips (either during or just after intercourse) is an additional aid to the sperm in reaching the cervix.

A little delayed gratification may also be helpful. "If the woman has an orgasm after the man," say Susan Curtis and Romy Fraser, authors of *Natural Healing for Women*, "the uterus acts like a vacuum to suck up the sperm into the fallopian tubes hundreds of times faster than they could swim there under their own steam."[41]

For more about **ovarian cysts**, see Chapter 4: Ovarian Cysts, pp. 138-156.

revealed that she had been trying for 20 years to get pregnant, had consulted nearly two dozen gynecologists and fertility specialists, and had undergone the full range of conventional treatments including surgeries, fertility drugs, and artificial insemination—all without success.

Annette's reproductive problems were longstanding and actually began when she started menstruating at age 12. From the beginning, her menstrual cycles were irregular, averaging every 30 to 45 days, with thick blood clots and bleeding so heavy that she would have to be put to bed with anemia due to blood loss. She went on birth control pills at age 13 to regulate her periods and stayed on them for ten years. During that time, she tried several times to get off the pill and have normal menses, but was unsuccessful. At age 25, Annette was diagnosed with polycystic ovaries, and underwent major surgery to remove the cysts. After the surgery, she no longer menstruated.

When she turned 27, Annette began to think about having children. Over the next four years, in an attempt to have regular menses and ovulation, she and her then-fiancé consulted 15 gynecologists and fertility specialists. During that time, Annette had more surgeries: D & Cs (dilatation and curettage, scraping of the uterine lining), laparoscopies, and a laparotomy (in which an incision is made through the abdominal wall and into the abdominal cavity). None of the procedures were successful in restoring her periods.

When the surgeries didn't work, the fertility specialists tried a string of fertility drugs, including Clomid for three years, none of which produced results. Annette had another surgery in which a uterine fibroid was removed, after which she was put on Pergonal, another fertility drug, for six months. She became violently ill from the side effects which included migraine headaches. At that point, Annette (by then in her mid-thirties) and her husband tried artificial insemination.

When that didn't work, Annette gave up trying to become pregnant. She was heartbroken, but by then she was 38 and figured there was no hope because she had tried everything. It wasn't until three years later, when her physician told her to see a nutritionist, that she realized she had tried everything *except* an alternative medicine approach.

After a comprehensive interview with Annette, Dr. Corsello ordered an immunological screen, a stress profile, and a thyroid gland evaluation. When the test results came back, no one was surprised to learn that Annette's immune system was not working properly. At that point, infertility was not even a question; Dr. Corsello was only concerned with restoring Annette's general health.

Annette's immune system problems were likely the result of a combination of factors, observes Dr. Corsello. "She had a high stress level from trying to succeed in the legal profession, a male-dominated field; she had deficiencies in antioxidants, essential fatty acids, and vitamin B6, all necessary for proper hormonal metabolism; and she had a probable genetic predisposition for immune system weakness." In addition, Annette was chronically constipated, which meant that toxins and an overgrowth of the yeast *Candida albicans* were not being eliminated promptly and so were building up in her intestinal tract.

"I decided, as I do with most of my patients, to start by cleaning Annette's gut," Dr. Corsello says. "I am well aware that 80% of the immune responses reside in the intestines and lymphatic system."

Dr. Corsello put Annette on a bowel cleansing program, the main element of which was a daily liquid concoction consisting of six ounces of water or plain seltzer, two ounces of fruit juice, 1 tsp of powdered vitamin C, and ½ to 1 tsp of Corsello Fiber-Max or Yerba Prima psyllium husks (powdered soluble and insoluble fibers). Annette drank the mixture first thing in the morning, following it with a cup of herbal tea or ten to 12 ounces of warm water containing a touch of lemon juice. The extra liquid is necessary to make sure the fiber flows smoothly through the digestive tract. Annette then waited 15 minutes to allow the fiber drink to be absorbed before having breakfast or other nutrients.

Dietary changes, an integral part of Dr. Corsello's treatment approach, were next in Annette's protocol. In all the years of her consulting doctor after doctor, no one had ever

To contact **Serafina Corsello, M.D.**, or for information on **Corsello Fiber Max**: The Corsello Centers for Nutritional Complementary Medicine, 200 West 67th Street, New York, NY 10019; tel: 212-399-0222; or 175 East Main Street, Huntington, NY 11743; tel: 516-271-0222 or 516-271-5992. **Yerba Prima psyllium husks** and **vitamin C powder** are available at health food stores.

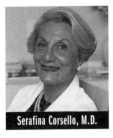

Serafina Corsello, M.D.

"I decided, as I do with most of my patients, to start by cleaning Annette's gut," Dr. Corsello says. "I am well aware that 80% of the immune responses reside in the intestines and lymphatic system."

QUICK DEFINITION

Biofeedback training is a method of learning how to consciously regulate normally unconscious bodily functions (such as breathing, heart rate, and blood pressure) through the use of simple electronic devices. These devices give immediate "feedback" or information about the biological system of the person being monitored, so that he or she can learn to consciously influence that system. Biofeedback is particularly useful to reduce stress, eliminate headaches, control asthmatic attacks, recondition injured muscles, and relieve pain.

asked Annette about her eating habits, states Dr. Corsello. With nutrition an important factor in fertility, this was a lamentable oversight. Under Dr. Corsello's guidance, Annette eliminated sugar and junk foods, and then dairy products after a food allergy test revealed her to be allergic to them.

To build her immune system and correct nutritional deficiencies, Annette received weekly intramuscular shots of folic acid, vitamins B12 and B6, zinc, and magnesium, among other vitamins and minerals. To help her manage stress more effectively, Dr. Corsello referred Annette to a course in biofeedback (SEE QUICK DEFINITION) which produced significant improvements in this area.

As the weeks went by, Dr. Corsello's assistants at the clinic kept close track of Annette's progress and monitored her nutrient levels. Three months after beginning treatment, Annette, to her amazement, was having more regular menstrual periods. That was exciting enough, but the real shocker came at the next evaluation several months later. Annette, now 42, was pregnant for the first time in her life. Annette maintained her dietary and nutritional program during the pregnancy and delivered a healthy baby boy.

Additional Alternative Medicine Therapies for Infertility

As mentioned throughout this chapter, natural therapies for infertility are not only considerably less expensive, they also are less invasive and work to correct the original imbalance that is making the woman or man infertile instead of artificially forcing conception. The numerous protocols already covered include acupuncture, herbal medicine, detoxification, nutritional support, thyroid strengthening, and aromatherapy.

The following section provides more information on thyroid support, offers herbal self-care remedies, and discusses another useful therapy for infertility—homeopathy.

Thyroid Support

If your thyroid gland is underactive, your alternative medicine physician may advise supplementing with natural thyroid hormone supplements, which are available by prescription. In that category, Armour Thyroid is widely prescribed because it contains three of the thyroid's four hormones (T4, T3, and di-iodothyronine).[44] Despite their effectiveness, thyroid supplements such as Armour Thyroid are viewed with some caution due to the likelihood that the person's system will become dependent on them and their own natural thyroid function will become lazy and even more sluggish.

Some practitioners prefer to find ways to stimulate the thyroid and its own production of thyroid hormones. This strategy may include supplements such as iodine and dietary additions such as kelp or dulse (all of which feed the thyroid), or animal-derived thyroid glandular extracts which have the actual hormone removed. These extracts do not take over the work of the thyroid, but instead serve to stimulate its activity.

Dr. Ralph Golan recommends the following foods to support the thyroid gland: iodine-rich foods such as fish, kelp, dulse, and seaweeds; zinc from beef, oatmeal, nuts, chicken, seafood, liver, and dried beans; copper from liver and other organ meats, eggs, yeast, legumes, nuts, and raisins; and tyrosine from soy products, beef, chicken, and fish.[45]

As nutritional supplement support, he typically suggests the following:

■ Iodine (as kelp or dulse supplements or in higher doses by prescription): 225-1,000 mcg daily

Diet and Supplements for Infertility

According to Ralph Golan, M.D., women with fertility problems should eat a whole foods diet, avoid highly processed and refined foods, and eliminate excess caffeine which can contribute to infertility.[42]

He also recommends taking the following supplements:[43]

■ Vitamin C: 1,000 mg three times daily

■ Zinc: 15-30 mg three times daily

■ Magnesium: at least 400 mg daily

■ Vitamin B complex: 25-50 mg daily

■ Beta carotene: 50,000 IU daily

■ Flaxseed oil: 1-2 teaspoons daily

■ Borage oil: 200-300 mg of gamma linolenic acid daily

■ Vitamin B6: 50 mg daily

■ Vitamin E: 400 IU daily

The Costs and Failures of *In Vitro* Fertilization

Unfortunately, the traditional alternative of *in vitro* fertilization (the implantation of a fertilized egg directly into the uterus) has proven to be an increasingly expensive process, without a corresponding increase in the success rate of the procedure. One study has shown that the more expensive *in vitro* fertilization and other high-technology procedures become, the longer it takes for a couple to conceive.

The 1994 study, which gathered data from six fertility clinics across the country, found that the average cost of a successful delivery with *in vitro* fertilization increased from $66,667 for the first cycle of *in vitro* fertilization to $114,286 by the sixth cycle. As the chances of successful pregnancy decrease over the six-month period, the cost of the procedure increases accordingly.[47]

In terms of the success rate of *in vitro* fertilization, *Fertility and Sterility* reports that despite significant improvements in fertility medication and techniques, the number of successful technology-assisted births has increased only slightly in recent years. The report documented that between 1993 and 1994, the success rate for *in vitro* procedures improved by less than 0.005%, even though fertility clinics performed about 4.4% fewer procedures in 1994 than in the previous year. Although there is no consensus as to why success rates have not significantly improved, some fertility doctors have attributed the problem to an overuse of *in vitro* procedures in couples who have little chance of a successful delivery.[48]

- Zinc: 15-30 mg daily
- Copper: 2-3 mg daily
- Selenium: up to 250 mcg daily
- Tyrosine: 300-1,000 mg daily
- Iron: for menstruating females, 18 mg daily
- Vitamin B complex: 25-50 mg daily
- Magnesium: up to 400 mg daily [46]

Herbal Remedies

As demonstrated by the case studies in this chapter, herbs can assist in correcting the underlying causes of infertility, such as hormonal imbalance, and can reverse some of the fertility-inhibiting conditions, such as irregular periods and anemia. Jill Stansbury, N.D., a naturopathic physician practicing in Battleground, Washington, makes these typical herbal recommendations for women experiencing fertility problems:

- **Chastetree berry** (*Vitex agnus-castus*)—Chastetree encourages ovulation by stimulating the production of luteinizing hormone (LH) which is vital to the release of the egg from the ovaries. In some cases, chastetree berry can restore normal menstrual cycles to women with amenorrhea (lack of menstrual periods).
- ***Dong quai*** (*Angelica*

sinensis)—Chinese women have long used *dong quai* to treat menstrual irregularities. This key fertility herb is known for its ability to regulate reproductive hormones, normalize the menstrual cycle, and tone the uterus.

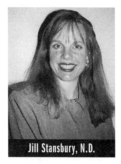

Jill Stansbury, N.D.

Herbs can assist in correcting the underlying causes of infertility, such as hormonal imbalance, and can reverse some of the fertility-inhibiting conditions, such as irregular periods and anemia, says Dr. Stansbury.

■ Red clover blossoms *(Trigolium pratense)*—Red clover contains the compounds coumestan and isoflavone, which have estrogen-like effects on the female reproductive system and thus work to enhance fertility. Women who are estrogen-deficient tend to benefit most from red clover.

■ **Licorice** *(Glycyrrhiza glabra)*—Research indicates that licorice-based remedies can improve menstruation in women with infrequent periods. Licorice also helps women with high testosterone and low estrogen, a hormonal imbalance often associated with health conditions such as polycystic ovary disease (multiple cysts on the ovaries) which can impede fertility.

■ **Siberian ginseng** *(Eleutherococcus senticosus)*—By enhancing a woman's overall health and vitality, ginseng also works to improve fertility. In addition, this herb has been shown to promote the proper regulation of reproductive hormones.[49]

Herbalist Susun Weed of Woodstock, New York, also cites red clover as beneficial for infertility because it draws blood to the uterus. She prefers the infusion form, using an ounce of the dried herb in a quart jar filled with boiled water (if you use the blossoms, brew by steeping two hours maximum; for leaves, four hours or more); drink from one cup to the whole quart daily.

Dr. Golan typically recommends the following to promote fertility, but cautions against taking them during menstruation:

■ Siberian ginseng: 100 mg twice daily before 4 p.m.

■ Royal jelly: 1,000-2,000 mg daily

■ False unicorn root and *Vitex agnus-castus* (equal parts as a tincture): 1 tsp three times daily

■ Alternate combination program—For the first half of the men-

Fertility Drugs Can Prevent Pregnancy

Research suggests that the use of fertility drugs can actually make it harder to become pregnant. This unlikely situation results from the fact that fertility drugs contribute to the formation of follicular cysts, a reproductive complication which may make it more difficult to conceive.

Most fertility drugs work by increasing the body's levels of FSH (follicle-stimulating hormone), a product of the pituitary gland. A woman taking fertility drugs, therefore, produces many extra follicles (the egg-containing sac which releases the egg during ovulation). When more than one egg is released, the chances of conception increase, at least in theory.

The difficulty is that not all of the extra follicles go on to ovulate, and when a follicle fails to rupture and remains attached to the ovary, a follicular cyst occurs—thereby decreasing your chances of becoming pregnant.

The medical journal *Fertility and Sterility* explored the relationship between follicular cysts and pregnancy rates in women attempting *in vitro* fertilization. Of the 18 women studied, none of the participants with a cyst larger than 15 mm became pregnant, compared with a 32% pregnancy rate for women without a cyst. Older women and women with the highest levels of FSH were at a greater risk of developing a follicular cyst during the fertility treatment.[54]

strual cycle (estrogen phase), take estrogen-building herbs in a tincture: licorice root (four parts), *Vitex* (one part), yarrow (one part), and *dong quai* (two parts); 1½ tsp three times daily. For the second half (progesterone phase), take: blessed thistle (three parts), milk thistle (three parts), sarsaparilla (one part), and *Vitex* (one part); 1 tsp three times daily. Don't take during menses.[50]

Other alternative medicine practitioners recommend these additional fertility-enhancing herbs: echinacea (to strengthen the pituitary which controls reproductive hormones);[51] black cohosh (to support the uterus); black haw (to relax and support the uterus); verbena and St. John's wort (to calm nerves, support *yin* or quiet cooling energy, and dispel anxiety and irritation); and garden sage (to keep blood flowing freely).[52]

Homeopathic Self-Care Remedies

As discussed in previous chapters, homeopathy (SEE QUICK DEFINITION) is unique in that the active ingredients in the remedies are not actual chemical substances, but bear the "holographic imprint" of an energetic aspect of that substance. This imprint can affect the energy of a woman and influence her fertility.[53]

Homeopaths Andrew Lockie, M.D., and Nicola Geddes, M.D., of England and Scotland, recommend the following remedies for infertility. All remedies are in dosages of 30C. They should not be viewed as long-term therapy, but should instead be considered temporary "fixes" until you can see a trained homeopath, who can prescribe a more precise remedy to fit your individual symptom and personality patterns.[55]

■ If you feel weepy, chilly, and irritable, lack sexual desire, and experience irregular periods with a "sensation that your womb is about to fall out," *Sepia* is recommended.

■ For vaginal dryness and tenderness in the lower abdomen over the right ovary, *Lycopodium clavatum* is helpful.

■ If you've had a previous miscarriage before the 12th week of pregnancy, use *Sabina*.

■ If your breasts are tender, with pockets of hard swellings, and if there is a loss of sex drive, try *Conium maculatum*.

QUICK DEFINITION

Homeopathy was founded in the early 1800s by German physician Samuel Hahnemann. Today, an estimated 500 million people worldwide receive homeopathic treatment; in Britain, homeopathy enjoys royal patronage. Homeopathy is now practiced according to two differing concepts. In classical homeopathy, only one single-component remedy is prescribed at a time, in a potency specifically adjusted to the patient; the physician waits to see the results before prescribing anything further. In complex homeopathy, typified by *Hepar compositum*, a prescription involves multiple substances given at the same time, usually in low potencies.

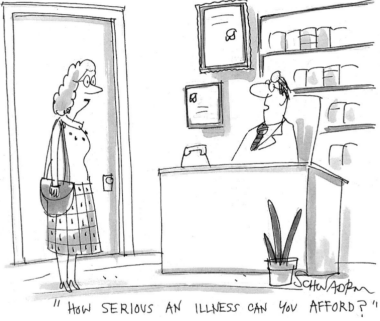

"HOW SERIOUS AN ILLNESS CAN YOU AFFORD?"

CHAPTER

6

Nearly every woman gets a

urinary tract infection at least once in

her life, but if you are having them

every year or more often,

it's time to strengthen your

immune system and balance your

body's internal environment

for lasting relief.

6 Cystitis

AND OTHER URINARY TRACT INFECTIONS

MOST WOMEN HAVE had at least one urinary tract or bladder infection in their lives. Anyone who has experienced the ailment's symptoms—searing, burning pain upon urinating and the constant sensation of needing to urinate even when you don't have to—isn't likely to forget it. Every year in the U.S., an estimated two million people, the majority of whom are women, suffer from bladder infection, also known as cystitis or, more generally, as urinary tract infection (UTI). In a *Prevention* magazine survey, UTI was the most common women's health problem reported.[1] Approximately 15% of those who contract cystitis develop a chronic case with frequent recurrences.[2]

Given that most cystitis is bacterial, conventional medicine's solution is antibiotics. While antibiotics stop the symptoms, providing welcome relief from the pain, their use actually perpetuates the problem and recurrence is likely (see sidebar: "Why Antibiotics Won't Cure Cystitis," p. 209). The better answer for UTIs, as you will learn from the patient success stories throughout this chapter, is natural treatments for the acute symptoms while introducing long-term preventive dietary and lifestyle changes. Those modifications will help you avoid future outbreaks by

---

14 Factors That Contribute to Cystitis/UTI

- Hygienic shortcomings
- Sexual intercourse (Honeymoon cystitis)
- Contraceptive devices
- Tampons
- Antibiotics
- Inadequate fluid intake
- Diet
- Chronic constipation
- Uterine prolapse
- Hormonal changes
- Underactive thyroid
- Acidic urine
- Energy blockages
- Unexpressed anger or resentment

improving hygiene, strengthening your immune system, and balancing your body's internal environment.

Before we turn to a case study illustrating some of these alternative medicine solutions, let's get clear on exactly what cystitis and UTIs are and how they are related.

A Quick Definition of Cystitis and Urinary Tract Infections

Cystitis is one kind of urinary tract infection, usually occurring when bacterial infection ascends the urethra (the tube from the bladder to the outside of the body through which urine is eliminated) to the bladder. The urinary tract itself is divided into two

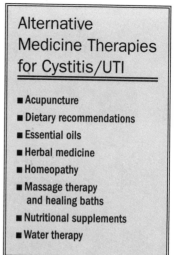

Alternative Medicine Therapies for Cystitis/UTI

- Acupuncture
- Dietary recommendations
- Essential oils
- Herbal medicine
- Homeopathy
- Massage therapy and healing baths
- Nutritional supplements
- Water therapy

UTIs are nearly ten times more common among women than men and about 15% of those who contract cystitis develop a chronic case with frequent recurrences.

sections: the lower tract, made up of the bladder and the urethra; and the upper tract, consisting of the two kidneys and their accompanying ureters (tubes that connect each kidney to the bladder). While infections can occur anywhere in the urinary tract, lower tract infections are by far the most common.

Urethritis is an infection of the urethra. It causes a burning sensation on urination, but no other symptoms. It is generated by bacteria or can be caused by a microorganism such as *Chlamydia trachomatis*, which is usually spread by sexual contact. Urethritis becomes cystitis when the bacteria work their way up the urethra and infect the bladder. Known as ascending UTI, this is a common occurrence. If the UTI is left untreated and works its way further up the urinary tract to the kidneys, it becomes pyelonephritis, which requires immediate medical care. This happens in about 10% of cystitis cases.[3] A descending UTI (far more serious) starts in the kidneys or bladder and moves down the urinary tract to the urethra.

In addition to the burning pain with urination and the false sensa-

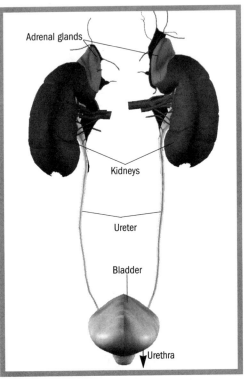

Adrenal glands

Kidneys

Ureter

Bladder

Urethra

URINARY TRACT INFECTION. An infection can develop anywhere in the urinary tract from the urethra to the kidneys. In most cases, however, the problem starts in the urethra and only moves further up the system in severe cases.

tion of needing to urinate, other UTI symptoms include increased urinary urgency and frequency, itching or a feeling of warmth during urination, fatigue, tenderness upon palpation over the bladder, lower back pain, increased nighttime urination, and sometimes bloody urine. Symptoms of kidney involvement include fever, chills, nausea, vomiting, and severe low back and/or pelvic pain.

Infections of the lower urinary tract involve contamination of the delicate membranes of the tract with one or more of six bacteria: *Escherichia coli, Klebsiella, Proteus, Enterobacter, Pseudomonas,* or *Serratia.* When the local immune defense system breaks down, any of these bacteria can invade the mucosal tissues of the urinary tract, multiply, and produce an infection. A UTI diagnosis is applied when there is a bacterial count in the urine of more than 100,000 bacteria/ml.

UTIs are nearly ten times more common among women than men. Most medical experts attribute the far higher incidence in women to the shortness of the female urethra (1¼" to 2" compared to 7¾" for the male urethra) and for its proximity to possible sources of contamination, such as the vagina and anus. Also, in men, the prostatic fluid is believed to act as an antibacterial shield against UTIs.

Nonbacterial cystitis can be caused by kidney stones, bladder protrusions into the vagina (cystoceles), or crevices that develop on the inside wall of the urethra (diverticula).[4] Another type of nonbacterial cystitis is interstitial cystitis (IC), which is not an infection but an inflammation of the bladder (specifically, of the interstitium or space between the bladder lining and bladder muscle).[5]

Characterized by tiny hemorrhages, scar tissue, or ulcers on the bladder wall, the result is bladder contraction which, in turn, produces frequent urination. While IC shares many of the symptoms of bacterial cystitis, the key symptoms to differentiate it are frequent muscle spasms, pain with movement, and no bacteria in the urine. This mysterious disorder affects more than 500,000 Americans, mostly middle-aged women.[6]

Now that you understand the different types of urinary tract infections you might have, here are two case studies illustrating successful alternative medicine treatment of cystitis. For these two women, herbal medicine and homeopathy produced lasting relief from acute and chronic UTI.

Success Stories: Reversing Acute and Chronic Cystitis With Herbal Medicine

When Miriam, 65, contracted acute cystitis for the first time in her life, she consulted naturopathic physician Jill Stansbury, N.D., who practices in Battleground, Washington. Miriam reported pelvic discomfort, and constantly feeling the need to urinate despite having little urine to pass. A urine analysis, showing a bacterial count of more than 100,000/ml, confirmed that she had bacterial cystitis.

Dr. Stansbury prescribed an herbal tea for Miriam to drink at the rate of three to five cups daily until her symptoms improved. The herbs included pipsissewa leaf (*Chimaphila umbellatum*, one ounce), marshmallow root (*Althea officinalis*, one ounce), pot marigold flowers (*Calendula officinalis*, ½ ounce), uva ursi or bearberry leaf (*Arctostaphylos uva ursi*, ½ ounce), and chamomile flowers (*Matricaria chamomilla*, one ounce). Miriam was to add one tablespoon total of these mixed herbs to a cup of just boiled water and steep for 20 minutes.

Dr. Stansbury notes that marshmallow root is a mucilaginous (soothing and coating) herb that can provide "quick symptomatic relief, sometimes so effectively that people feel the complaint is entirely resolved and discontinue treatment before the infection is completely cleared up." She adds that pipsissewa and uva ursi have properties that work against the bacterial infection in cystitis. In Miriam's case, she reported the next day that her discomfort was more than 50% reduced; all of her symptoms were relieved within a few

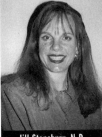

Jill Stansbury, N.D.

Marshmallow root is a soothing and coating herb that can provide "quick symptomatic relief, sometimes so effectively that people feel the complaint is entirely resolved and discontinue treatment before the infection is completely cleared up," says Dr. Stansbury.

days. "A follow-up visit and urinalysis ten days later showed the infection to be completely resolved," says Dr. Stansbury.

Cases of chronic urinary tract infections require a slightly different herbal approach, Dr. Stansbury advises. For example, you need to rule out certain causes that would require a more serious intervention. Underlying diabetes or a high sugar intake can contribute to chronic UTIs; conditions such as asthma, hay fever, chemical sensitivity, and multiple food allergies can irritate the bladder.

Dr. Stansbury further explains that a person with constipation, a generally poor diet, or toxic intestines can develop a UTI as the kidneys try to help the intestines eliminate waste. Finally, a person who is immune deficient or has chronic fatigue, fibromyalgia (chronic muscle pain), or a yeast overgrowth of *Candida albicans* can also manifest a UTI as part of their symptom picture.

Una, 38, was into her third bout of acute cystitis in five months when she consulted Dr. Stansbury. Additionally, Una had undergone several other UTIs in the past eight years for which she had been treated with antibiotics. She complained of frequent urination and a constant burning sensation in her pelvis; as a self-prescribed remedy, Una had been drinking copious amounts of water and cranberry juice.

Dr. Stansbury suggested an herbal formula consisting of six herbs, to be taken as a tea (three cups daily). These herbs included agrimony leaf (*Agrimonia spp.*, ½ ounce), pot marigold flowers (*Calendula officinalis*, ½ ounce), cleavers leaf (*Galium aperine*, ½ ounce), uva ursi or bearberry leaf (*Arctostaphylos uva ursi*, ½ ounce), desert mallow (marshmallow) root (*Althea officinalis*, one ounce), and peppermint leaf (*Mentha piperita*, one ounce).

The cleavers leaf was added to the formula as "a nourishing immune tonic that stimulates lymphatic flow and filtration and waste elimination by the kidneys," says Dr. Stansbury. She also gave Una a commercially prepared immune-support formula which included echinacea, garlic, vitamin C, beta carotene, and zinc.

Finally, Dr. Stansbury advised Una to "drastically reduce" her high intake of sugars and caffeine, and to cut way back on her water and cranberry juice consumption for a week to give the herbs a chance to work. A week later, Una reported that her symptoms were "dramatically reduced." The pain upon urination had diminished over the seven days and her urinary frequency had subsided. At this point, Dr. Stansbury prescribed a homeopathic remedy (SEE QUICK DEFINITION) called *Nux vomica* (poison nut) to help remove the energetic traces of the UTI bacteria.

At least six other homeopathic remedies can be helpful with UTIs, depending on the specific symptoms. *Apis*, for example, is indicated when the urine is highly colored, scanty, and painful at the last drops; *Cantharis* is given when there is a constant, almost intolerable urge to urinate, but the urine passes in drops, with cutting pains. Una continued to improve over the next months and when new UTI symptoms occasionally reappeared in the next few years, Dr. Stansbury repeated the herbal tea procedure. "No antibiotics have been required in the last eight years," she reports.[7]

Homeopathy was founded in the early 1800s by German physician Samuel Hahnemann. Today, an estimated 500 million people worldwide receive homeopathic treatment; in Britain, homeopathy enjoys royal patronage. Homeopathy is now practiced according to two differing concepts. In classical homeopathy, only one single-component remedy is prescribed at a time, in a potency specifically adjusted to the patient; the physician waits to see the results before prescribing anything further. In complex homeopathy, typified by *Hepar compositum*, a prescription involves multiple substances given at the same time, usually in low potencies.

As the cases of Miriam and Una illustrate, cystitis can be effectively treated using only natural therapies. Here, herbal medicine and homeopathy accomplished everything antibiotics would have—that is, symptom relief and killing of the bacteria behind the cystitis—without the detrimental side effects or the perpetuation of the cycle of infection.

These alternative medicine methods actually accomplish *more* than antibiotics because they address the fundamental imbalances and deficiencies that allowed the bacteria to grow. For example, some of the herbs Dr. Stansbury included in her formulas were immune enhancers, strengthening a weakened immune system and restoring the body's self-healing capacities. In order to fully treat your UTI and prevent recurrences, you need to identify and address or eliminate the factors that are contributing to creating an environment in your body in which UTI can flourish.

Alternative medicine methods accomplish more than antibiotics because they address the fundamental imbalances and deficiencies that allowed the bacteria to grow in the first place.

14 Factors That Contribute to Cystitis/UTI

The following 14 factors begin with outer behaviors or practices that increase your chances of contracting a urinary tract infection and progress to internal contributing causes. You can take steps today to change the behavioral factors present in your life. Depending on the degree of their contribution, these modifications, such as dietary changes and more thorough hygienic practices, may be enough to prevent future UTIs. However, if some of the deeper causes are involved, an alternative medicine physician can help you correct them.

1) Hygienic Shortcomings

How the bacteria get into your urethra in the first place is often a matter of hygiene. Women who wipe from back to front after a bowel movement can inadvertently introduce bacteria into the urinary tract. To avoid this, it is advisable to wipe from front to back. Irritating chemicals from commercial douches can also create problems. Getting into the urinary tract during vaginal douching, they can cause inflammation which leaves the tissues vulnerable to infection. Bacteria can also be introduced as a result of swimming in a body of water in which the bacterial content is high. Most experts recommend urinating after swimming to flush any harmful bacteria from the urethra.

Retired urologist Larrian Gillespie, M.D., of Beverly Hills, California, who specialized for many years in the treatment of cystitis, says bacteria must be flushed out of the urinary tract by an adequate stream of urine. Dr. Gillespie, who is the author of *You Don't Have to Live With Cystitis*, states: "A urinary tract infection is not a problem of bacteria getting into the bladder. It is a problem of bacteria not getting out."

Dr. Gillespie cites a study in which a group of medical students had samples of fecal material introduced into their bladders. They were then told to urinate several times. By the time all had urinated twice, no trace of bacteria from the fecal matter remained in their urine. Dr. Gillespie applies this simple standard for "adequate" urination: "If you can move 'dirt on the sidewalk' with your stream, instead of 'tinkling' drops out, you will not get a bladder infection," she says.[8]

2) Sexual Intercourse or "Honeymoon Cystitis"

Cystitis is common in sexually active women for a variety of reasons. (The euphemistic label of "honeymoon cystitis" for sex-related cystitis refers to the supposed increase in sexual activity on a honeymoon). Sexual intercourse, during which bodily fluids are intermingled, can lead to the transmission of bacteria from the intestines or the vagina to the urethra and urinary tract.

Additionally, if the woman is not sufficiently aroused and her vagina is too dry prior to penetration, the vaginal passage can be bruised during intercourse. Unfriendly bacteria, introduced via the penis, can find a breeding ground in small cuts in the vagina. Similarly, sexual activities or positions that are too rough can also cause bruising and irritation, again allowing unfriendly bacteria to proliferate.

You can take practical steps to ensure cleanliness. Urinating before and after sexual intercourse is cited by many physicians as a preventive step for UTI. A strong stream of urine will flush out any bacteria that may have been transmitted to the urethra during intercourse. Be sure you and your sexual partner keep your genital and anal areas clean. Wash your hands before foreplay and intercourse. If your partner is uncircumcised, have him clean under the foreskin before sex. If you engage in anal intercourse, be sure your partner uses a condom, throws it away, and washes his penis before engaging in vaginal intercourse. Use vaginal lubricants such as K-Y Lubricating Jelly to minimize irritation.[9]

3) Contraceptive Devices

If your contraceptive diaphragm is too big, so that it not only covers the cervix (entrance of the uterus) but also juts out and presses on the adjacent bladder neck, it could prevent you from emptying your bladder after intercourse. Having the fit of your diaphragm checked by your gynecologist and getting a smaller size if it is indeed too large or using a cervical cap instead is a wise precaution. The contraceptive sponge is also problematic in this way, so it is best to avoid this form of birth control if you are prone to UTIs.

Contraceptive jelly can create problems by providing a medium for bacteria to get into the vagina and from there into the urethra.[10] As with the chemicals in commercial douches, chemicals in contraceptive creams can also get into the urinary tract and inflame the tissues, opening the way for bacterial infection.

"Women who use tampons may have a higher incidence [of cystitis] than women who just use a pad," states Dr. Grant Mulholland. The warm, moist string on a tampon is also an excellent breeding ground for bacteria and provides a means of easy entry into the body.

Friendly bacteria, or probiotics, refer to beneficial microbes inhabiting the human gastrointestinal tract where they are essential for proper nutrient assimilation. The human body contains an estimated several trillion beneficial bacteria comprising over 400 species, all necessary for health. Among the more well known of these are *Lactobacillus acidophilus* and *Bifidobacterium bifidum*. Overly acidic bodily conditions, chronic constipation or diarrhea, dietary imbalances, consumption of highly processed foods, and the excessive use of antibiotics and hormonal drugs can interfere with probiotic function and even reduce the number of these microbes, setting up conditions for illness.

For more about **yeast infections**, see Chapter 7: Vaginitis, pp. 244-245. For more about **yeast overgrowth**, see "Anti-*Candida* Diet," this chapter, p. 221.

4) Tampons

According to Grant Mulholland, M.D., chair of the Department of Urology at Jefferson University Medical College in Philadelphia, Pennsylvania, the use of tampons, which introduces foreign materials and chemicals into the vagina's delicate lining, can irritate the vagina, leaving it more vulnerable to bacterial overgrowth which can then travel to the urethra.

"Women who use tampons may have a higher incidence [of cystitis] than women who just use a pad," states Dr. Mulholland.[11] The warm, moist string on a tampon is also an excellent breeding ground for bacteria and provides a means of easy entry into the body. If you do use tampons, it is advisable to change them frequently—although not frequently enough to dry out the vagina and cause irritation.[12]

5) Antibiotics

The use of antibiotics as a treatment for cystitis or other infections contributes to the creation of a climate in which bacteria can flourish. Antibiotics accomplish this by killing off *all* the bacteria in the body, not just the targeted "bad" bacteria. By killing off the "friendly" bacteria (SEE QUICK DEFINITION) which ordinarily protect the body against invading microorganisms, the stage is set for overgrowth in the intestines and vagina of infectious bacteria and the yeast-like fungus *Candida albicans*, which provides a fertile bacterial breeding ground. From there, it is a short trip to the urethra and a full-blown UTI. As you can see, the use of antibiotics, the preferred conventional medicine prescription for cystitis, can actually lead to further UTI incidence (see sidebar: "Why Antibiotics Won't Cure Cystitis," p. 209).

6) Inadequate Fluid Intake

A low fluid intake may contribute to UTIs by preventing the bladder

Why Antibiotics Won't Cure Cystitis

Prescription antibiotics, the conventional medical treatment for cystitis, can seem like a quick fix for many women. To be sure, the antibiotics can relieve the symptoms of burning pain with urination, urinary urgency and frequency, and pelvic pain. They do this by killing the infecting bacteria. But the quick fix comes with a high price tag: your immune system is weakened. There are two reasons why this happens.

First, the antibiotics work by suppressing your symptoms. While this affords you temporary relief, ultimately this suppression drives the original imbalance or disturbance (the one that allowed the infection in the first place) deeper into your body, according to homeopathic scholar George Vithoulkas. As a result, on the surface you may seem symptom-free and thus healthy, but in reality the "center of gravity of susceptibility has moved into more vital regions of the organism." The disappearance of symptoms following conventional medication is, to Vithoulkas, "not a sign of improvement in health but rather a sign of degeneration." Vithoulkas also says the drugs create their own type of disease, which conventional medicine usually labels as "side effects."[13]

Secondly, the antibiotics destroy the "friendly" bacteria, or probiotics, in the digestive tract that are vital for keeping the intestinal microflora in a healthy balance. These probiotics perform numerous important tasks to strengthen the body's immune system. Without their protection, there are no restraints on infecting bacteria, so your urinary tract infection can persist. Some of the protective and therapeutic roles of the probiotics include:

■ They manufacture some of the B vitamins, including niacin (B3), pyridoxine (B6), folic acid, and biotin.[14]

■ They manufacture the milk-digesting enzyme lactase, which helps digest calcium-rich dairy products.[15]

■ They actively produce antibacterial substances which kill or deactivate hostile disease-causing bacteria. They do this by changing the local levels of acidity, by depriving pathogenic (disease-causing) bacteria of their nutrients, or by actually producing their own antibiotic substances which can kill invading bacteria, viruses, and yeasts.[16]

■ They improve the efficiency of the digestive tract—when they are weakened, bowel function is poor.[17]

■ They help to recycle estrogen (a female hormone) which reduces the likelihood of menopausal symptoms.[18]

These two factors—symptom suppression and eradication of the friendly bacteria—are the reasons your immune system becomes weakened when you use antibiotics. The more weakened your immune system, the more vulnerable you are to developing chronic, recurring cystitis.

from being flushed and kept free of infectious agents. Delaying urination can also be a contributing factor because when the urine stays in

Practical Ways to Cleanse Your Colon

The following natural internal cleansing products are available without prescription, enabling you to accomplish a self-care detoxification program to cleanse your intestines as a preventive measure against digestive impairment and the growth of bacteria which can lead to UTIs.

A.M./P.M. Ultimate Cleanse™—This program is set up as a two-part vegetarian detoxification formula. It involves 29 cleansing herbs, amino acids, antioxidants, digestive enzymes, vitamins, and minerals, and five kinds of fiber. Both formulas are taken in the morning and evening, in gradually increasing dosages, for several weeks. Positive signs that the detoxification program is working include flu-like sensations, runny nose, transient pimples, headaches, "brainfog," and/or fatigue, all of which will pass in a day or two. "The goal is to stimulate, feed, and detoxify the complete internal body, not just the bowel," states the manufacturer.

Nature's Pure Body Program™—This program is a blend of 27 herbs specifically chosen for their ability to flush toxins out of the organs and old fecal matter from the intestines. There are two sets of pills: colon and whole-body blends. Users start with one colon and three whole-body pills taken twice daily with water,

30 minutes before breakfast and 30 minutes before dinner.

The colon pills can be increased to three or more pills twice a day, until the bowels move twice daily; the whole-body pills are increased to 4-7, taken two times daily. Users need to double their intake of pure water (to at least 64 ounces daily), take one day off from the pills every week, and take a daily multivitamin. The program is designed to last about 30 days, although first-time users may find that three courses are required for complete inner cleansing and detoxification.

Cleanse Thyself™—This self-care colon cleansing program from Arise & Shine enables you to "clean your entire alimentary canal from your tongue to your stomach, to your organs, all the way down to your colon," says its manufacturer. The results of a saliva test to determine pH dictate the user's starting point among the program's four progressively more intense detoxifying phases. The program includes liquid bentonite shakes (a purifying clay), psyllium husk powder (a fibrous bulking agent), liquid vitamins and minerals, an herbal laxative (containing plantain, Cascara sagrada, barberry, peppermint, sheep sorrel, fennel seed, ginger root, myrrh gum, red raspberry, rhubarb root, goldenseal, and lobelia), dietary restrictions, and copious amounts of pure water.

For more about **A.M./P.M. Multi-Cleanse™**, contact: Nature's Secret, 4 Health, Inc., 5485 Conestoga Court, Boulder, CO 80301; tel: 303-546-6306; fax: 303-546-6416. For **Nature's Pure Body Program™**, contact: Pure Body Institute of Beverly Hills, 423 East Ojai Avenue #107, Ojai, CA 93023; tel: 800-952-7873 (orders) or 805-653-5448 (customer service); fax: 805-653-0373. For **Cleanse Thyself™**, contact: Arise & Shine, 401 Berry Street, P.O. Box 1439, Mt. Shasta, CA 96067; tel: 916-926-0891 or 800-688-2444; fax: 916-926-8866.

the bladder too long, it gives bacteria a chance to build up, says Agatha Thrash, M.D., a medical pathologist in Seale, Alabama.[19] Therefore, as preventive measures, it is advisable to urinate at the first urge, rather than to hold it, and to drink sufficient fluids.

For women who are prone to UTIs, many experts define "sufficient" as two quarts of water daily. A portion of that amount can consist of unsweetened cranberry or blueberry juice. In addition to providing fluid, these juices contain hippuric acid, a natural antibiotic which keeps problem bacteria from adhering to the wall of the bladder.[20] Coffee, tea, and alcohol should not be factored into the two-quart requirement because they have the opposite effect of water and other flushing fluids; they cause dehydration and concentrate the urine, making it more acidic.

Foods that foster the overgrowth of the yeast *Candida albicans* in the intestines can also contribute to cystitis by weakening the immune system and making the intestines a breeding ground for bacteria.

Drinking two quarts of fluid daily is a good preventive practice to establish. At the first sign of infection, you should increase your water intake immediately. Drink at least six to eight 8-ounce glasses of water daily if you are under 50 years old, increase to ten glasses daily if you are older than 50, and 12 glasses daily if you are over 60, advises Dr. Thrash.

For more about **cranberry juice**, see this chapter, pp. 219-222. For more about the **anti-*Candida* diet** and for **general anti-cystitis dietary suggestions**, see this chapter, pp. 218-222. For more about **bowel detoxification**, see "Practical Ways to Cleanse Your Colon," this chapter, p. 210.

7) Diet

Foods and beverages that are too spicy or acidic can irritate the bladder, making it more susceptible to infection. Foods linked to a worsening of cystitis include tomatoes, citrus fruits, strawberries, red grapes, potatoes, asparagus, raw carrots, spinach, dairy products, and red meat, among others.[21] Coffee and alcohol are the worst acidic offenders among beverages.

Foods that foster the overgrowth of the yeast *Candida albicans* in the intestines can also contribute to cystitis by weakening the immune system and making the intestines a breeding ground for bacteria. Yeast feeds on sugar, refined carbohydrates such as baked goods, and fermented foods such as vinegar and pickles. If *Candida* is a factor in your cystitis, it would be a good idea to eliminate these foods from your diet.

8) Chronic Constipation

When toxins build up in your intestinal tract, as happens with chronic constipation, your immune function is impaired, thereby making you susceptible to infection. The intestines are an integral part of the immune system, containing more immune (lymphoid) tissue than any other organ in the body. The lining of the intestines is the immune system's first line of defense; it acts as a filter for disease-causing microorganisms.

With chronic constipation, the filter cannot operate well and bacteria and other invaders are able to permeate the intestinal wall and enter the bloodstream. The immune system is then kept in a state of heightened activity, working to eliminate the foreign substances. Chronic constipation also further weakens immunity by contributing to nutritional deficiencies. Poor digestion of food results in poor absorption of nutrients by the body. Without the proper nutrients, the immune and other body systems cannot function at their full capacity.

Fecal buildup in the intestines can contribute to cystitis in a directly physical way as well, by putting pressure on the nearby bladder wall, impairing the bladder's ability to empty properly.[22] As mentioned previously, urine that sits in the bladder too long creates a bacterial breeding ground and opens the way for cystitis to develop.

9) Uterine Prolapse

If the pelvic floor muscles are weakened by pregnancy or surgery, it can lead to prolapse (sagging) of the uterus. As with chronic constipation or a contraceptive diaphragm that is too large, the pressure this exerts on the bladder wall can result in incomplete emptying of the bladder. Once again, stagnant urine in the bladder creates an ideal climate for bacteria.[23]

10) Hormonal Changes

Women in menopause have a tendency to develop cystitis; the incidence of UTIs increases by 1% to 25% each decade after menopause.[24] The reason is that as estrogen levels decline, bacteria are more prone to adhere to the bladder lining and vaginal tissue (from where they are easily transferred to the urethra). Hormonal changes can also lead to vaginal dryness, affecting the mucous membranes and making infection more likely.[25]

When estrogen levels drop, the pH (SEE QUICK DEFINITION) of the vagina alters and the number of good bacteria declines, says Kimberly Workowski, M.D., assistant professor of medicine in the Department of Infectious Diseases at Emory University in Atlanta. As stated earlier, subnormal levels of friendly bacteria open the way for disease-causing bacteria to flourish.

11) Underactive Thyroid

If your thyroid (see sidebar: "The Thyroid," p. 214) is sluggish (a condition called hypothyroidism) and not producing its normal level of hormones, it has a serious impact on your immune system, says Lita Lee, Ph.D., who frequently treats thyroid-generated problems.

Since adequate thyroid hormone is required for proper immune system function, frequent infections are common in people who have low thyroid function. It is not surprising, says Dr. Lee, that hypothyroid people are subject to chronic infections, including frequent colds, respiratory infections, bronchitis and pneumonia, chronic sore throats, sinusitis, recurrent otitis media (middle ear infection), tonsillitis, and recurrent bladder infections.

Female problems—infertility, miscarriage, fibrocystic breast disease, ovarian fibroids, cystic ovaries, endometriosis, PMS, menopausal symptoms—are usually caused by or aggravated by hypothyroidism which leads to hormonal imbalances such as estrogen dominance. Generally, a woman needs about ten times more progesterone than estrogen to avoid the toxic side effects of estrogen dominance. This can occur even with a normal estrogen level if progesterone is low, or with normal progesterone if the estrogen is high, says Dr. Lee.

What is the thyroid-estrogen connection? "Estrogen inhibits thyroid secretion. Progesterone stimulates it. Progesterone is made in the body from cholesterol if there is adequate thyroid hormone. Low thyroid function and the resulting estrogen dominance, no matter what the cause, has far-reaching consequences," Dr. Lee explains. This is why a weak immune system cannot mobilize the necessary resources to prevent bacteria from multiplying, making you susceptible to all kinds of infection, including UTIs.

12) Acidic Urine

There is presently no definitive word on the exact role of urine pH (SEE QUICK DEFINITION) in UTIs, although many practitioners suspect there is a connection.[26] However, it is clear that more acidic urine worsens the symptoms of urethritis and cystitis. It is the acid in urine which causes the burning sensation with urination. In addition, some patients have found that eating an acidic diet causes a flare-up of their symptoms.[27]

As a result, most alternative medicine physicians, such as noted natural medicine specialist Michael Murray, N.D., of Bellevue, Washington, recommend that you

QUICK DEFINITION

The term **pH**, which means "potential hydrogen," represents a scale for the relative acidity or alkalinity of a solution. Acidity is measured as a pH of 0.1 to 6.9, alkalinity is 7.1 to 14, and neutral pH is 7.0. The numbers refer to how many hydrogen atoms are present compared to an ideal or standard solution. Normally, blood is slightly alkaline, at 7.35 to 7.45; urine pH can range from 4.8 to 8.0, but is usually somewhat acidic, with a normal reading between 5.0 and 6.0.

The Thyroid

The thyroid gland, one of the body's seven endocrine glands, is located just below the larynx in the throat, with interconnecting lobes on either side of the trachea. The thyroid is the body's metabolic thermostat, controlling body temperature, energy use, and, for children, the body's growth rate. The thyroid controls the rate at which organs function and the speed with which the body uses food; it affects the operation of all body processes and organs. Of the hormones synthesized in and released by the thyroid, T3 (triiodothyronine) represents 7%, and T4 (thyroxine) accounts for almost 93% of the thyroid's hormones active in all of the body's processes. Iodine is essential to forming normal amounts of thyroxine. The secretion of both these hormones is regulated by thyroid-stimulating hormone, or TSH, secreted by the pituitary gland in the brain. The thyroid also secretes calcitonin, a hormone required for calcium metabolism.

Hypothyroidism is a condition of low or underactive thyroid gland function that can produce numerous symptoms. Among the 47 clinically recognized symptoms: fatigue, depression, lethargy, weakness, weight gain, low body temperature, chills, cold extremities, general inappropriate sensation of cold, infertility, rheumatic pain, menstrual disorders (excessive flow, cramps), repeated infections, colds, upper respiratory infections, skin problems (itching, eczema, psoriasis, acne, dry, coarse, or scaly skin, skin pallor), memory disturbances, concentration difficulties, paranoia, migraines, oversleep, "laziness," muscle aches and weakness, hearing disturbances, burning/prickling sensations, anemia, slow reaction time and mental sluggishness, swelling of the eyelids, constipation, labored or difficult breathing, hoarseness, brittle nails, and poor vision. A resting body temperature (measured in the armpit) *below* 97.8° F indicates hypothyroidism; menstruating women should take the underarm temperature only on the second and third days of menstruation.

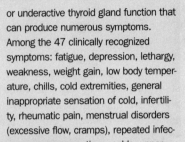

For more about **hypothyroidism,** see Chapter 5: Infertility, pp. 163-165, and Chapter 1: Menstrual Problems, pp. 24-26.

keep your urine alkaline (normal urine pH is slightly acidic). "The more alkaline your urine, the better," say homeopaths Andrew Lockie, M.D., of London, England, and Nicola Geddes, M.D., of Edinburgh, Scotland. They prescribe a teaspoon of baking soda (an alkaline) in a glass of water twice a day to accomplish this. A bowl of vegetable broth

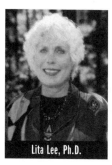

Lita Lee, Ph.D.

"Low thyroid function and the resulting estrogen dominance, no matter what the cause, has far-reaching consequences," Dr. Lee explains. **"This is why a weak immune system cannot mobilize the necessary resources to prevent bacteria from multiplying."**

or a glass of Effercitrate (available at pharmacies), taken daily, will produce the same effect, according to Drs. Lockie and Geddes.[28]

People who have high blood pressure or heart conditions should not take baking soda because of its high salt content. Try the other natural remedies or consult your practitioner.

Larrian Gillespie, M.D., concurs with the effort to alkalinize the urine as treatment for UTI, and prescribes a strict low-acid diet—avoiding red meat, alcohol, citrus fruits, sugar, coffee, and spicy foods. For cystitis prevention, she recommends drinking a glass of water with a half teaspoon of baking soda in it before eating a meal that includes any known bladder irritants. Baking soda can neutralize acid foods.[29] Carolyn Dean, M.D., of New York City, author of several women's health books, uses baking soda for acute cystitis relief. As soon as symptoms begin, drink a glass of water containing ¼ to ½ teaspoon of baking soda, and repeat every 30 minutes until symptoms are relieved, advises Dr. Dean.[30]

Not all acid foods create acidic urine and not all alkaline foods create alkaline urine. Orange juice, for example, is acid when you drink it, but it makes your urine more alkaline.[31] To bypass the confusion and because foods react individually in each person's body, urologist Kristene Whitmore, M.D., of Philadelphia, Pennsylvania, suggests that cystitis sufferers monitor their own urine pH by dipping litmus paper or nitrazine paper strips (available from pharmacies) into a sample of their urine several times a day. The papers turn different colors to indicate relative pH values. Pink litmus paper, for example, will turn blue if the urine is alkaline. In this way, cystitis sufferers can see what effect different foods have on their urine and change their diets to achieve a more alkaline pH.[32]

13) Energy Blockages

If you hold back on urinating even when your bladder is full, or if you wear underclothing that is too tight, this prevents the normal circula-

As soon as cystitis symptoms begin, drink a glass of water containing ¼ to ½ teaspoon of baking soda, and repeat every 30 minutes until symptoms are relieved, advises Dr. Carolyn Dean.

tion of energy in the body. The same is true of chronic stress and anxiety, which create tense muscles, irregular breathing, and blockages of the flow of energy to important organs such as the stomach. Energy blockages mean those body parts or organs will not have the normal vitality or *qi* (SEE QUICK DEFINITION) available to defend themselves against infection.[33]

QUICK DEFINITION

Qi (pronounced *CHEE*) is a Chinese word variously translated to mean "vital energy," "essence of life," and "living force." In Chinese medicine, the proper flow of *qi* along energy channels (meridians) within the body is crucial to a person's health and vitality. There are many types of *qi*, classified according to source, location, and function (such as activation, warming, defense, transformation, and containment). Within the body, *qi* and blood are closely linked, as each is considered to flow along with the other. The manipulation and readjustment of *qi* to treat disease and ensure maximum health benefit is the basic principle of acupuncture, although other remedies and therapies can be used to influence *qi*.

Acupuncture meridians are specific pathways in the human body for the flow of life force or subtle energy, known as *qi* (pronounced *CHEE*). In most cases, these energy pathways run up and down both sides of the body, and correspond to individual organs or organ systems, designated as Lung, Small Intestine, Heart, and others. There are 12 principal meridians and eight secondary channels. Numerous points of heightened energy, or *qi*, exist on the body's surface along the meridians and are called acupoints. There are more than 1,000 acupoints, each of which is potentially a place for acupuncture treatment.

This concept is a basic principle of energy medicine, a practice that uses energy fields—electrical, magnetic, sonic, acoustic, microwave, and infrared—to screen for or treat health conditions. Several different alternative therapies fall under the category of energy medicine, including acupuncture (SEE QUICK DEFINITION), which is based on a network of energy channels called meridians. Therapeutic touch, which is increasingly employed in hospitals, is also an energy medicine. Here, practitioners use their hands to sense and correct energy blockages in the patient's body; their hands are conduits for healing energy.

In addition to creating energy blockages, stress and anxiety deplete your energy reserves by increasing nervous system activity. This places more demand on the kidneys to filter adrenaline. Adrenaline is the hormone produced by your adrenal glands (one gland rests atop each kidney) in stressful situations to stimulate your "fight or flight" response. Designed to mobilize your body resources in the presence of danger, this response is meant to be a short-term event. However, with the constant stress and anxiety of modern life, many people are living in a near-constant state of "fight or flight." Under these circumstances of tremendous demand, your body becomes fatigued and your systems begin to break down, increasing the chance of infection.[34]

14) Unexpressed Anger or Resentment

Many practitioners, especially those versed in either homeopathy or

For more about **acupuncture and how blockages in energy flow create illness**, see "Success Story: Acupuncture Helps Couple Conceive," Chapter 5: Infertility, pp. 181-183.

Chinese medicine, emphasize that along with bacterial infection, there is an emotional component to cystitis, especially when it recurs. The colloquial expression "pissed off" may be more true than vulgar in describing the nature of this emotional component.

Often there is unexpressed, even unacknowledged, anger and resentment underlying cystitis, as if these strong emotions tainted the urine, making it burn as physical compensation for the unarticulated anger. Many times these emotions are focused upon a sexual partner or close friend. In the body's wisdom, the woman's UTI not only metaphorically expresses her irritation, but also conveniently punishes her partner by making it too painful to have sexual intercourse. Getting in touch with emotions you may not be acknowledging is an important first step in disarming this factor in your illness.

While many holistic physicians have observed that anger and resentment are commonly linked to UTIs, there is no formula to the emotional component of an individual's illness. The following case from women's health expert Christiane Northrup, M.D., of Yarmouth, Maine, illlustrates how another repressed emotion helped create chronic urinary tract infections and how uncovering the emotion led to reversing the condition.

Success Story: The Emotion Behind the Cystitis

Elaine, in her early thirties, came to Dr. Northrup complaining of recurrent cystitis and herpes outbreaks whenever she had sexual relations with her new boyfriend. The UTIs and herpes were in addition to a long history of vaginal and pelvic pain, including pain with sexual intercourse (dyspareunia). Elaine had divorced her husband a few years earlier. During her marriage and afterward, she had tried minor surgical treatments, standard medical care, a macrobiotic diet, and yoga, but the vaginal pain persisted. Now, with the cystitis and herpes, she was upset and uncertain as to what kinds of changes—nutrition, lifestyle, treatments—she should make to have a healthy sex life.

Elaine already had medications for the current case of cystitis and herpes, so Dr. Northrup let her continue with those to alleviate the symptoms. In the meantime, she counseled Elaine to "stay with the despair she was feeling and not instantly jump to the what-should-I-do-to-fix-it mode," to just let herself experience the depth of her feelings over the next few weeks. One day, spontaneously, Elaine had a flashback image from when she was in the womb. "She remembered the feeling of her father's penis against the amniotic sac," says Dr. Northrup.

Often there is unexpressed, even unacknowledged, anger and resentment underlying cystitis, as if these strong emotions tainted the urine, making it burn as physical compensation for the unarticulated anger.

"She felt clearly and viscerally her mother's disgust and 'just get this over with' indifference. Elaine told me, 'I feel as though I inherited my mother's sexual revulsion before I was born.'" Over the next few days, Elaine allowed herself to experience the emotions stimulated by the womb memory. Then, gradually, she began to notice her pelvic pain and vaginal pain with intercourse were easing. Over the next few months, the pain greatly diminished and it continued to do so after that.

Dr. Northrup states that the deeper healing sometimes takes months or years, due to the programming that gets embedded in the body from such memories. But the important first step, which Elaine took, is to become more in touch with your feelings.[35]

Alternative Medicine Therapies for Cystitis/UTI

Once you have an idea of the factors which may be contributing to your urinary tract infection, you can begin taking steps to correct these factors. As you learned in the previous section, some steps can be accomplished on your own. Others will require the assistance of a practitioner. This section provides information on a range of alternative medicine therapies which can help you eliminate your UTIs and prevent a recurrence. Included are natural self-help techniques which can give you fast relief of your symptoms without detrimental side effects.

Dietary Changes

As discussed under factors that contribute to urinary tract infections, intake of plenty of fluids along with a diet that avoids urine-acidifying foods and emphasizes urine-alkalinizing foods are recommended for both the elimination and prevention of UTIs. However, Drs. Lockie and Geddes caution that if a *Candida albicans* (SEE QUICK DEFINITION) overgrowth is an element in your urethritis or cystitis, you may not want to alkalinize your diet too much, as the yeast thrive in an alkaline environment.[36]

In addition to acidic foods, foods which are high in the amino acids phenylalanine, tryptophan, tyrosine, and tyramine can also irritate the bladder of patients with hypersensitive symptoms, according to Dr. Larrian Gillespie. She suggests avoiding bananas, cranberries, pineapple, avocados, aspartame, figs, yogurt, chocolate, and citrus fruits.

For UTI sufferers, Joseph E. Pizzorno, Jr., N.D., a naturopathic physician and president of Bastyr University, a naturopathic medical college in Seattle, Washington, recommends a diet in which you restrict your calorie intake, avoid all simple sugars, refined carbohydrates (white breads and pasta), and full-strength fruit juices, and eat generous amounts of garlic and onion. Dr. Pizzorno also recommends drinking at least 64 ounces of pure water or unsweetened liquid daily. This can include 16 ounces of unsweetened cranberry or blueberry juice.[37]

The refined carbohydrate restrictions are also part of the anti-*Candida* diet recommended by William G. Crook, M.D., author of *The Yeast Connection and the Woman*. In addition to eliminating simple sugars, soft drinks, ready-to-eat cereals, corn syrup, and white bread and other white flour products, Dr. Crook advises avoiding the following foods: hydrogenated and partially hydrogenated oils; yeast-feeding foods and beverages, including dried fruits, mushrooms, condiments, alcohol, juices (except for freshly squeezed), leavened breads, bagels, pastries, pretzels, and pizza. Instead, eat vegetables and grain alternatives (such as amaranth and quinoa) and use unrefined oils such as flaxseed, canola, and olive.[38] (For more anti-yeast dietary recommendations, see sidebar: "Anti-Candida Diet," p. 221.)

Cranberry Juice: To Drink or Not to Drink?

Cranberry juice is prescribed by many physicians for urinary tract infections. However, there is slight disagreement over this practice. Some say the juice is to be avoided because it increases urine acidity. Larrian Gillespie, M.D., a proponent of this view, states that hippuric acid (a component of cranberries) "only adds more acid to the urine, which in turn, increases the burning sensation." She claims that cranberry juice may be helpful to prevent an infection, but if you already have one, it only makes matters worse.

Michael Murray, N.D., refutes this, maintaining that you would have

QUICK DEFINITION

Candida albicans is a yeast-like fungus found widely in nature, in the soil, on vegetables and fruits, and in the human body. It is frequently present in small quantities in the intestines and in a woman's vagina. When its numbers are few, *Candida* is generally not harmful to the human body. A *Candida* overgrowth, a condition called candidiasis, can become pathogenic and cause allergic reactions throughout the body. These reactions can lead to a wide range of symptoms, including depression, fatigue, weight gain, anxiety, rashes, headaches, and muscle cramping.

For more about **acidic conditions within the body**, see "Inadequate Fluid Intake," pp. 208-211, "Diet," p. 211, and "Acidic Urine," pp. 213-215, this chapter. For more about *Candida*, see Chapter 2: Endometriosis, pp. 76-77. For more about **antibiotics**, see "Why Antibiotics Won't Cure Cystitis," this chapter, p. 209.

A Purifying Fast for Cystitis

A diet to purify the kidneys, bladder, and urethra can be useful in the treatment of both acute and chronic cystitis, according to acupuncturist and psychologist Jacqueline Young. She recommends the following regimen which is best conducted under the guidance of a qualified practitioner:[40]

Stage 1: Liquid Fast

For five to seven days, eat no solid foods and drink the following daily:

- Parsley tea (diuretic, i.e., increases urine flow): as desired
- Watermelon seed tea (purifies): according to thirst
- Unsweetened cranberry juice (diuretic; prevents bacteria from sticking to the walls of the bladder and urethra): up to 250 ml twice a day
- Apple cider vinegar, water, and pure honey (for general cleansing): one cup three times daily

Stage 2: Reintroduction of Solids

For the next seven to ten days, or until, condition clears, eat and drink according to the following regimen:

- Continue to drink eight or more glasses of the liquids listed above, while refraining from tea, coffee, alcohol, or carbonated drinks. Freshly made vegetable juices can be added because they help alkalinize the body.
- Avoid all dairy and animal products, including eggs; stick to vegetarian foods.
- Avoid salt; use garlic for flavor.
- Eat plenty of the following: fresh vegetables steamed or simmered, especially asparagus, celery, parsnips, and carrots; whole grains; salads including parsley and watercress; baked potatoes; kidney and adzuki beans.

After this period, reintroduce other foods gradually. Continue to avoid large amounts of animal protein as it overtaxes the kidneys.

Reprinted from *The Natural Way: Cystitis* by Jacqueline Young. Copyright © Jacqueline Young, 1997. Used by permission of Element Books, Inc.

to drink at least a quart of cranberry juice at one time for it to acidify the urine. He affirms cranberry juice's effectiveness in cystitis treatment, but dispels a view commonly held by cranberry supporters—that it works because hippuric acid prevents the growth of bacteria. "The concentration of hippuric acid in the urine as a result of drinking cranberry juice is not sufficient to inhibit bacteria," he says. Instead, it works by preventing unwanted bacteria (typically *E. coli*, a fecal bacteria) from adhering to the bladder lining and initiating infection.[39]

More support for cranberry juice as a cystitis preventative comes from a study published in the *Journal of the American Medical Association*. The study tracked 153 women—all chronic UTI sufferers—over the course of six months; one group drank ten ounces daily of a commercially

Anti-*Candida* Diet

Acupuncturist and clinical psychologist Jacqueline Young, of Hertfordshire, England, outlines a diet designed to eliminate an overgrowth of *Candida albicans*:[43]

Eliminate from your diet for at least one month:

- All foods containing yeast, including bread, biscuits, and cakes. (Substitute rye crackers or 100% rye bread.)

- All fermented foods, such as vinegar, soy sauce, and pickled foods. (Make salad dressings with freshly squeezed lemon juice instead.)

- All forms of sugar and sugar products, including sweets, chocolates, honey, maple syrup, sweetened drinks, and sweetened yogurt.

- Milk and dairy products. (Use soy products instead.)

- All refined white flour products. (Use brown flour and whole grains instead.)

- All moldy foods, including mushrooms and old food. (Prepare fresh food whenever possible.)

- Alcohol, tea and coffee. (Use herbal teas and mineral water instead.)

- Foods with artificial sweeteners, colorings, preservatives, and additives. (Eat unadulterated fresh foods instead.)

Include in your diet:

- Plenty of fresh vegetables, salads, and whole grains.

- Garlic, crushed or finely sliced on salads or vegetables.

- Extra virgin, cold-pressed olive oil should be the only oil used.

- Moderate your intake of fruit: have none for the first week or so (due to the high sugar content) and then reintroduce gradually; limit to two fruits per day and avoid citrus and very sweet fruits.

Reprinted from *The Natural Way: Cystitis* by Jacqueline Young. Copyright © Jacqueline Young, 1997. Used by permission of Element Books, Inc.

---

available cranberry juice, while a control group drank a non-cranberry beverage. At the end of the study, the cranberry juice drinkers had reduced their chances of developing a urinary tract infection by 73%, as compared with the non-cranberry drinkers.[41]

Only unsweetened cranberry juice or a dry extract of cranberry juice in capsules should be used, according to Dr. Murray. Sweetened cranberry juice should be avoided since the sugars will enhance bacterial growth. Dr. Murray advises drinking 16 ounces of unsweetened cranberry juice (or the capsules as directed) at the *first* sign of symptoms.[42]

Nutritional Supplements

Joseph Pizzorno, Jr., N.D., typically recommends the following supplements in the event of a cystitis outbreak: vitamin C (500 mg every

Two Ways to Support Your Friendly Bacteria

The following are potent probiotic supplements which can help restore the healthy bacteria in your body.

Nature's Biotics™—Life Science Products of St. George, Utah, developed this blend of 61 nutrients, including at least six selectively bred strains of soil-based probiotic organisms. In addition, this supplement contains amino acids, phytoplanktons, plant pigments and enzymes, minerals, trace elements, essential fatty acids, and starches. Once the mixture makes contact with water, the friendly bacteria become active.

The product is intended to help remove waste, debris, and toxins from the intestines; it improves digestion and assimilation; it works against harmful molds, yeasts, fungi, and viruses; and it stimulates the immune system which in turn releases more B-lymphocytes. Researchers at the University of Washington School of Medicine found that microorganisms with therapeutic properties (probiotics) can be used successfully to treat and prevent select-ed urinary tract, vaginal, and intestinal infections including candidiasis.[44]

NutraFlora® (FOS)—A new approach to restoring the balance of intestinal flora was developed in Japan in the mid-1980s and is called prebiotics. It involves introducing nutrients that directly feed the beneficial bacteria already in place in a person's large intestine, most typically, *Bifidobacteria* and *Lactobacilli*. Japanese researchers determined that a naturally occurring form of carbohydrate, called fructo-oligosaccharides (FOS), found in certain foods in minute amounts, could be a perfect food for *bifidobacteria*.

FOS acts like an intestinal "fertilizer," selectively feeding the friendly microflora in the large intestine so that their numbers can usefully increase which, in turn, discourages the growth of unfriendly bacteria. Feeding the friendly bacteria is a crucial step in maintaining the correct balance of intestinal microflora. NutraFlora contains 95% pure FOS in dry powder form or as a syrup to be used as a dietary supplement.

For **Nature's Biotics™**, contact: Life Science Products, Inc., 321 North Mall Drive, Building F-201, St. George, UT 84790; tel: 801-628-4111 or 800-713-3888; fax: 801-628-6114. For more about **FOS** and **NutraFlora®**, contact: GTC Nutrition Company, 1400 West 122nd Avenue, Suite 110, Westminster, CO 80234; tel: 303-254-8012; fax: 303-254-8201.

For more about **probiotics**, see Chapter 7: Vaginitis, pp. 250-251.

two hours); vitamin A (50,000 IU daily); zinc (30 mg daily); uva ursi, also known as bearberry or upland cranberry (¹/₂ tsp fluid extract or 1¹/₂ tsp tincture); and goldenseal (*Hydrastis canadensis*, ¹/₂ tsp fluid extract or 1¹/₂ tsp tincture).

Several other physicians recommend even higher doses of vitamin C. Robert Atkins, M.D., of New York City, and Ralph Golan,

M.D., of Seattle, Washington, suggest taking 1,000 mg every hour when a cystitis infection hits. Lower the dose slightly if you get diarrhea. Australian naturopath Judy Jacka, N.D., Grad.Dip.H.R.E. (England), recommends taking iron phosphate to reduce inflammation in the urethra, and sodium phosphate to promote alkalinity in the urine.[45]

Lactobacillus acidophilus and other friendly bacteria (SEE QUICK DEFINITION) are also useful supplements. They can help restore the bacterial balance in the urinary tract and vagina, which can in turn help drive out the infectious bacteria causing your UTI. In a study of 41 women with acute UTI, of those given vaginal suppositories of 500 mg of *acidophilus* twice a week for two weeks, then once a month for two months, only 21% had a recurrence of the infection compared to 47% given a placebo.[46] You can also add *acidophilus* to your diet by eating yogurt with live or active cultures.

Acupuncture

Acupuncture works well to relieve the pain and other symptoms of cystitis, as well as to correct underlying organ and energy imbalances. In a 1988 study reported in the *Journal of Urology*, 22 of 26 cystitis patients treated with acupuncture reported improvement of their symptoms. The study involved 52 women who had urinary frequency, urinary urgency, and pain with urination (dysuria).

Half the women received a sham acupuncture treatment; meaning, an acupuncture needle was inserted at a site on the body that was not a legitimate acupuncture point. For the other half of the study subjects, acupuncture needles were inserted at traditional acupuncture points specific to urinary problems. The women who received the legitimate acupuncture treatment had better and more efficient urinary function and a reduction in other symptoms. The researchers concluded that "acupuncture could be used as a simple and effective method to treat female patients with frequency, urgency, and dysuria."[47]

QUICK DEFINITION

Friendly bacteria, or probiotics, refer to beneficial microbes inhabiting the human gastrointestinal tract where they are essential for proper nutrient assimilation. The human body contains an estimated several trillion beneficial bacteria comprising over 400 species, all necessary for health. Among the more well known of these are *Lactobacillus acidophilus* and *Bifidobacterium bifidum.* Overly acidic bodily conditions, chronic constipation or diarrhea, dietary imbalances, consumption of highly processed foods, and the excessive use of antibiotics and hormonal drugs can interfere with probiotic function and even reduce the number of these microbes, setting up conditions for illness.

Acupuncture is an integrated healing system developed by the Chinese over 5,000 years ago and introduced in the United States in the mid-1800s. The treatment is administered by an acupuncturist using hair-thin, stainless-steel needles, generally presterilized and disposable; these are lightly inserted into the skin at any of over 1,000 locations on the body's surface, known as acupoints. Acupoints are places where vital energy, or *qi* (pronounced *CHEE*), can be accessed by acupuncturists to reduce, enhance, or redirect its flow. These acupoints exist on meridians, which are the body's specific pathways for the flow of energy. In most cases, these energy pathways relate to individual organs or organ systems, designated as Lung, Small Intestine, Heart, and others. There are 12 principal meridians and eight secondary channels. Acupuncture is employed for a wide variety of conditions (the World Health Organization counts 104), including pain relief, asthma, migraines, and arthritis.

Essential Oils

Aromatherapy's essential plant oils yield a practical solution for UTIs. The healing properties of the plants are powerfully concentrated in these oils, which can be utilized in massages and baths or taken orally.

Massage and Baths

Several essential plant oils can help ease your cystitis symptoms. At the first sign of symptoms, draw a hot bath, add 20 drops each of eucalyptus and sandalwood essential oils, and soak in the tub for ten minutes, advises Judith Jackson, an aromatherapist in Greenwich, Connecticut. Alternately, depending on your scent preference, juniper and thyme essential oils can be substituted for the eucalyptus and sandalwood oils (use the same dosage), says Jackson.[48]

Essential oils can also provide symptomatic relief through massage. A good massage oil combination for cystitis is three to four drops each of tea tree, sandalwood, and bergamot (or lavender) oils added to five teaspoons of a basic light massage oil such as sweet almond or grapeseed. Massage the mixture gently into your lower abdomen and back at least twice daily.[49]

Another good cystitis first-aid technique is to wipe the opening of your urethra after you urinate with a mixture of ten to 12 drops of tea tree oil in $3\frac{1}{2}$ ounces of cooled, boiled water. Shake the solution well before using, and apply with a soaked cotton swab.[50]

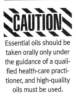

Essential Oils Taken Orally

Under careful supervision, essential oils can also be used orally to reverse urinary tract infections. This method worked well for Barbara, 43, a patient of Victor Marcial-Vega, M.D., of Coral Gables, Florida. She telephoned him one day, desperate for relief from a urinary tract infection accompanied by fevers, chills, and excruciating pain. Her condition had been growing worse for a week, she told him, and another doctor had already phoned in an antibiotic prescription to her pharmacy. Since Dr. Marcial-Vega prefers that his patients refrain from taking antibiotics whenever possible, he offered Barbara an alternative: a combination of essential oils taken orally, used in a bath, and inhaled.

On his instructions, Barbara added six drops each of lavender, tea tree, and myrrh essential oils to her bath water, then immersed herself in the solution for 20 minutes. By the time her husband returned from the pharmacy with the prescription antibiotics, Barbara was symptom free. Over the next few days, she took a blend of the oils of onion and garlic orally, a single drop on her tongue two to three times daily, and continued the aromatherapy baths, once daily. Four times a day, she also daubed a few drops of the lavender, tea tree, and myrrh oils on her palms and inhaled the aroma. To date, Barbara has not had a recurrence of the urinary tract infection, reports Dr. Marcial-Vega.

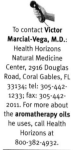

To contact **Victor Marcial-Vega, M.D.**: Health Horizons Natural Medicine Center, 2916 Douglas Road, Coral Gables, FL 33134; tel: 305-442-1233; fax: 305-442-2011. For more about the **aromatherapy oils** he uses, call Health Horizons at 800-382-4932.

Herbal Medicine

Herbs in forms other than as essential oils can also be useful for bladder infections. At the first sign of cystitis accompanied by pain and burning, David L. Hoffmann, B.Sc., M.N.I.M.H., of Sebastopol, California, past president and a founding member of the American Herbalist Guild in Boulder, Colorado, suggests taking 1 tsp, three times daily of a mixture of three herbal tinctures. The mixture includes one part each of tinctures of corn silk, bearberry (uva ursi), and buchu.

Tinctures are elixirs that result when fresh plant materials are steeped for six weeks or more in alcohol, allowing the essence and healing properties of the plant to be extracted by the liquor. They are available from herbalists or at health food stores. You can also make your own tinctures, says Hoffman. Chop up the fresh plants, put them in a jar, and fill it with 100-proof vodka or grain alcohol, he explains. Cap the jar tightly and let it stand for six weeks. Remove the plants and use the tincture as per the directions above or instructions from your herbalist.[51]

Alternately, you can drink a hot herbal infusion to ease symptoms, says Hoffmann. An infusion is a beverage—like a tea but stronger—made from large amounts of dried herbs brewed for a long time (see sidebar: "How to Prepare an Herbal Infusion," p. 229). For cystitis, Hoffmann recommends combining equal parts of dried marshmallow leaf, corn silk, couch grass, and bearberry and drinking a cup of the infusion four to five times a day.

Dr. Larrian Gillespie recommends corn silk as well, in the form of tea. Its effectiveness for cystitis is due to the fact that it contains silica which acts as a soothing coating to inflamed bladder tissue, she says. During the acute phase of the cystitis, drink three to four cups of corn silk tea daily (spaced three hours apart) to help reduce burning with

Home Remedies
for Urinary Tract Infections

If you've ever had a urinary tract infection (UTI), chances are that someone—a friend, a co-worker, your mother—has suggested drinking cranberry juice. Cranberry is now widely recognized as an effective remedy for UTIs, but it was the Pequot Indians of New England who first used the berries to promote urinary tract health. In *Natural Health Secrets From Around the World*, authors Glenn Geelhoed, M.D., and Jean Barilla, M.S., list additional "home remedies" for UTIs:[53]

Nasturtium—In Germany, infections of the urinary tract and bladder are treated with the flower of the nasturtium plant, believed to work as an antibiotic.

Sandalwood—Pakistanis have long used sandalwood to ease the often painful symptoms of urinary tract infection; add a few drops of sandalwood to a warm bath to soothe external itching and irritation.

Parsley—Although Dutch men often drink parsley tea to avoid prostate problems, the vegetable can also help prevent UTIs. Parsley acts as a diuretic, promoting frequent urination and thus flushing excess bacteria from the urinary tract.

Bearberry (uva ursi)—Native Americans originally used the leaf of this plant to treat inflammation of the bladder and kidneys. Bearberry is now available in leaf, powder, and capsule form.

Raspberries—This old English remedy for UTIs consists of douching with a blend of red raspberry tea, black currant, witch hazel leaves, and powdered myrrh. This herbal douche acts as an antifungal and antiseptic.

urination, she suggests.

Ralph Golan, M.D., of Seattle, Washington, author of *Optimal Wellness*, recommends taking herbal and vitamin capsules called Arbu-Tone from PhytoPharmica (one or two capsules, five to seven times a day when UTI symptoms are acute). Arbu-Tone contains vitamin B6 and magnesium to support kidney and bladder function, and potassium and sodium for fluid regulation and balance. The formula also contains the diuretic herbs bearberry and goldenrod, which help to flush bacteria out of the urinary system.[52]

Carolyn DeMarco, M.D., of Toronto, Ontario, prefers an herbal tincture designed by the European herbalist Alfred Vogel. The tincture, distributed to health food stores by the Bioforce company, is called CYS Complex and contains a mixture of St. John's wort, berberi, echinacea, fragrant sumach, balm, yarrow, belladonna, aspen, and flowering oat. At the first sign of symptoms, start taking 15 drops, three times daily, 15 minutes before meals, and continue the treatment for two weeks, says Dr. DeMarco.

Fresh parsley, eaten raw or brewed as a tea, is "a time-honored remedy for cystitis," say Julian and Susan Scott, in *Natural Medicine for Women*. They recommend eating fresh parsley chopped or grated as a garnish. Dried parsley is less effective.[54] Parsley tea, which is diuretic and thus flushes out the urinary system, can be made by steeping a bunch of fresh parsley in several quarts of boiling water for about 20 minutes, then removing the parsley and drinking the tea hot or cold. Chinese diuretic and antibacterial herbs can also be helpful. For example, a common Chinese medicine herb prescribed for UTIs is akebia, which is available in a potent herbal formula called Akebia 14 (from Seven Forests), among other preparations.

Homeopathy

In using homeopathy (SEE QUICK DEFINITION) to permanently eliminate your cystitis, you will need to consult a classical homeopath who can prescribe a constitutional remedy, which is one that corrects imbalances in all aspects—from physiological to emotional and even genetic—of your individual make-up. However, for relief of acute cystitis, you can try the following remedies, according to homeopaths Andrew Lockie, M.D., and Nicola Geddes, M.D. Take them in the 30C potency every half hour for up to ten dosages:[55]

■ For cystitis symptoms that are worse before menstrual periods, with fluid retention and joint pain—*Pulsatilla*

■ For cystitis symptoms that are worse before menstrual periods—*Sepia, Lycopodium*

■ For cystitis symptoms and weakness that are worse before menstrual periods—*Calcarea*

■ For cystitis symptoms and weakness, fluid retention, and chilliness—*Arsenicum*

■ For cystitis symptoms and fluid retention with joint pains—*Nux vomica*

■ For cystitis symptoms and fluid retention—*Mercurius, Belladonna*

■ For cystitis symptoms and weakness—*Causticum, Conium*

■ For cystitis symptoms that are worse with heat and better with cold—*Apis*

Carolyn Dean, M.D., N.D., recommends taking the homeopathic remedy *Staphasagria* in the 6C or 30C potency every hour at the first sign of cystitis-like irritation or other symptoms after sexual

For **Arbu-Tone**, contact: PhytoPharmica, 825 Challenger Drive, Green Bay, WI 54311; tel: 800-553-2370 (practitioners) or 800-376-7889 (consumers). For **Akebia 14** by Seven Forests (available by prescription only through licensed Chinese medicine practitioners), contact: Institute for Traditional Medicine, 2017 S.E. Hawthorne Blvd., Portland, OR 97214; tel: 800- 544-7504 or 503-233-4907; fax: 503-233-1017.

QUICK DEFINITION

Homeopathy was founded in the early 1800s by German physician Samuel Hahnemann. Today, an estimated 500 million people worldwide receive homeopathic treatment; in Britain, homeopathy enjoys royal patronage. Homeopathy is now practiced according to two differing concepts. In classical homeopathy, only one single-component remedy is prescribed at a time, in a potency specifically adjusted to the patient; the physician waits to see the results before prescribing anything further. In complex homeopathy, typified by *Hepar compositum*, a prescription involves multiple substances given at the same time, usually in low potencies.

intercourse. For general cystitis symptoms, take the remedies *Cantharis* or *Causticum* in the 6C or 30C potency, every hour after urinary problems begin, Dr. Dean advises.[56]

To contact **Tori Hudson, N.D.:** A Woman's Time: Menopause Options and Natural Medicine, 2067 N.W. Lovejoy Street, Portland, OR 97209; tel: 503-222-2322; fax: 503-222-0276.

Tori Hudson, N.D., author of *Gynecology and Naturopathic Medicine* (TK Publications, 1992) and the forthcoming *Encyclopedia of Women's Health and Natural Medicine* (Keats Publishing, 1998), is also a featured physician in *An Alternative Medicine Definitive Guide to Cancer* (Future Medicine Publishing, 1997; ISBN 1-887299-01-7); to order, call 800-333-HEAL.

Water Therapy

Contrast sitz baths (pelvic immersion in shallow tubs of alternating hot and cold water) can relieve cystitis pain and improve circulation in the pelvic area, states Tori Hudson, N.D., a naturopathic physician and director of A Woman's Time: Menopause Options and Natural Medicine clinic in Portland, Oregon.

To prepare the baths, find two basins or tubs that you can sit in comfortably (you need to be able to immerse your pelvis in water). Fill one with hot water to about the level of your navel, and the other with cold water to the same level. Soak first in the hot bath for three to five minutes; then in the cold water for 30 seconds. Repeat three times, finishing with cold water. (Hot and cold compresses can be substituted if you don't have the tubs). Perform this treatment once or twice daily.[57]

Bottle Washing— A Simple Hygienic Technique

Good hygiene can be useful not only for preventing cystitis but also for treating it. By keeping the body as clean as possible, you can prevent additional bacteria from reaching the affected area and compounding an existing infection. The following cleansing routine should be performed after every bowel movement if possible:[58]

1) Using soft toilet paper (to avoid chemicals in dyes, white is preferable), wipe your bottom from front to back.

2) Wash your hands.

3) Lather the fingers of one hand with a non-perfumed soap. Use your lathered fingers to wash your anal (not vaginal) area. Leave the soap on.

4) Wash your hands.

5) Fill a small bottle with warm water. Then, sitting on the toilet, lean back, and slowly pour the water over the urethral and vaginal openings, using your free hand to wash inside the folds of skin.

6) Pat dry with a soft towel after all the soap has been washed away. Don't use a towel that is also available for general drying; use a special towel kept only for this procedure.

How to Prepare an Herbal Infusion

You can buy dried herbs at many health food stores or herb shops. It's helpful to know what part of the plant—root, bark, leaves, flowers, or seeds or berries—you're buying because some parts require longer brewing times than others. Noted herbalist Susun Weed of Woodstock, New York, recommends that you prepare the infusions in pint or quart jars with tight lids. A teapot can also be used but is not as effective. Boil the water, pour it into a jar, add herbs, and cover tightly. Let it brew for the specified time. Remove the herbs and drink. The following are brewing guidelines:[59]

- For roots and bark of plant: add 1 oz dried herb to a pint of water and brew for at least eight hours.
- For leaves of a plant: add 1 oz dried herb to a quart of water and brew for at least four hours.
- For flowers of a plant: Add 1 oz dried herb to a quart of water and brew for no more than two hours.
- For seeds and berries of a plant: Add 1 oz herb to a pint of water and brew for no more than 30 minutes.

Interstitial Cystitis Requires Its Own Treatment

As mentioned previously, interstitial cystitis (IC) is not a bacterial infection, but an inflammation in the bladder walls. As such, treatment requires a different approach. While many of the symptoms are the same as bacterial cystitis, IC is also characterized by frequent muscle spasms and pain with movement.

The condition may have started with a bladder infection, or have a bladder infection occurring at the same time, but once IC develops, antibiotics do not alleviate the symptoms. Curiously, IC may also be accompanied by endometriosis, another painful condition, in which cells from the lining of the uterus migrate to abnormal locations and bleed with menstruation.

Given the symptomatic overlap with cystitis and further confusion created by a concurrent bacterial infection, diagnosis of IC is often difficult. A standard conventional method of diagnosis is an uncomfortable procedure called bladder hydrodistention (literally, distension with water). The bladder is filled with water to greater-than-normal capacity via a cytoscope (an instrument with two tubes—one for transfering fluids and the other having a light and viewing lenses). The patient holds the water in the bladder for two to seven minutes, and then releases it. After

Arginine for Interstitial Cystitis Relief

Research has found that the amino acid L-arginine can significantly reduce the symptoms of interstitial cystitis (IC). Ten patients with IC took 1.5 g of L-arginine orally every day for six months. At the end of that period, they reported a significant decrease in the discomfort accompanying urination, a decrease in urinary frequency both during the day and at night, and less pain in the lower abdomen, vagina, and urethra. IC patients may lack a urinary substance called nitric oxide synthase, a chemical that manufactures nitric oxide from L-arginine. Nitric oxide is a vasodilator (opens up and relaxes the blood vessels) and possibly affects immune reaction as well.[60]

Both of those functions are important to interstitial cystitis patients, to reduce inflammation and the painful spasms in the pelvic area. Supplementing with L-arginine appears to replenish the body's stores of nitric oxide synthase which may account for the positive results, the researchers conclude.[61]

CAUTION

If you have herpes, taking L-arginine is inadvisable because it can exacerbate herpes symptoms.

the water drains, the physician uses the viewing tube in the cytoscope to inspect the bladder wall for hemorrhages (called glomerulations), scarring, or ulcers, which typify interstitial cystitis.

The conventional medical treatment for IC is equally invasive and uncomfortable. It involves delivering DMSO (dimethyl sulfoxide, a liquid anti-inflammatory agent) into the patient's bladder via a catheter on a weekly basis for six weeks or more. The DMSO solution is actually a chemical "cocktail," containing steroids and pain-killing drugs as well. It must be held in the bladder for 30 minutes.

Alternative medicine practitioners prefer to avoid such invasive techniques, relying instead on symptom patterns to reach an IC diagnosis and treatment programs addressing the underlying imbalances rather than focusing only on pain relief. Interstitial cystitis is a complex disorder and therefore often requires a complex, multilayered treatment approach. However, once the underlying imbalances and toxicities in the body are identified and the right combination of therapies are applied, the results can be dramatic, as demonstrated by the following case.

Success Story: Supplements and Diet Reverse Interstitial Cystitis

When Suzanne, 47, consulted Diana Brady, M.A., C.N.C. (certified nutritional consultant), a health counselor at the Ultimate Health

Center in Asheville, North Carolina, she had been experiencing constant severe pelvic pain and spasms for over two years. The pain was located over her bladder and along the right and left sides of her abdomen. Suzanne also felt the urge to urinate every 15 to 30 minutes during the day and every 15 minutes at night. Laboratory urine tests had revealed a bladder infection of *E. coli* and *Enterococcus* bacteria.

Suzanne also had abdominal cramping, spasms, pain and bloating after meals, and was in a constant state of exhaustion. Emotionally, she alternated between depression and anxiety and had frequent panic attacks. Her breasts were tender and sore, she had vaginal bleeding, and she was sensitive to chemicals in the environment. These three symptoms are indicative of an estrogen excess (too much estrogen in ratio to progesterone), says Brady, adding that the majority of her IC patients have this imbalance. Suzanne was menopausal and had been on estrogen in the form of an estrogen patch, which delivers hormones through the skin.

She had taken repeated courses of antibiotics and steroids, with little alleviation of her symptoms. As a result of her condition, Suzanne was unable to work or travel, had no desire for food or sexual intercourse, and had trouble maintaining relationships, including her marriage.

Brady, who works under the supervision of David S. Bate, M.D., at the Ultimate Health Center, explains that Suzanne's condition was interstitial cystitis, with an accompanying bacterial infection. "Most interstitial cystitis patients have accompanying bacterial infections," says Brady. "In fact, experts think the bacterial infection *triggers* the interstitial cystitis, which may be a type of autoimmune reaction. It's frustrating for the patients because they can't tell which symptoms are the IC and which are the bacterial infection."

The IC diagnosis was established by Suzanne's symptom pattern, particularly the telltale bladder pain and spasms that she experienced with any jarring movement, such as jogging. Due to the obviousness of her symptoms, Brady concluded that testing through hydrodistention (see above) was not necessary. Along with the added complication of a bacterial infection, Brady suspected Suzanne had irritable bowel syndrome, based on her symptoms of abdominal bloating and cramping after meals, and candidiasis (an overgrowth of the yeast-like fungus *Candida albicans*), as evidenced by her exhaustion and overall discomfort. Her repeated antibiotic use probably contributed to all of these conditions.

At Brady's suggestion, the following tests were ordered for Suzanne:

Interstitial cystitis often requires a complex, multilayered treatment approach. However, once the underlying imbalances and toxicities in the body are identified and the right combination of therapies applied, the results can be dramatic.

For more about **endometriosis**, see Chapter 2: Endometriosis, pp. 68-98.

■ Great Smokies Diagnostic Laboratory Digestive Stool Analysis and *Candida* (blood) Serum Analysis: to assay digestive function and test for yeast antibodies and parasites

■ Trace Elements Inc. Tissue and Mineral Analysis of the Hair: to test for toxic metals, tissue mineral levels, and metabolic type

■ Great Smokies Diagnostic Laboratory Secretory IgA Saliva Test: to determine immune system status

Meanwhile, Brady started Suzanne on a special IC diet, eliminating foods containing the amino acids tyrosine, tryptophan, aspartate, and phenylalanine, and the compound tyramine (from tyrosine). These substances are precursors for the neurotransmitters (SEE QUICK DEFINITION) serotonin and norepinephrine, explains Brady. In IC, both serotonin and norepinephrine irritate the damaged bladder and cause pain.

The foods eliminated under this category included: broad beans, turkey, foods high in vitamin B3 and vitamin B6 such as white potatoes and peanuts (supplements containing these vitamins were eliminated as well), fermented foods, aged or ripened foods, sprouted foods, chocolate, and vitamins buffered with aspartate. Brady also eliminated other bladder-irritating foods: saccharine, the nightshade family (tomatoes, potatoes, eggplants), foods high in potassium such as bananas, foods containing MSG or oxalic acid (spinach, broccoli), and foods containing preservatives such as benzoic acid, sulfites, sulfates, nitrites, and nitrates.

Citrus fruits, coffee, alcohol, and carbonated beverages were cut out of Suzanne's diet to prevent acid "burn" in the bladder. Due to the possible candidiasis, Brady recommended that she limit her intake of refined and natural sugars and foods high in yeast. Suzanne was encouraged to eat: alkaline ash foods such as dark green vegetables, watermelon, and legumes; vegetable oils high in monounsaturated fats (olive and canola); whole grains such as brown rice, quinoa, millet, amaranth, spelt, and buckwheat; legumes such as garbanzo beans, northern beans, kidney beans, adzuki beans, pinto beans, and split peas; dairy products such as ricotta, cream cheese, and Armenian string cheese; nuts such as pine and pecan; organically grown chicken, veal, lamb, and beef as well as fish. Brady instructed her to drink aloe vera juice, chamomile or mint herbal teas, and eight glasses of pure water daily.

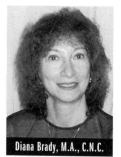

Diana Brady, M.A., C.N.C.

"Most interstitial cystitis patients have accompanying bacterial infections," says Diana Brady. "In fact, experts think the bacterial infection *triggers* the interstitial cystitis, which may be a type of autoimmune reaction."

In addition to the specific IC recommendations and the avoidance of bladder-irritating foods, the dietary changes were aimed at creating a more alkaline environment in Suzanne's body. An acid environment predisposes the body to develop a UTI and fosters the growth of an existing infection. The dietary plan would be subject to modification according to Suzanne's test results.

Next, Suzanne started the basic interstitial cystitis program as devised by the Ultimate Health Center, consisting of the following elements:

■ DMSO (SEE QUICK DEFINITION) gel with aloe vera: ½ to one teaspoon applied twice daily on the skin of the lower abdomen directly above the pubic hairline (the area over the bladder); the skin area should be cleansed first with hydrogen peroxide or alcohol to prevent any surface bacteria from being absorbed into the body.

■ Lehning's Anti-Anxiety Homeopathic Drops (a combination of about 20 homeopathic remedies by PhytoPharmica): ten to 30 drops as needed to relieve symptoms of urinary frequency, urinary urgency, and pelvic spasms; also useful for irritable bowel symptoms.

■ Amni's Fundamental Sulfur or MSM (SEE QUICK DEFINITION): one tablet three times daily, six days a week; for reduction of inflammation, detoxification, and cellular repair.

■ Floressence tea (contains eight herbs, including burdock root, watercress, kelp, turkish rhubarb, and slippery elm, among others): two

A **neurotransmitter** is a brain chemical with the specific function of enabling communications to happen between brain cells. Chief among the 100 identified to date are acetylcholine, gamma-aminobutyric acid (GABA), serotonin, dopamine, and norepinephrine. Acetylcholine is required for short-term memory and all muscle contractions. GABA works to stop excess nerve signals and thus keeps brain firings from getting out of control; serotonin does the same and helps produce sleep, regulate pain, and influence mood, although too much serotonin can produce depression. Norepinephrine is an excitatory neurotransmitter.

ounces of tea mixed with two ounces of distilled water, taken on an empty stomach, morning and night, six days a week; for pain reduction and cleansing the digestive tract.

For more about **antibiotics**, see "Why Antibiotics Won't Cure Cystitis," this chapter, p. 209. For more about **acid/alkaline balance**, see "Acidic Urine," this chapter, pp. 213-215.

DMSO, or dimethyl sulfoxide, is a simple by-product of wood, used to help relieve pain, reduce swelling and inflammation, slow bacterial growth, relax muscles, increase circulation, repair tissue damage, and enhance healing. It is believed able to penetrate living tissues without causing damage and to speed up certain chemical reactions. DMSO was first synthesized in 1866 by a Russian scientist; it was first widely publicized in the U.S. in 1964, when it was touted as "the closest thing to a wonder drug produced in the 1960s." The FDA opposed its use for nearly 20 years, finally relenting in 1979.

MSM (methyl sulfonal methane) is a natural form of sulfur found in all living organisms. Sulfur is vital to many body functions including carbohydrate metabolism, cell respiration, and maintaining pH balance. MSM in supplement form is derived from DMSO (dimethyl sulfoxide), a by-product of wood. MSM helps the body utilize vitamins, aids in detoxifying, improves blood circulation, and stabilizes blood sugar.

■ Inflazyme (contains magnesium carbonate, vitamin C, the digestive enzyme bromelain, mixed bioflavonoids [SEE QUICK DEFINITION], quercetin, and the amino acid L-cysteine): one tablet, twice daily on an empty stomach, seven days a week; for relief of urinary frequency and urgency and reduction of scar tissue in the bladder wall

■ Freeze-dried aloe vera capsules: 1,200 mg, three times daily; to heal the bladder lining.

■ Anti-bacterial supplements: colloidal silver (3 tsp, three times daily); Garlicinpro (one tablet, two times daily); powdered *acidophilus* (¼ tsp) plus powdered *bifidus* (¼ tsp) taken with Probioplex (½ tsp) three times daily before meals.

■ Epsom salt baths: one to 1½ cups of Epsom salt and 40 to 60 drops of grapefuit seed extract (a natural disinfectant) in a tub of hot water; baths as needed to soothe sore muscles and relieve achiness.

■ Capsin-HP Lotion (contains 0.075% capsaicin, the active ingredient of cayenne): applied on the back, from the base of the tailbone up along the spine to the top of the neck, every few hours until pain subsides; for pain relief, especially during a spasmodic attack. (If skin irritation results, over-the-counter capsaicin creams may be preferable as they usually contain only 0.025% capsaicin).

■ Ice packs: applied for 15 minutes to an hour on the lower abdomen, the area over the bladder, with paper towels between the ice pack and skin to avoid skin "burning;" for pain relief. (Ice packs are especially effective for the painful spasmodic attacks triggered by the jolts of traveling in a vehicle or on an airplane—jolting movements irritate the nerve endings in the already inflamed bladder. Attacks can occur up to five or six hours afterwards.)

After following this program for a few days, Suzanne felt better, reporting that she felt "normal" for two days in a row for the first time in two years, but she still had an "uncomfortable feeling" in her pelvic region. When the original laboratory test results came back two weeks later, they revealed that Suzanne had:

■ High levels of *Candida albicans* antibodies in the blood.

■ High levels of mercury and aluminum which deplete

the body of precious nutrients, tax the immune system, and cause a general bodywide weakening, all of which make it difficult for the body to heal infection and inflammation.

■ High levels of calcium and magnesium, but low levels of manganese, chromium, sodium, potassium, and silicon. Chromium and manganese are important minerals to fight yeast overgrowth. Sodium and potassium depletion can indicate adrenal and thyroid exhaustion. Silicon is important for immune function and bone strength. High levels of calcium and magnesium indicate a "slow" metabolic type.

■ Insufficient digestive enzymes; *Candida* and pollen in the stool, and high levels of the enzyme beta-glucuronidase (SEE QUICK DEFINITION), indicating imbalance in intestinal flora.

■ A strong immune system, in spite of all of the above.

On the basis of these test results, Brady added the following items to Suzanne's program:

■ Chlorella (green algae): two capsules, three times daily before meals (chlorella is difficult for some IC patients to tolerate); helps in elimination of mercury and other heavy metals

■ Inflazyme Forte (digestive enzymes): two with meals, three times daily

■ Flaxseed oil: 3 tsp, three times daily

■ Manganese: 20 mg daily

■ Trace EPD (a supplement with trace minerals such as selenium, chromium, and molybdenum): one capsule daily

■ Silica: 405 mg, two tablets daily

■ Pycnogenol (antioxidant): 20 mg, three times daily

■ Beta carotene: 50,000 IU, two capsules, twice daily

■ Cal Apatite (calcium and mineral formula from Metagenics): 100 mg, twice daily

■ Esterol (buffered vitamin C): 675 mg capsule, twice daily

■ ProGest cream (natural progesterone): ¼ tsp applied topically, twice daily for three weeks out of the month

Suzanne's symptoms of pelvic pain, bloating, irritable bowel, bladder pain and spasms, frequent urination, and anxiety began to improve dramatically. Her breast soreness, vaginal bleeding, and chemical sensitivity had lessened considerably as well. Under physician supervision, Suzanne had gradually stopped using the estrogen patch.

After six weeks on the program, Suzanne said she "felt like a new woman." She continued on the program for another five months, at which time Suzanne felt well enough to begin working part-time

QUICK DEFINITION

A **bioflavonoid** is a pigment within plants and fruits that acts as an antioxidant to protect against damage from free radicals and excess oxygen. In the body, bioflavonoids enhance the beneficial activities of vitamin C, and are often formulated with this vitamin in supplement form. Originally called vitamin P (until 1950), these vitamin C "helper" substances include citrin, hesperidin, rutin, quercetin, epicatechin, flavones, and flavonols. When taken with vitamin C, bioflavonoids increase the absorption of vitamin C into the liver, kidneys, and adrenal glands. Acting as antioxidants, they also protect vitamin C from destruction by free radicals.

To contact **Diana Brady, M.A. C.N.C.:** The Ultimate Health Center, 31 College Place, Asheville, NC 28801; tel: 800-268-6905 or 704-669-1053. For **Digestive Stool Analysis, Candida Serum Analysis,** and **Fecal Secretory IgA Analysis** (saliva test is no longer available), contact: Great Smokies Diagnostic Laboratory, 63 Zillicoa Street, Asheville, NC 28801; tel: 800-522-4762 or 704-253-0621; fax: 704-253-1127. For **Trace Elements Inc. Tissue and Mineral Analysis of the Hair,** contact: Trace Elements, Inc., P.O. Box 514, Addison TX 75001; tel: 800-824-2314. For **Lehning's Anti-Anxiety Homeopathic Remedy, Inflazyme,** and **pycnogenol,** contact: PhytoPharmica, P.O. Box 1745, Green Bay, WI 54305; tel: 800-555-2370; fax: 414-469-4418. For **Amni's Fundamental Sulfur, MSM, manganese, ProGest Cream, DMSO gel with aloe vera,** and **Garlicinpro,** contact: Emerson Ecologics Inc., 18 Lomar Park, Pepperell, MA 01463; tel: 800-654-4432; fax: 800-718-7238. For **freeze-dried aloe vera,** contact: Special Harvest Inc., P.O. Box 49552, Colorado Springs, CO 80949; tel: 800-688-9977; fax: 719-598-8918. For **Probioplex, Cal-apatite,** and refrigerated powdered *acidophilus,* contact: Metagenics West, 12445 East 39th Avenue, Suite 402, Denver, CO 80239; tel: 800-647-6100 or 303-371-6848; fax: 303-371-9303. For **Capsin-HP Lotion,** contact: Nu Biologics (formerly Lewis-Gitomer Labs), 30 West 100 Butterfield Road, Warrenville, IL 60555; tel: 800-332-3130 or 800-645-6016; fax: 630-393-7547. For **Floressence tea** and **flaxseed oil,** contact: Flora, 805 East Badger Road, Lynden, WA 98264; tel: 360-354-2110 or 800-498-3610; fax: 360-354-5355. For **colloidal silver,** contact: Source Naturals, 19 Janis Way, Scotts Valley, CA 95066; tel: 800-815-2333. For **Trace EPD** and **Esterol-buffered Vitamin C,** contact: Allergy Resources, 557 Burbank Street, Suite K, Broomfield, CO 80020; tel: 800-873-3529 or 303-438-0600 ext. 108; fax: 303-438-0700. For **Inflazyme Forte,** contact: American Biologics, 1180 Walnut Avenue, Chula Vista, CA 91911; tel: 800-227-4473; fax: 619-429-8004.

QUICK DEFINITION

Beta-glucuronidase is an enzyme produced by various bacteria in the colon. Elevated levels may result from bacterial overgrowth, an abnormal intestinal pH, too much dietary fat (especially from meat), or low levels of beneficial bacteria. Elevated levels can increase bioactivation of carcinogens in the bowel, thus increasing the risk of colon cancer.

again. She was able to do some traveling without worrying about urinary problems. Suzanne's husband wrote to Brady thanking her for "giving me my wife back."

A month later—six months after Suzanne started the program—follow-up stool, blood, urine, and hair analyses showed that Suzanne's yeast and toxic metal levels had improved, her digestive enzymes were in the normal range, her beta-glucunronidase level had decreased significantly, and the *Enterococcus* and *E. coli* bacteria were completely gone.

Vaginitis is a common disorder
and relatively easy to treat. However, the relief
of symptoms obtained by conventional
vaginal creams or other methods does nothing
to prevent a recurrence. For lasting
and permanent relief from this highly
uncomfortable condition, it is necessary
to eliminate the contributing factors
through alternative medicine therapies and
attention to lifestyle.

CHAPTER

7

Vaginitis

(VAGINAL INFECTION OR INFLAMMATION)

AGINITIS, AN INFECTION or inflammation of the vagina or vulva (folds of skin surrounding the vaginal opening), accounts for nearly 7% of all visits to gynecologists.[1] The uncomfortable itching and pain (often worse on urination and during sexual intercourse) associated with vaginitis prompt many women to consult their physicians. Unfortunately, others are embarrassed by the abnormal or foul-smelling vaginal discharge, which also signals vaginitis, and are therefore reluctant to seek medical help. This is inadvisable because, if left untreated, vaginitis can lead to more serious conditions, such as endometrial (uterine lining) or cervical inflammation, pregnancy complications (such as ectopic pregnancy, the implantation of a fertilized egg outside the uterus), and pelvic inflammatory disease (PID), a condition which can scar the fallopian tubes and cause infertility.[2] If you have the above symptoms and/or a bright reddish color to your vulva,[3] it would be best not to delay treatment.

A variety of causal factors contribute to vaginal infections. Bacterial vaginosis, for example, is caused by harmful bacteria such as *Neisseria gonorrhea* and *Chlamydia trachomatis*, while vaginal candidiasis (also called candidal vaginitis) results from an overgrowth of the yeast *Candida albicans*. About 90% of vaginitis is caused by such infectious organisms, particularly bacteria, *Candida*, and the parasitic protozoan *Trichomonas vaginalis*.[4] Other factors in vaginitis include local irritants (such as

---

Causes of Vaginitis

- Vaginal environment
- Weakened immune system
- Bacterial infection
- *Candida* (yeast) overgrowth
- Parasites
- Hormonal imbalance
- Diet and nutritional deficiencies
- Irritants and foreign objects

---

tight clothing or nylon pantyhose), hormonal changes, and emotional or psychological issues, among others.

As vaginitis may be caused by different infectious agents, it is important to determine the source of the infection before proceeding with any kind of treatment. Once the cause is identified, alternative medicine therapies such as those covered in this chapter can then be implemented to not only treat existing vaginitis but to prevent this often painful condition from recurring. In the next section, women's health specialist Jesse Hanley, M.D., of Malibu, California, demonstrates how natural treatments can be used to heal vaginitis by restoring balance in the body.

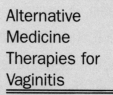

Alternative Medicine Therapies for Vaginitis

- Dietary recommendations
- Herbal medicine
- Nutritional supplements
- Homeopathy
- Vaginal suppositories and douches

Success Story: Two Years of Vaginitis Cured With Diet, Herbs, and Supplements

Charlotte, 36, came to Dr. Hanley after suffering with vaginitis for two years. During this time, Charlotte had experienced yellowish vaginal discharges, often of a strong odor, and sensations of burning and discomfort during sexual intercourse. Despite numerous rounds of antibiotics, her vaginitis symptoms kept returning. Her medical history included many years of taking birth control pills and various antibiotics, and recurrent vaginal yeast infections.

In Dr. Hanley's view, Charlotte had a chronic yeast infection which had set the stage for *Streptococcus* bacteria to proliferate. Her conventional physicians kept giving her antibiotics to try and wipe out the *Streptococcus*, but this failed to produce any lasting benefits because it did not address the underlying yeast infection.

Dr. Hanley put Charlotte on an anti-*Candida* diet. This consisted of: the complete elimination of all sugars, both refined and natural (as in fruit and fruit juices), as these feed the yeast; restriction of carbohydrate intake to no more than 100 g daily; avoidance of all dairy products, refined white flour products, mushrooms, and all fermented foods, including wine and vinegar. "When the immune system is this hyperactive, it acts as if it is allergic to the yeast in these foods,"

When the population of "friendly" bacteria in the vagina becomes depleted, through overly acidic pH, poor diet or a diet high in processed foods, or the excessive use of antibiotics and hormonal drugs, conditions are set for vaginitis unless steps are taken to replenish those bacteria.

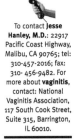

To contact **Jesse Hanley, M.D.:** 22917 Pacific Coast Highway, Malibu, CA 90765; tel: 310-457-2016; fax: 310- 456-9482. For more about **vaginitis**, contact: National Vaginitis Association, 117 South Cook Street, Suite 315, Barrington, IL 60010.

Friendly bacteria, or probiotics, refer to beneficial microbes inhabiting the human gastrointestinal tract where they are essential for proper nutrient assimilation. The human body contains an estimated several trillion beneficial bacteria comprising over 400 species, all necessary for health. Among the more well known of these are *Lactobacillus acidophilus* and *Bifidobacterium bifidum*. Overly acidic bodily conditions, chronic constipation or diarrhea, dietary imbalances, consumption of highly processed foods, and the excessive use of antibiotics and hormonal drugs can interfere with probiotic function and even reduce the number of these microbes, setting up conditions for illness.

comments Dr. Hanley. Charlotte began eating a diet based on fresh vegetables and protein, with a small amount of carbohydrates from whole grains or beans.

Next, Dr. Hanley prescribed a series of herbs to combat the fungal overgrowth. For this, Dr. Hanley often uses tea tree oil (*Maleluca alternafolla*), goldenseal (*Hydrastis canadensis*), and garlic (*Allium sativum*). She also started Charlotte on a *Lactobacillus acidophilus* supplement and, for a short time, Sporanox, a fast-acting conventional drug given for fungal infections and taken once daily. During the first few weeks of treatment, Dr. Hanley advised Charlotte to douche four nights in a row with a combination of *L. acidophilus* and aloe vera gel.

"Aloe is soothing, nourishing, and healing to the vaginal tissue, while mixing in *acidophilus* speeds up the replenishment of normal, healthy flora in the vagina and discourages the unwanted ones," explains Dr. Hanley. Vaginitis is usually marked by a change in the ratio of beneficial to unbeneficial microflora in the vagina. Through applying *acidophilus*, "friendly" bacteria (SEE QUICK DEFINITION) were reintroduced into Charlotte's body both systemically, by the oral *acidophilus*, and locally, via the douches. Dr. Hanley adds that the combination of *acidophilus* and aloe vera can be prepared either as a watery douche or as a paste to insert in the vagina.

Within two months, Charlotte was symptom free; she noticed that other symptoms of which she had been barely aware due to the primacy of her vaginal discomfort disappeared as well. "Her mind became clearer, her energy got better, and she had less bloating and fatigue," says Dr. Hanley. In the two years since then, Charlotte has not had a recurrence of vaginitis, despite being highly sexually active and therefore potentially exposed to new sources of infections.

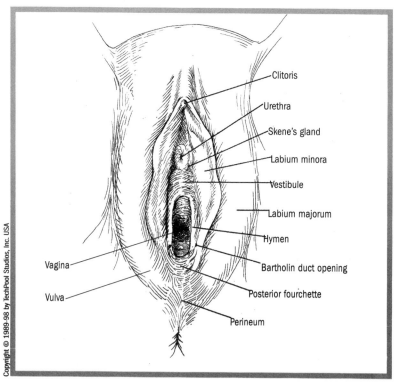

WHERE VAGINITIS DEVELOPS. Vaginitis is an infection or inflammation of the vagina or vulva (pictured above).

Eight Causes of Vaginitis

Various stressors on the body, such as the repeated courses of antibiotics and long-term use of birth control pills in the case above, can, over time, weaken the body which allows infection by microorganisms usually held in abeyance. Once the infections and stressors are recognized and addressed, however, even recurrent vaginitis can be eliminated, as was the case with Charlotte. The following eight factors are known to contribute to vaginitis.

1) Vaginal Environment

Imbalances in the vaginal environment can result in vulnerability to infection. The pH (SEE QUICK DEFINITION) level of vaginal tissues, blood sugar (glucose) level, and the presence of organisms such as the

241

In a study of women with bacterial vaginosis, only 25% had sufficient amounts of the friendly bacteria *L. acidophilus* and *L. plantarum* in their vaginas. Among the healthy study participants, 87% had enough beneficial bacteria.

yeast *Candida albicans* and the parasitic protozoa *Trichomonas vaginalis* are components of the vaginal environment. These factors have an impact on the development of vaginitis and are often interrelated, according to naturopathic physician Paul Reilly, N.D.

For example, a more acidic pH (resulting from excess progesterone or poor diet, among other factors) makes the vagina particularly hospitable to the growth of *Trichomonas vaginalis.*[5] Parasitic infection and *Candida* overgrowth (as you saw in the case of Charlotte) create an ideal climate for proliferation of vaginitis-producing bacteria. High levels of blood sugar (glucose), such as found in diabetes or excessive sugar consumption, contribute to vaginitis because the sugar feeds yeast.

Another important component of the vaginal environment is the population of "friendly" bacteria which normally reside there and help to keep both harmful bacteria and *Candida albicans* in check. When the population becomes depleted, through overly acidic pH, poor diet or a diet high in processed foods, or the excessive use of antibiotics and hormonal drugs, among other factors, conditions are set for vaginitis, unless steps are taken to replenish those bacteria. Once the balance in vaginal flora has been disrupted, a self-perpetuating cycle is set in motion: as numbers of harmful bacteria increase (leading to vaginitis), the numbers of friendly bacteria decrease, creating an environment even more vulnerable to infection.

In a study of women with bacterial vaginosis, only 25% (30 of 120) had sufficient amounts of the friendly bacteria *L. acidophilus* and *L. plantarum* in their vaginas. Among the healthy study participants, 87% (47 of 53) had enough beneficial bacteria.[6] These results reflect the importance of maintaining the proper balance of vaginal microflora as a preventive measure against vaginal infection.

As mentioned earlier, antibiotics kill both beneficial and pathogenic (disease-causing) bacteria. The standard conventional medicine approach of treating vaginitis with antibiotics means that if an imbalance in vaginal flora was not originally behind your vaginitis, it soon will be. Another product of modern medicine, spermacides such as nonoxynol 9 (an ingredient in contraceptive sponges, creams, and gels) also inhibit the growth of friendly bacteria[7] and thus contribute to vaginitis.

In addition to pH levels and the microflora population, the vaginal environment is influenced by a woman's overall health and immune status.

2) Weakened Immune System

Perhaps the most common predisposing condition for vaginitis is weakened immunity, which can occur from nutritional deficiencies, medications, pregnancies, chronic stress, and toxic overload, among many other causes, as discussed throughout this book. A weakened immune system obviously does not have the same ability to fight off the many infectious agents to which we are exposed every day and which a healthy immune system is able to dispatch without difficulty. Weakened immunity leaves every system in the body, including the reproductive, vulnerable to opportunistic infections. Vaginitis is a simple outgrowth of this condition.

3) Bacterial Infection

Various bacteria can infect the vagina, causing bacterial vaginosis (also called vaginal bacteriosis). The discharge in bacterial vaginosis is white or gray and fishy-smelling. Some bacteria that cause this type of vaginitis, such as *Neisseria gonorrhea*, are sexually transmitted (the vaginitis caused by this bacteria is actually a symptom of the venereal disease gonorrhea). Of non-sexually transmitted bacteria, the most common is *Gardnerella vaginalis*.

Bacterial vaginosis can also result from bowel bacteria (such as *Escherichia coli*) migrating into the vagina. Normally, the vagina's mucosal lining provides immunological protection against such bacterial infiltration, but if this lining is deficient, an infection may develop, according to Dr. Jesse Hanley. A deficiency may be caused by poor health, aggressive intercourse, declining hormone levels, poor diet, or abnormal microflora populations, she says.

E. coli is not life-threatening or even particularly invasive, says Dr. Hanley, which is why she prefers treating it directly in the vagina through douches or suppositories rather than by taking oral medicines which have to find their way through the body to the targeted tissues.

4) *Candida* (Yeast) Overgrowth

In the past 20 years, infection by the yeast *Candida albicans* has increased two-and-a-half times due to several factors, chief among them the increased use of antibiotics.[8] As mentioned previously, *Candida albicans*, the yeast-like fungus normally found in the intestinal tract and vagina, is usually held in check by friendly bacteria. However, when the immune system is weakened, the friendly bacteria have been wiped out by antibiotics, or when yeast are transmitted from a partner during sexual intercourse, *Candida* can proliferate in the vagina and result in candidal vaginitis. This type of vaginitis is characterized by a thick, white, odorless discharge accompanied by intense itching.

One of the foremost authorities on yeast infections is William G. Crook, M.D., author of multiple books on the subject. Dr. Crook explains that antibiotics open the door to yeast growth, while birth control pills, cortisone, and other drugs and a diet rich in sugar stimulate the yeast to grow. In addition, your immune system becomes weakened by toxins from excess yeast, nutritional deficiencies, and by exposure to environmental molds and chemicals, including formaldehyde, petrochemicals, perfume and tobacco, he says.[9] As noted above, immune dysfunction is often accompanied by a depletion in the vaginal flora which keep *Candida* in check.

Chronic vaginitis can also be the result of a toxic bowel, according to Ralph Golan, M.D. If the intestines are clogged, as in chronic constipation, they are not eliminating the excess yeast and other toxic organisms, he explains. Over time, these toxins build up in the intestines and can then migrate to the vagina.[10]

In addition to food allergies, insufficient digestive secretions, such as deficient stomach acid or lack of pancreatic enzymes or bile, contribute to *Candida* overgrowth, as can anti-ulcer drugs such as Tagamet and Zantac.[11]

If a yeast infection is recurrent, it is important to consult a qualified health practitioner to identify the sources of the problem, advises naturopathic physician Tori Hudson, N.D., founder of A Woman's Time: Menopause Options and Natural Medicine clinic in Portland, Oregon. "Sometimes there are systemic health problems that cause it—diabetes, for instance—and more worrisome these days is that chronic yeast vaginitis is the primary presenting symptom of women who are HIV positive." One should also test for food, chemical, and environmental sensitivities, as allergic reactions can disturb the balance of vaginal and intestinal flora, says Dr. Hudson.

For more about *Candida*, see Chapter 2: Endometriosis, pp. 76-77.

Conventional medicine relies on antifungal drugs which, while eliminating the immediate infection, do not address the underlying cause and therefore do nothing to prevent a recurrence. Also, some people may experience side effects, such as headaches, nausea, and stomach pain, from these medications.

5) Parasites

As mentioned previously, approximately 90% of vaginitis cases are caused by bacteria, *Candida*, or a parasite, *Trichomonas vaginalis*. Like the gonorrhea bacteria, *Trichomonas* is commonly transmitted through sexual intercourse. These parasites, called trichomonads, grow best in an acidic pH climate (optimum is a pH of 5.5 to 5.8).[12] *Trichomonas* vaginitis produces a yellowish-green or reddish-yellow, foul-smelling discharge. In most cases, viewing cervical mucus under a microscope can identify this type of vaginal infection.

If a microscope is not available to diagnose *Trichomonas*, you can use the hydrogen peroxide test: Mix a drop of 3% hydrogen peroxide with vaginal secretions on a microscope slide; if there are trichomonads, bubbles will form due to the presence of white blood cells (not present with *Candida* or bacterial vaginosis).[13] *Trichomonas* infections are conventionally treated with the prescription antibiotic metronidazole or Flagyl.

6) Hormonal Imbalance

Vaginitis occurs more frequently among women who take birth con-

Vaginitis Relief in Three Days With Grapefruit Seed Extract

Physicians in Monterrey, Mexico, found that out of 20 patients with vaginal yeast infection, 15 experienced relief of their symptoms in three days after douching with grapefruit seed extract every 12 hours.[14] The extract, prepared from the ground seeds and membranous material of the grapefruit, works as a multipurpose germ killer, or natural antibiotic, for bacteria, viruses, and yeast (*Candida albicans*).

In the years since its discovery in 1964, grapefruit seed extract has been tested and validated by the U.S. Food and Drug Administration and the Department of Agriculture, the Pasteur Institute in France, and numerous physicians. The extract is concentrated—a little goes a long way. It is also nontoxic and produces no side effects. However, approximately 3% to 5% of people will be sensitive to the substance and may not be able to tolerate its acidity. There are different strengths and preparations of grapefruit seed extract, according to application.

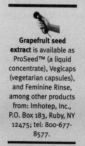

Grapefruit seed extract is available as ProSeed™ (a liquid concentrate), Vegicaps (vegetarian capsules), and Feminine Rinse, among other products from: Imhotep, Inc., P.O. Box 183, Ruby, NY 12475; tel: 800-677-8577.

trol pills, states John R. Lee, M.D., of Sebastopol, California. Dr. Lee suggests that one reason for this is that birth control pills work by suppressing hormones and the vaginal mucus production that goes along with the hormones is also suppressed.[15] (As already noted, taking birth control pills promotes vaginal yeast overgrowth).

Another type of vaginitis, called atrophic vaginitis, is caused by hormonal changes during and after menopause. These hormonal changes, chiefly lack of estrogen, cause vaginal dryness. The vaginal mucosa becomes pale, thin, and powdery, and sexual intercourse can be painful as a result. The reduced mucus and vaginal dryness predispose a woman to vaginal infection, Dr. Lee says.

The discharge in atrophic vaginitis is thin, white or blood-streaked, and foul-smelling. Treatment is application of a topical vaginal estrogen cream.

7) Diet and Nutritional Deficiencies

Deficiencies in zinc and vitamins A, C, E, and B complex invite vaginitis.[16] Zinc and vitamin A are necessary for proper cell repair and the normal growth of tissues, including the vaginal mucosa. Zinc and vitamins A, C, and E all support immune response and thus increase your resistance to infection. In addition, vitamin C strengthens connective tissue and vitamin E helps regulate hormones. The B vitamins are needed for almost every metabolic function in the body; vitamin B1 and pantothenic acid enhance the action of estradiol (a form of estrogen) and may thus help with atrophic vaginitis, a condition caused by relative lack of estrogen.

Diet is most directly implicated in candidal vaginitis; specifically, sugar, refined carbohydrates, a high-fat diet, processed foods, milk and dairy products, and mold- and yeast-containing foods (alcoholic beverages, cheese, dried fruits, peanuts) can all contribute to *Candida* overgrowth.

Researchers have found a link between vaginal candidiasis and low levels of beta carotene in the body. According to a recent study, the amount of beta carotene in vaginal cells was significantly reduced in women with vaginal candidiasis. Beta carotene is a precursor to

For more about **diet and Candida**, see "Anti-Candida Diet," Chapter 6: Cystitis, p. 221.

vitamin A; reduced beta carotene levels may thus affect the body's immune response, altering the bacterial climate of the vagina and encouraging *Candida* to flourish. Women can boost their beta carotene levels by eating more carrots, green leafy vegetables, and other beta carotene–rich foods, or by taking supplements.[17]

8) Irritants and Foreign Objects

The vagina can become irritated or inflamed by tight pants or under-wear, douches, perfumes or other chemicals, allergic reactions, soaps, or medications such as spermicidal creams and gels.[18] Such irritation is called irritant vaginitis, and usually creates a watery, purulent (pus-containing) discharge.

Another type of vaginitis, foreign-body vaginitis, or inflammation caused by a foreign object in the vagina, creates a foul-smelling, watery, and sometimes blood-streaked discharge. It is usually caused by a tampon left in the vagina for too long.

Alternative Medicine Therapies for Vaginitis

If you do get a vaginal infection, irritation, or itching, it is wise to consult a health-care practitioner; first, in order to identify or rule out pathologies such as gonorrhea or herpes; and second, because, as stated earlier, untreated vaginal infections can spread to other areas of the reproductive system and cause more serious problems.

Rather than using conventional drugs which can actually deepen the problem, you can employ a variety of alternative medicine therapies to eliminate your vaginitis, prevent a recurrence, and in the process improve your overall health by strengthening your body so infectious agents are dispatched with ease. Dietary recommendations, nutritional and herbal supplements, homepathy, and vaginal sup-positories and douches can all be effective in this comprehensive treatment approach.

> ## 42% of Women Used Alternative Medicine for Vaginitis
>
> In a study of 105 women with chronic vaginitis, 73% reported self-med-icating for their condition and, of those, 42% report-ed using alternative medi-cine to treat it. Therapies used included acupunc-ture, herb teas, garlic, natural douches, and oral and topical forms of probi-otics. Of the women who used alternative thera-pies, the greatest number had the candidal variety of vaginitis.[19]

Dietary Recommendations

Like all conditions, vaginitis can be greatly influenced by nutrition. A basic diet for vaginitis is low in fats, sugars, and refined foods.[20] Tori Hudson, N.D., of Portland, Oregon, suggests different dietary guide-lines depending on the type of vaginitis. Vaginitis caused by

Tips for the Prevention and Treatment of Vaginitis

The following are simple steps you can take to help eliminate vaginitis and prevent its recurrence.[21]

Prevention:

- Shower daily to keep vulval area clean.
- Wipe from front to back after a bowel movement.
- Keep vaginal area dry.
- Wear cotton underwear and avoid nylon pantyhose.
- Avoid using perfumed chemical douches or other perfumed or chemical products in the vaginal area.
- Use condoms during sexual intercourse to reduce transmittal of infection.

Treatment:

- If your vaginitis is a recurring problem, make sure your sexual partner gets treated as well.
- To avoid reinfection and to protect your sore vaginal tissues against more injury, it is best to refrain from sexual activity while you are being treated for vaginitis.

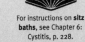

For instructions on **sitz baths**, see Chapter 6: Cystitis, p. 228.

- A warm sitz bath, either in plain water or with a cup or two of Epsom salts added to the bath water, can help relieve the itching and burning of vaginitis. (Don't alternate with a cold sitz bath, however, as is done in other female health conditions.)
- For all types of vaginitis, take *Lactobacillus acidophilus* capsules (three daily is the average dose) or eat one portion of yogurt with active cultures daily at least until the vaginitis is completely eliminated. (Consult with your health-care practitioner on a preventive maintenance dosage.)

Trichomonas responds best to fasting, while treatment of bacterial vaginosis requires eliminating all foods which may produce an allergic reaction, says Dr. Hudson.

For candidal vaginitis, she recommends following a yeast-free diet and avoiding fermented foods and sugar which feed yeast growth. The anti-*Candida* diet generally also involves avoiding dairy products and refined flour, as these encourage *Candida* overgrowth as well. Dr. Hudson advises increasing intake of garlic and live-culture yogurt, as these act as antifungals and help restore your body's natural defenses against yeast infection.

According to an Israeli study, eating as little as one-half cup of yogurt (enriched with *Lactobacillus acidophilus* or "active" bacterial cultures) daily may help prevent recurring episodes of vaginitis. The study, which tracked 46 women over a period of six months, revealed that eating enriched yogurt significantly reduced the incidence of vaginitis as compared with eating pasteurized yogurt or no yogurt at all. Researchers noted that eating *Lactobacillus*-containing yogurt resulted in a clear increase in beneficial bacteria in the vagina and rectum, and therefore a significant decrease in the form of bacteria which causes vaginosis.[22]

Herbal Medicine

Herbal medicine's versatility is particularly apparent in its application to vaginitis. Tinctures, teas, swabs, and phytoestrogens are all helpful in treating the disorder.

A tincture of herbal extracts consisting of two parts goldenseal (*Hydrastis canadensis*), two parts echinacea (*Echinacea augustifolia*), and one part phytolacca (*Phytolacca amercana*), taken at a dosage of 20 to 60 drops every two to four hours, can help relieve vaginitis, according to Dr. Paul Reilly. The goldenseal acts as an antifungal, echinacea builds immune strength, and phytolacca helps draw toxins from the body. This tincture can also be taken as a tea (1 tsp of the mixture to one cup of hot water). Drink one cup of the tea every two to four hours until symptoms are relieved.[23]

For candidal vaginitis, one herbal remedy is to swab the vagina with an extract of gentian violet (*Gentiana macrophylla*). Dr. Reilly considers this plant, which has fungicidal properties, to be "as close to a specific treatment for *Candida*" as can be found in herbal medicine. Susun Weed, an herbalist based in Woodstock, New York, concurs. Here are her instructions: use cotton swabs to apply a 1% solution of gentian violet (mixed with water) to the vulva, vaginal walls, and cervix every night before going to bed; use a sanitary pad to avoid staining clothing or bedding; repeat four to six times over a two-week period.

Certain herbs, called phytoestrogens, can help balance hormones and thus assist in treating atrophic vaginitis (when vaginal tissues become thin and dry). Phytoestrogens have very weak estrogenic activity (as little as 2% of hormonal estrogen), but they can attach to estrogen receptor sites in the cells and therefore fulfill the role of estrogen. The estrogen content of phytoestrogens is primarily estriol, the least carcinogenic of the three main estrogens in the body (the other two are estradiol and estrone). Thus phytoestrogens can increase estrogen activity without the risks associated with synthetic estrogen replacement drugs, which have been known to cause breast and uterine cancer.

Phytoestrogenic herbs include fennel (*Foeniculum vulgare*), anise (*Pimpinella anisum*), ginseng (*Panax quinquefolius*), alfalfa (*Medicago sativa*), dong quai (*Dang gue*), and red clover (*Trifolium pratense*). Certain foods, such as soy, are phytoestrogenic as well.

For more about **fennel, anise, and other herbs**, contact: Country Herbs, 4709 Colleyville Blvd., #560, Colleyville, TX 76034; tel: 817-498-8055; fax: 817-428-8637.

For other herbal aid in hormonal balancing, oral doses of black cohosh (*Cimicifuga racemosa*), wild yam (*Dioscorea villosa*), and vitamin E can be used in conjunction with herbal suppositories (see sidebar: "Natural Vaginal Suppositories," p. 253) or a vitamin E topical cream.

Nutritional Supplements

Correcting nutritional deficiencies is most important with the infectious types of vaginitis. Bacteria, yeast, or protozoa (*Trichomonas*), can only take hold in a woman's body if her immune system is weakened or if her gastrointestinal flora are out of balance. Vitamins and minerals that boost immune function and promote healthy tissues help strengthen the vaginal mucosa so that these delicate tissues can shield themselves against infiltration by infectious organisms.

As mentioned previously, deficiencies in zinc, beta carotene, and vitamins A, B complex, C, and E have been linked with vaginitis. Supplementation can help correct this contributing factor.

Dr. Paul Reilly typically recommends the following supplements and dosages for vaginitis:[24]

- Vitamin A: 25,000 IU (or beta carotene, 200,000 IU) daily
- Vitamin C: 500-1,000 mg every four hours
- B complex: a good quality tablet or capsule, averaging 20-50 mg of the major components, daily
- Zinc: 10-15 mg daily
- Vitamin E: 200 IU daily
- *Lactobacillus acidophilus*: $\frac{1}{2}$ tsp twice daily

For more about **Nature's Biotics™**, contact: Life Science Products Inc., 321 North Mall Drive, Building F-210, St. George, UT 84790; tel: 800-713-3888 or 801-628-4111; fax: 801-628-6114. Another source of **probiotics** (available to qualified health-care professionals) is Spectra Probiotic, available from: NF Formulas, 9775 S.W. Commerce Circle, C-5, Wilsonville, OR 97070-9602; tel: 800-547-4891 or 503-682-9755; fax: 503-682-9529.

Friendly bacteria—Supplementation with friendly bacteria (probiotics, which include *Lactobacillus acidophilus* and *Bifidobacteria bifidum*) is the most commonly recommended treatment for candidal vaginitis. Probiotics help suppress the growth of yeast, improve digestion by increasing the production of some enzymes, produce acids that fight bacteria, and manufacture nutrients such as vitamins K, B1, B2, B3, B12, and folic acid.

Researchers at the University of Washington School of Medicine report that probiotics can successfully treat and prevent selected vaginal, urinary tract, and intestinal infections such as candidiasis, diarrhea associated with antibiotic use, and infantile diarrhea. Probiotics "may offer an alternative to conventional antimicrobials to which many pathogenic microorganisms eventually develop resistance," states Gary W. Elmer, Ph.D., author of the report.[25]

Life Science Products of St. George, Utah, has developed a probiotics supplement, Nature's Biotics™, which is a blend of 61 nutrients, including at least six selectively bred strains of soil-based probiotic organisms, amino acids, phytoplanktons, plant pigments and enzymes, minerals, trace elements, essential fatty acids, and starches. Once the mixture makes contact with water in your stomach, the friendly bacteria become active. The intent is to "steer your digestive system toward proper absorption, thereby increasing your body's ability to stay healthy from the inside," says David Dodart, company president. According to Dodart, the product helps to remove waste, debris, and toxins from the intestines; improves digestion and assimilation; works against harmful molds, yeasts, fungi, and viruses; and stimulates the immune system which, in turn, releases more B lymphocytes.

When you first start using Nature's Biotics, Dodart says, it's advisable for the first week to take one capsule 30 minutes before the evening meal with ten ounces of pure water. Then in the second week, Dodart recommends taking one capsule 30 minutes before lunch and dinner; in the third week, one capsule before breakfast, lunch, and dinner.

Homeopathy

Homeopaths Andrew Lockie, M.D., of London, England, and Nicola Geddes, M.D., of Edinburgh, Scotland, typically suggest the following homeopathic (SEE QUICK DEFINITION) remedies as emergency, short-term treatment for vaginal yeast (*Candida albicans*) infections (6C potency, to be taken six times daily for up to five days):[26]

■ For yeast infection with dryness of the vagina—*Aconite, Arsenicum, Belladonna, Berberis, Ferrum, Graphites, Lycopodium, Natrum muriaticum, Sepia*

■ For yeast infection with intense itching in the vagina—*Caladium, Kreosotum, Lilium*

■ For yeast infection with creamy vaginal discharge—*Calcarea phosphorica, Natrum phosphoricum, Pulsatilla, Secale*

■ For yeast infection with burning pains in the vagina—*Belladonna, Berberis, Calcarea phosphorica, Cantharis, Chamomilla, Chelidonium, Graphites, Kali bichrom, Kreosotum, Mercurius, Natrum muriaticum, Nitricum acidum, Petroleum, Pulsatilla, Sulphur, Thuja*

QUICK DEFINITION

Homeopathy was founded in the early 1800s by German physician Samuel Hahnemann. Today, an estimated 500 million people worldwide receive homeopathic treatment; in Britain, homeopathy enjoys royal patronage. Homeopathy is now practiced according to two differing concepts. In classical homeopathy, only one single-component remedy is prescribed at a time, in a potency specifically adjusted to the patient; the physician waits to see the results before prescribing anything further. In complex homeopathy, typified by *Hepar compositum*, a prescription involves multiple substances given at the same time, usually in low potencies.

Homeopathic first-aid remedies are not intended to take the place of treatment which addresses the underlying causes of vaginitis. To accomplish that, consult a homeopath who can prescribe a constitutional remedy.

■ For yeast infection with burning pain in the vagina during intercourse—*Kreosotum*, *Lycopodium*, *Sulphur*

Vaginal Suppositories and Douches

Natural vaginal suppositories and douches are frequently a component in alternative medicine treatment programs for vaginitis. They are most effective when used in conjunction with the dietary, nutritional, and lifestyle changes outlined elsewhere in this chapter.

Suppositories can be herbal or vitamin-based, mixtures of friendly bacteria or essential oils. Which one you use depends on what type of vaginitis you have. Some of the suppositories are also used for other conditions, such as sexually transmitted diseases or cystitis. Consult with your health-care practitioner as to which one would be best for you.

The suppository that Dr. Tori Hudson typically prescribes for vaginitis consists of powdered boric acid mixed with three herbs—*Berberis*, goldenseal (*Hydrastis canadensis*), and marigold (*Calendula officinalis*), all antifungals—prepared in capsule form. "This works so well," says Dr. Hudson, "that I no longer prescribe douches for this condition." Dr. Hudson has been a pioneer in the use of a suppository called a Vaginal Depletion Pack, which contains ingredients similar to those in the Essential Oils Plus suppository (see sidebar: "Natural Vaginal Suppositories," p. 253), such as goldenseal and tea tree oil. She recommends it for bacterial vaginitis and *Trichomonas* vaginitis (use every evening before bed for ten days; use the Herbal suppository in the mornings—see sidebar).

Dr. Ralph Golan usually suggests the following garlic suppository which you can make yourself: peel a clove of garlic, being careful not to nick it. Wrap it in a piece of gauze, lubricate with vegetable oil, and insert it as a tampon suppository, leaving a tail of gauze externally. Change every 12 hours for three to five days or more. It may be used for all infectious agents.[27]

Julian Whitaker, M.D., often suggests treating candidal vaginitis by using a boric acid capsule (500-600 mg) twice daily as a vaginal suppository. He cautions not to do this for more than a week, as it could be irritating. Dr. Whitaker also recommends a daily douche of tea tree oil and water (one teaspoon of 20% tea tree oil in a pint of warm water).[28] Another technique is to saturate a tampon in a 1% solution of tea tree oil, insert it into the vagina, and leave in for 24 hours; do this once a week for four to six weeks, in addition to the daily douche.[29]

CAUTION

Tea tree oil and grapefruit seed extract are both caustic to the skin and therefore must be handled carefully and used in small amounts.

Natural Vaginal Suppositories

Earth's Botanical Harvest in Sandy, Oregon, makes a line of herbal (and vitamin) vaginal suppositories recommended by numerous alternative medicine practitioners. The suppositories have a cocoa butter base which melts at body temperature; it is advisable to use a sanitary pad to protect clothing and bedding (nighttime use is generally prescribed). The following are some of the suppositories available:

■ Herbal—for bacterial vaginitis and *Trichomonas*; contains antimicrobial and astringent herbs, and herbs that are soothing to the vaginal tissues: calendula (*Calendula officinalis*), echinacea (*Echinacea augustifolia*), bearberry (*Arctostaphylos uva ursi*), milfoil (*Achillea millefolium*), althea (*Althea officinalis*), manzanita (*Arctostaphylos tomentosa*), Oregon grape (*mahonia aquifolium*), and comfrey (*Symphytum officinale*)

■ Essential Oils Plus—for bacterial vaginosis and *Trichomonas* infection; contains hydrastis and lomatium and essential oils of tea tree, thuja, and bitter orange

■ Goldenseal (*Hydrastis canadensis*)— for bacterial and *Candida* infections; contains berberine, an alkaloid which is said to be effective against bacteria, fungi, and protozoa

■ Calendula and Vitamin A—for vaginitis caused by irritations or ulcerations; calendula (marigold) and vitamin A heal wounds and tissue

■ Tea Tree Oil—for *Candida*, *Trichomonas*, and bacterial vaginal infections

Herbal vaginal suppositories are available (to licensed health-care professionals only) from Earth's Botanical Harvest, 14385 S.E. Lusted Road, Sandy, OR 97055; tel: 800-428-3308 or 503-668-4120; fax: 503-668-3227.

■ Vitamin E—for vaginal dryness and atrophic vaginitis; vitamin E helps regulate hormones

■ Black Cohosh (*Cimicifuga racemosa*), Wild Yam (*Dioscorea villosa*), and Vitamin E—for vaginal dryness and atrophic vaginitis; like vitamin E, Wild Yam and black cohosh are hormone regulators (both herbs can also be taken as teas or in capsule form in conjunction with the suppositories, and with 400-800 IU of oral vitamin E daily)

Other practitioners recommend douches as well. Silena Heron, R.N., N.D., of Sedona, Arizona, often prescribes a douche of antiseptic herbs such as St. John's wort, goldenseal, echinacea, fresh plantain, garlic, and calendula along with herbs like comfrey leaves and self heal to soothe the inflamed membranes. Calendula is both antiseptic and reparative.

Other douche recommendations from Dr. Julian Whitaker include: apple cider vinegar (two tablespoons to one quart water), *acidophilus* (two opened capsules to one quart water), or a solution of water and garlic from capsules or fresh juice. Topical pau d'arco, black walnut, and tea tree oil are also options and vitamin E cream may relieve itching. Betadine, or povidone iodine, is effective as a douche in several kinds of vaginitis, including yeast infections and *Trichomonas* vaginitis. The typically recommended mix is one part Betadine to 100 parts water, douching twice daily for two weeks.[30] A douche of grapefruit seed extract (ten to 20 drops in two cups of water) may also be used.

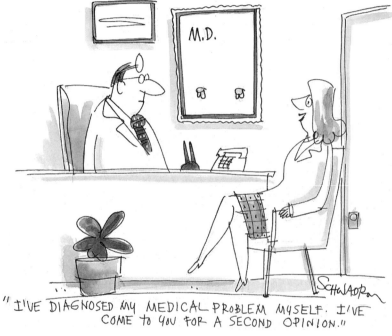

"I'VE DIAGNOSED MY MEDICAL PROBLEM MYSELF. I'VE COME TO YOU FOR A SECOND OPINION."

Endnotes

Chapter I
Menstrual Problems

1 Toni Weschler, M.PH. *Taking Charge of Your Fertility: The Definitive Guide to Natural Birth Control and Pregnancy Achievement* (New York: HarperCollins, 1995).

2 Centers for Disease Control and Prevention, Division of Reproductive Health, Women's Health and Fertility Branch, Fertility and Epidemiology Section, Atlanta, Georgia.

3 Betsy Thompson, M.D., et al. "Trends in Hospitalizations for Abnormal Uterine Bleeding in the United States, 1980-1992." *Journal of Women's Health* 6:1 (1997), 73.

4 J. Claude Bennett, M.D., and Fred Plum, M.D. *Cecil Textbook of Medicine*, 20th Ed. (Philadelphia, PA: W.B. Saunders, 1996), 1301-1302.

5 Linaya Hahn, L.N.C. *PMS: Solving the Puzzle* (Chicago: Spectrum Press, 1995), 132-133.

6 Kathleen A. Head, N.D. "Premenstrual Syndrome: Nutritional and Alternative Approaches." *Alternative Medicine Review* 2:1 (1997), 19-20.

7 John R. Lee. *What Your Doctor May Not Tell You About Menopause* (New York: Warner, 1996), 230.

8 J.M. Hershman. "Clinical Application of Thyrotropia-Releasing Hormone." *New England Journal of Medicine* 290 (1974), 886-890.

9 C.T. Sawin. "Clinical Use of Thyrotropin-Releasing Hormone." *Pharmacology and Therapeutics* (1976), 351-366.

10 Linaya Hahn, L.N.C. *PMS: Solving the Puzzle* (Chicago: Spectrum Press, 1995), 130.

11 Ibid., 99.

12 Ralph Golan M.D. *Optimal Wellness* (New York: Ballantine Books, 1995), 407.

13 R.L. Siblerud. "The Relationship between Mercury from Dental Amalgam and Mental Health." *American Journal of Psychotherapy* 43:4 (1989), 575-587.

14 Linaya Hahn, L.N.C. *PMS: Solving the Puzzle* (Chicago: Spectrum Press, 1995), 87.

15 K. Griffin. "Good News for Java Junkies." *Hippocrates* (November/December 1989), 18-22.

16 Linaya Hahn, L.N.C. *PMS: Solving the Puzzle* (Chicago: Spectrum Press, 1995), 112.

17 E. Bass and L. Davis. *The Courage to Heal: A Guide for Women Survivors of Child Sexual Abuse* (New York: Harper Perennial, 1992).

18 Michael Reed Gach. *Acupressure's Potent Points: A Guide to Self-Care for Common Ailments* (New York: Bantam Books, 1990), 168-169.

19 Melvyn Werbach, M.D. "Premenstrual Syndrome: Magnesium." *Townsend Letter for Doctors* (June 1995), 26.

20 Erich Keller. *The Complete Home Guide to Aromatherapy* (Tiburon, CA: H.J. Kramer, 1991). Available from: H.J. Kramer, P.O. Box 1082, Tiburon, CA 94920; tel: 415-435-5367.

21 Marla Ahlgrimm. "PMS Management: Self-Care and Hormone Options." *American Journal of Natural Medicine* 4:10 (December 1997), 19-21.

22 Alan R. Gaby, M.D. *Nutrition and Healing* 1:3 (October 1994), 6.

23 M.J. Williams et al. "Controlled Trial of Pyridoxine in The Premenstrual Syndrome." *Journal of Internal Medical Research* 13 (1985), 174-179.

24 Research abstracts provided by Reflexology Research, Kevin and Barbara Kunz, P.O. Box 35820, Station D, Albuquerque, NM 87176; tel: 800-713-6711. See also: B. Flocco. "Reflexology and Premenstrual Syndrome Research Study." A paper presented at the International Council of Reflexologists Conference: Reflexology Around the World. Virginia Beach, VA (1991).

25 Terrence Oleson, Ph.D., and Bill Flocco. "Randomized Controlled Study of Premenstrual Symptoms Treated With Ear, Hand and Foot Reflexology." *Obstetrics and Gynecology* 82 (1993), 906-911.

26 Lynne McTaggart. "Sorting Out Period Problems Naturally." *What Doctors Don't Tell You* 8:6 (September 1997), 4.

27 J. Noel Hulmston. "Case Studies: PMS." *International Journal of Aromatherapy* 6:4 (1995), 24-25. Available from: The American Alliance of Aromatherapy, P.O. Box 750428, Petaluma, CA 94975; tel: 800-809-9850; fax: 800-809-9808; 4 issues/$40.

28 Nancy Lonsdorf, M.D., et al. *A Woman's Best Medicine: Health, Happiness, and Long Life Through Maharishi Ayur-Veda* (New York: Jeremy P. Tarcher/Putnam, 1995).

29 J.T. Salonen et al. "High Stored Iron Levels are Associated with Excess Risk of Myocardial Infarction in Eastern Finnish Men." *Circulation* 86:3 (1992), 803-811. S. Hite. *The Hite Report* (New

York: Macmillan, 1976), 351.

30 Nancy Lonsdorf, M.D., et al. *A Woman's Best Medicine: Health, Happiness, and Long Life Through Maharishi Ayur-Veda* (New York: Jeremy P. Tarcher/Putnam, 1995).

31 Kathleen A. Head, N.D. "Premenstrual Syndrome: Nutritional and Alternative Approaches." *Alternative Medicine Review* 2:1 (1997), 12-25.

32 C. Peters-Welte and M. Albrecht. "Menstrual Abnormalities and PMS: *Vitex agnus-castus.*" *Quarterly Review of Natural Medicine* (Winter 1994), 313-318.

33 Michael Murray, N.D. "A Comprehensive Evaluation of Premenstrual Syndrome." *American Journal of Natural Medicine* 4:2 (1997), 10.

34 Ibid., 11.

35 Z. Harel et al. "Supplementation with Omega-3 Polyunsaturated Fatty Acids in the Management of Dysmenorrhea in Adolescents." *American Journal of Obstetrics and Gynecology* 174 (1996), 1335-1338.

36 Alan R. Gaby, M.D. *Nutrition and Healing* 1:3 (October 1994), 6.

37 B.R. Golding et al. "Estrogen Excretion Patterns and Plasma Levels in Vegetarian and Omnivorous Women." *New England Journal of Medicine* 307 (1982), 1542-1547.

38 A.M. Rossignol and H. Bonnlander. "Caffeine-Containing Beverages, Total Fluid Consumption, and Premenstrual Syndrome." *American Journal of Public Health* 80:9 (1989), 67-69.

39 Melvyn Werbach, M.D. *Nutritional Influences On Illness* (Tarzana, CA: Third Line Press, 1996), 539.

40 J.B. Stebbing et al. "Reactive Hypoglycaemia and Magnesium." *Magnesium Bulletin* 4:2 (1982), 131-134.

41 G.E. Abraham et al. "Effect Of Vitamin B6 on Plasma and Red Blood Cell Magnesium Levels in Premenopausal Women." *Annals of Clinical Laboratory Science* 11:4 (1981), 333-336.

42 Melvyn Werbach, M.D. *Nutritional Influences On Illness* (Tarzana, CA: Third Line Press, 1996), 539-540.

43 E. Block. "The Use of Vitamin A in Premenstrual Tension." *Acta Obstetricia et Gynecologica Scandinavica* 39 (1960), 586-592.

44 S. Pilar. "Amelioration of Premenstrual Depressive Symptomatology With L-Tryptophan." *Journal of Psychiatry and Neuroscience* 19:2 (1994), 114-119.

45 Melvyn Werbach, M.D. *Nutritional Influences On Illness* (Tarzana, CA: Third Line Press, 1996), 540.

46 G. Lague et al. "Idiopathic Cyclic Edema: The Role of Capillary Hyperpermeability and Its Correction by *Ginkgo biloba* Extract." *Presse Medicale* 31 (1986), 1550-1553.

47 J. Argonz and C. Albinzano. "Premenstrual Tension Treated With Vitamin A." *Journal of Clinical Endocrinology* 10 (1950), 1579-1589.

48 D.V. Jones. "Influence of Dietary Fat on Self-Reported Menstrual Symptoms." *Physiology and Behavior* 40:4 (1987), 483-487.

49 Melvyn Werbach, M.D. *Nutritional Influences On Illness* (Tarzana, CA: Third Line Press, 1996), 540.

50 M.Y. Dawood. "Current Concepts in the Etiology and Treatment of Primary Dysmenorrhea." *Acta Obstetricia et Gynecologica Scandinavica* 138:Suppl. (1986), 7-10.

51 S.M. Lark, M.D. *Menstrual Cramps: A Self-Help Program* (Los Altos, CA: Westchester Publishing, 1993), 12.

52 J.E. Pizzorno and M.T. Murray, eds. *A Textbook of Natural Medicine* (Seattle, WA: John Bastyr College Publications, 1988-1989).

53 S.M. Lark, M.D. *Menstrual Cramps: A Self-Help Program* (Los Altos, CA: Westchester, 1993), 12.

54 Ibid.

55 Bob Flaws. "Endometriosis." *Endometriosis, Infertility, and Traditional Chinese Medicine* (Boulder, CO: Blue Poppy Press, 1997), 39-42.

56 From the patient records of Judith Lewis, R.N., N.D., of Mill Valley, California.

57 Susan Lark, M.D. *Heavy Menstrual Flow and Anemia* (Berkeley, CA: Celestial Arts, 1995), 7.

58 M.L. Taymor et al. "The Etiological Role of Chronic Iron Deficiency in Production of Menorrhagia." *Journal of the American Medical Association* 187:5 (1964), 323-327.

59 Jason Elias and Katherine Ketcham. *Feminine Healing: A Woman's Guide to Healthy Body, Mind and Spirit* (New York: Warner Books, 1997), 241-255.

60 Jake Fratkin. *Chinese Herbal Patent Formulas* (Boulder, CO: Shya Publications, 1986), 133.

61 "Going With the Flow: What to Do About Heavy Menstrual Periods." *Dr. Christiane Northrup's Health Wisdom for Women* 3:6 (June 1996), 1-4. Available from: Philips Publishing, Inc., P.O. Box 60042, 7811 Montrose Road, Potomac, MD 20859; tel: 800-211-8561; 12 issues/$69.

62 Jacques Jouanny, M.D., et al. *Homeopathic Therapeutics. Possibilities in Chronic Pathology* (France: Editions Boiron, 1994), 189-190.

63 Ralph Golan, M.D. *Optimal Wellness* (New York: Ballantine Books, 1995), 329.

64 Ibid.

65 Sarah Berga. "Stress and Amenorrhea." *The Endocrinologist* 5:6 (1995), 416-421.

66 Paul Callinan. *Family Homeopathy: A Practical Handbook for Home Treatment* (New Canaan, CT: Keats Publishing, 1995), 184-185.

Chapter 2
Endometriosis

1 "The Estrogen Complex." *Newsweek* (March 21, 1994), 77.

2 Susan M. Lark, M.D. *The Women's Health Companion: Self-Help Nutrition Guide and Cookbook* (Berkeley, CA: Celestial Arts, 1995), 106.

3 J.S. Bernstein et al. *Hysterectomy: A Literature Review and Rating of Appropriateness* Publication No. JR-04 (Santa Monica, CA: Rand, 1992), 7-8.

4 Endometriosis Association, International Headquarters, 8585 N. 76th Place, Milwaukee, WI 53223.

5 Mary Lou Ballweg. *The Endometriosis Sourcebook* (Chicago: Contemporary Books, 1995), 11-12.

6 Joseph Anthony. "A Potential Test for Endometriosis." *American Health* (May 1996), 61.

7 *Physicians' Desk Reference* (Montvale NJ: Medical Economics, 1995), 2205.

8 Mary Lou Ballweg. *The Endometriosis Sourcebook* (Chicago: Contemporary Books, 1995), 188.

9 Alice D. Domar, Ph.D., and Henry Freher. *Healing Mind, Healthy Woman* (New York: Henry Holt, 1996), 366-367.

10 Susan M. Lark, M.D. *Fibroid Tumors and Endometriosis Self-Help Book* (Berkeley, CA: Celestial Arts, 1995), 243-244.

11 Vicki Hufnagel, M.D. *No More Hysterectomies* (New York: Penguin Books, 1989), 91.

12 Alice D. Domar, Ph.D., and Henry Dreher. *Healing Mind, Healthy Woman* (New York: Henry Holt, 1996), 364.

13 Christiane Northrup, M.D. *Women's Bodies, Women's Wisdom* (New York: Bantam Books, 1994), 158.

14 A. Gibbons. "Dioxin Tied to Endometriosis." *Science* 262 (1993), 1373.

15 "The Estrogen Complex." *Newsweek* (March 21, 1994), 77.

16 W.P. Dmowski et al. "The Role of Cell-mediated Immunity in Pathogenesis of Endometriosis." *Acta Obstetricia et Gynecologica Scandinavica* Supplement 159 (1994), 7-14.

17 Donald M. Portz, M.D., et al. "Oxygen Free Radicals and Pelvic Adhesion Formation in an Endometriosis Model." *International Journal of Fertility* 56:1 (1991), 39-41.

18 *Allergy Hotline* (1996), 6.

19 Christiane Northrup, M.D. *Women's Bodies, Women's Wisdom* (New York: Bantam Books, 1994), 158-159.

20 Alice D. Domar, Ph.D., and Henry Dreher. *Healing Mind, Healthy Woman* (New York: Henry Holt, 1996), 365.

21 Ibid.

22 Carolyn Myss, Ph.D. *The Creation of Health* (Walpole, NH: Stillpoint Publishing, 1993), 98.

23 Ibid., 376.

24 From the patient records of Robert Milne, M.D., Milne Medical Center, Las Vegas, Nevada.

25 Hugh Macpherson and Ted J. Kaptchuck, eds. "Shouting For Sympathy." *Acupuncture in Practice: Case History Insights From the West* (London, England: Churchill Livingstone, 1997), 169-179.

26 Daniel Gagnon. *Liquid Herbal Drops in Everyday Use* (Santa Fe, NM: Botanical Research and Education Institute, 1996), 60.

27 John R. Lee, M.D., with Virginia Hopkins. *What Your Doctor May Not Tell You About Menopause* (New York: Warner Books, 1996).

28 From the patient records of Carolyn DeMarco, M.D., Toronto, Ontario, Canada.

29 *International Journal of Aromatherapy* 6:3 (1995), 29.

30 Marc T. Goodman et al. "Association of Soy and Fiber Consumption With the Risk of Endometrial Cancer." *American Journal of Epidemiology* 146:4 (1997), 294-306.

31 Susan M. Lark, M.D. *Fibroid Tumors and Endometriosis Self-Help Book* (Berkeley, CA: Celestial Arts, 1995), 121.

32 Shiva Barton, N.D. "Endometriosis." *The Naturopathic Physician* (Summer 1994).

33 Susan M. Lark, M.D. *Fibroid Tumors and Endometriosis Self-Help Book* (Berkeley, CA: Celestial Arts, 1995), 75, 125, 131-134.

34 Susan M. Lark, M.D. *The Women's Health Companion: Self-Help Nutrition Guide and Cookbook* (Berkeley, CA: Celestial Arts, 1995). Susan M. Lark, M.D. *Fibroid Tumors and Endometriosis Self-Help Book* (Berkeley, CA: Celestial Arts, 1995), 125, 131-134.

Chapter 3
Fibroids

1 F.H. Stuart. *My Body, My Health: The Concerned Woman's Book of Gynecology* (New York: John Wiley & Sons, 1979), 422

2 Vicki Hufnagel, M.D. *No More Hysterectomies* (New York: Penguin Books, 1989).

3 Susan Lark, M.D. *Fibroid Tumors and Endometriosis Self-Help Book* (Berkeley, CA: Celestial Arts, 1995), 8.

4 National Center for Health Statistics, U.S. Centers for Disease Control and Prevention, Hyattsville,

Maryland. Eileen Hoffman, M.D. *Our Health, Our Lives* (New York: Pocket Books, 1995), 219. Vicki Hufnagel, M.D. *No More Hysterectomies* (New York: Plume/Penguin, 1989), 66.

5 Eileen Hoffman, M.D. *Our Health, Our Lives* (New York: Pocket Books, 1995), 219.

6 The Burton Goldberg Group. *Alternative Medicine: The Definitive Guide* (Tiburon, CA: Future Medicine Publishing, 1995), 667.

7 Vicki Hufnagel, M.D. *No More Hysterectomies* (New York: Plume/Penguin, 1989), 66.

8 Ibid., 108.

9 *Family Practice News* (November 1995).

10 T. Smith. *Homeopathic Medicine for Women* (Rochester, VT: Healing Arts Press, 1989).

11 Christiane Northrup, M.D. *Women's Bodies, Women's Wisdom* (New York: Bantam Books, 1994), 180.

12 Kate M. Brett, Ph.D., Jane Marsh, B.A., and Jennifer Madans, Ph.D. "Epidemiology of Hysterectomy in the United States: Demographic and Reproductive Factors in a Nationally Representative Sample." *Journal of Women's Health* 6:3 (1997), 309-315.

13 L.M. Marshall et al. "Variation in the Incidence of Uterine Leiomyoma Among Premenopausal Women by Age and Race." *Obstetrics and Gynecology* 90:6 (December 1997), 967-973.

14 Ibid.

15 John R. Lee, M.D. *What Your Doctor May Not Tell You About Menopause* (New York: Warner Books, 1996), 40.

16 National Institutes of Health, National Cancer Institute. *What You Need to Know About Cancer of the Uterus* Publication No. 93-1562 (Washington, DC: National Institutes of Health, 1991).

17 Ann Louise Gittleman. *Super Nutrition for Menopause* (New York: Pocket Books, 1993), 87.

18 John R. Lee, M.D. *What Your Doctor May Not Tell You About Menopause* (New York: Warner Books, 1996), 110.

19 Hugh MacPherson and Ted Kaptchuk, eds. *Acupuncture in Practice* (New York: Churchill Livingstone, 1997), 193-203.

20 Jason Elias and Katherine Ketcham. *Feminine Healing: A Woman's Guide to a Healthy Body, Mind, and Spirit* (New York: Warner Books, 1997).

21 *Townsend Letter for Doctors* (May 1994), 432-434. See also: *Explore! for the Professional* 4:5 (1993), 17-19.

22 Susun Weed. *Menopausal Years: The Wise Woman Way* (Woodstock, NY: Ash Tree Publishing, 1992), 12-13.

23 Andrew Lockie, M.D., and Nicola Geddes, M.D. *The Women's Guide to Homeopathy* (New York: St. Martin's Press, 1994), 227.

24 Susan M. Lark, M.D. *Fibroid Tumors and Endometriosis Self-Help Book* (Berkeley, CA: Celestial Arts, 1995), 121-144.

25 Robert C. Atkins. *Dr. Atkins' Health Revelations* 2:9 (September 1994), 5.

26 Carolyn Dean, M.D. *Complementary Natural Prescriptions for Common Ailments* (New Canaan, CT: Keats Publishing, 1994), 87.

Chapter 4
Ovarian Cysts

1 Ralph Golan, M.D. *Optimal Wellness* (New York: Ballantine Books, 1995), 399.

2 Ibid.

3 Christiane Northrup, M.D. *Women's Body, Women's Wisdom* (New York: Bantam Books, 1994), 173.

4 John R. Lee, M.D., with Virginia Hopkins. *What Your Doctor May Not Tell You About Menopause* (New York: Warner Books, 1996), 239.

5 G. Wyshak et al. "Smoking and Cysts of the Ovary." *International Journal of Fertility* 33:6 (November-December 1988), 398-404.

6 Susan E. Brown, Ph.D. *Better Bones, Better Body* (New Canaan, CT: Keats Publishing, 1996), 154.

7 Ibid.

8 Kristy Fassler. "Ovarian Cysts." *New England Journal of Homeopathy* 3:1 (1994), 11-14.

9 Hugh MacPherson and Ted Kaptchuk, eds. *Acupuncture in Practice: Case History Insights from the West* (New York: Churchill Livingstone, 1997), 93-100.

10 John R. Lee, M.D., with Virginia Hopkins. *What Your Doctor May Not Tell You About Menopause* (New York: Warner Books, 1996), 273-274.

11 Ralph Golan, M.D. *Optimal Wellness* (New York: Ballantine Books, 1995), 399-400.

12 Tori Hudson, N.D. *Gynecology and Naturopathic Medicine: A Treatment Manual* (Aloha, OR: TK Publications, 1992), Chap. 11, p. 1.

13 Paul Callinan. *Family Homeopathy* (New Canaan, CT: Keats Publishing, 1995), 189.

14 Ralph Golan, M.D. *Optimal Wellness* (New York: Ballantine Books, 1995), 400.

Chapter 5
Infertility

1 Theo Colborn, Dianne Dumanoski, and John Peterson Myers. "Altered Destinies." *Our Stolen Future* (New York: Dutton, 1996), 178-179.

2 Associated Press. "Fertility Clinic Touts Refunds." (1995).

3 Theo Colborn, Dianne Dumanoski, and John Peterson Myers. "Altered Destinies." *Our Stolen Future* (New York: Dutton, 1996), 178-179.

4 J. Claude Bennet, M.D., and Fred Plum, M.D. *Cecil Textbook of Medicine*, 20th Ed. (Philadelphia, PA: W.B. Saunders, 1996), 1308.

5 Ralph Golan, M.D. *Optimal Wellness* (New York: Ballantine Books, 1995), 385.

6 J. Claude Bennet, M.D., and Fred Plum, M.D. *Cecil Textbook of Medicine*, 20th Ed. (Philadelphia, PA: W.B. Saunders, 1996), 1308.

7 Ralph Golan, M.D. *Optimal Wellness* (New York: Ballantine Books, 1995), 385.

8 *New England Journal of Medicine* (July 23, 1997).

9 Joseph Anthony. "Endometriosis: The Hidden Epidemic." *American Health* (May 1996), 61.

10 From the clinic information of enzyme specialist Lita Lee, Ph.D., of Lowell, Oregon.

11 Broda O. Barnes, M.D., and Lawrence Galton. *Hypothyroidism: The Unsuspected Illness* (New York: Harper and Row, 1976), 126-127.

12 Ibid., 128-129.

13 Ralph Golan, M.D. *Optimal Wellness* (New York: Ballantine Books, 1995), 385.

14 Anita Singh, M.D., et al. "Presence of Thyroid Antibodies in Early Reproductive Failure: Biochemical Versus Clinical Pregnancies." *Fertility and Sterility* 63:2 (February 1995), 277-281.

15 Melvyn Werbach, M.D. "Female Infertility." *Townsend Letter for Doctors* (August/September 1995), 34.

16 Gary Null, Ph.D. *The Woman's Encyclopedia of Natural Healing* (New York: Seven Stories Press, 1996), 213.

17 D.W. Dawson and A.H. Sawers. "Infertility and Folate Deficiency: Case Reports." *British Journal of Obstetrics and Gynaecology* 89 (1982), 872-875.

18 G.E. Abraham and J.T. Hargrove. *Medical World News* (March 19, 1979).

19 G.H. Rushton et al. "Ferritin and Fertility." *The Lancet* 337:8756 (June 1991), 1554.

20 B.B. Green, N.S. Weiss, and J.R. Daling. "Risk of Ovulatory Infertility in Relation to Body Weight." *Fertility and Sterility* 50:9 (1988), 621-626.

21 Voukje M. Zaadstra et al. "Fat and Female Fecundity: Prospective Study of Effect of Body Fat Distribtuion on Conception Rates." *British Medical Journal* 306 (February 20, 1993), 484-487.

22 Sherry Boschert. "Diet May Be a Factor in Female Infertility." *Family Practice News* (December 15, 1995), 58.

23 Theo Colborn, Dianne Dumanoski, and John Peterson Myers. *Our Stolen Future* (New York: Dutton/Penguin Group, 1996).

24 S.C. Freni. "Exposure to High Fluoride Concentrations in Drinking Water is Associated With Decreased Birth Rates." *Journal of Toxicological and Environmental Health* 42:1 (May 1994), 109-232.

25 Barbara Seaman. *The Doctors' Case Against the Pill* (Alameda, CA: Hunter House, 1995), 212.

26 Ibid., 213.

27 Ibid.

28 Ibid.

29 Gary Null, Ph.D. *The Woman's Encyclopedia of Natural Healing* (New York: Seven Stories Press, 1996), 218.

30 Donna Day Baird, Ph.D., et al. "Vaginal Douching and Reduced Fertility." *American Journal of Public Health* 86:6 (June 1996), 844-850.

31 E. Alderete, B. Eskenazi, and R. Sholtz. "Effect of Cigarette Smoking and Coffee Drinking on Time to Conception." *Epidemiology* 6:4 (July 1995), 403-408.

32 D.J. Rowlands et al. "Smoking and Decreased Fertilization Rates *In Vitro*." *The Lancet* 340 (December 5, 1992), 1409-1410.

33 C.K. Stanton and R.H. Gray. "Effects of Caffeine Consumption on Delayed Conception." *American Journal of Epidemiology* 142:12 (December 15, 1995), 1322-1329.

34 Melvyn Werbach, M.D. "Female Infertility." *Townsend Letter for Doctors* (August/September 1995), 34.

35 "Infertility's Dark Moods." *Science News* 148 (Dec. 16, 1995), 409.

36 Samuel K. Wasser, Ph.D. "Psychosocial Stress as the Cause of Infertility." *Fertility and Sterility* 59:3 (March 1993), 685-689.

37 Excerpted from: Stephanie Marohn. "Designing Healthy Women." *Alternative Medicine Digest* 12 (1996), 40-42, 74.

38 Gary Null, Ph.D. *The Woman's Encyclopedia of Natural Healing* (New York: Seven Stories Press, 1996), 216.

39 From the patient records of Roger C. Hirsh, O.M.D., L.Ac., of Beverly Hills, California.

40 Jason Elias and Katherine Ketcham. *Feminine Healing* (New York: Warner Books, 1995), 219.

41 Susan Curtis and Romy Fraser. *Natural Healing for Women* (London, England: Pandora, 1991), 136.

42 Ralph Golan, M.D. *Optimal Wellness* (New York: Ballantine Books, 1995), 386.

43 Ibid., 385.

44 Linaya Hahn. *PMS: Solving the Puzzle* (Chicago: Spectrum Press, 1995), 41.

45 Ralph Golan, M.D. *Optimal Wellness* (New York: Ballantine Books, 1995), 384.

46 Ibid.

47 Peter J. Neumann, Sc.D., et al. "Cost of a Successful Delivery With *In Vitro* Fertilization." *New England Journal of Medicine* 331:4 (July 1994), 239-243.

48 "Rates of Births via Assisted-Reproductive

Technologies Have Improved Only Slightly." *Medical Tribune* (January 1997), 8.

49 Jill Stansbury. "Fortifying Fertility With Vitamins and Herbs." *Nutrition Science News* 2:12 (December 1997), 606-612.

50 Ralph Golan, M.D. *Optimal Wellness* (New York: Ballantine Books, 1995), 386.

51 Glenn W. Geelhoed, M.D. *Natural Health Secrets From Around the World* (New Canaan CT: Keats Publishing, 1995), 321.

52 Jason Elias and Katherine Ketcham. *Feminine Healing* (New York: Warner Books, 1995), 220.

53 William Collinge, M.P.H., Ph.D. *The American Holistic Health Association Complete Guide to Alternative Medicine* (New York: Warner Books, 1996), 137.

54 M.D. Keltz et al. "Baseline Cyst Formation After Luteal Phase Gonadotropin-Releasing Hormone Agonist Administration is Linked to Poor *In Vitro* Fertilization Outcome." *Fertility and Sterility* 64:3 (September 1995), 568-572.

55 Andrew Lockie, M.D., and Nicola Geddes, M.D. *Women's Guide to Homeopathy* (New York: St. Martin's Press, 1994), 127.

Chapter 6
Cystitis and Other Urinary Tract Infections

1 Bill Gottlieb. *New Choices in Natural Healing* (Emmaus, PA: Rodale Press, 1995), 545.

2 Rebecca Chalker and Kristene Whitmore, M.D. *Overcoming Bladder Disorders* (New York: Harper and Row, 1990), 3.

3 Ellen Michaud. *Total Health for Women* (Emmaus, PA: Rodale Press, 1995), 63.

4 *PDR Family Guide to Women's Health and Prescription Drugs* (Montvale, NJ: Medical Economics, 1994), 92-93.

5 Carolyn DeMarco, M.D. "Bladder Blues." *Take Charge of Your Body* (Aurora, Ontario, Canada: Well Women Press, 1995), 78-79.

6 Rebecca Chalker and Kristene Whitmore, M.D. *Overcoming Bladder Disorders* (New York: Harper and Row, 1990), 3. *Taber's Cyclopedic Medical Dictionary* (Philadelphia: F.A. Davis, 1993).

7 Jill Stansbury, N.D. "Lower Urinary Tract Infections." *Medical Herbalism* 9:1 (Spring 1997), 1, 5-11. Available from: Medical Herbalism, P.O. Box 20512, Boulder, CO 80308; tel: 303-541-9552; 4 issues/$36.

8 Larrian Gillespie, M.D. *You Don't Have to Live with Cystitis* (New York: Avon Books, 1996).

9 *PDR Family Guide to Women's Health and Prescription Drugs* (Montvale, NJ: Medical Economics, 1994), 91-92.

10 Ellen Michaud. *Total Health for Women* (Emmaus, PA: Rodale Press, 1995), 63.

11 Ibid., 61.

12 Rebecca Chalker and Kristene Whitmore, M.D. *Overcoming Bladder Disorders* (New York: Harper and Row, 1990), 121.

13 George Vithoulkas. *The Science of Homeopathy* (New York: Grove Press, 1980), 110.

14 L. Alm et al. "Effect of Fermentation on B Vitamin Content of Milk in Sweden." *Journal of Dairy Science* 65 (1982), 353-359.

15 L. Alm. *Journal of Dairy Science* 64:4 (1981), 509-514.

16 B. Friend and M.K. Shahani. "Nutritional and Therapeutic Aspects of *Lactobacilli*." *Journal of Applied Nutrition* 36, 125-153.

17 K. Shehani. "Role of Dietary *Lactobacilli* in Gastrointestinal Microecology." *American Journal of Clinical Nutrition* 33 (1980), 2248-2257.

18 M. Speck. "Interactions Among Lactobacilli and Man." *Journal of Dairy Science* 59:2 (1976), 338-343.

19 Bill Gottlieb. *New Choices in Natural Healing* (Emmaus, PA: Rodale Press, 1995), 546.

20 I. Ofek et al. "Anti-*Escherichia coli* Adhesion Activity of Cranberry and Blueberry Juices." *New England Journal of Medicine* 324:22 (1991), 1599.

21 Andrew Lockie, M.D., and Nicola Geddes, M.D. *The Women's Guide to Homeopathy* (New York: St. Martin's Press, 1994), 87.

22 Jacqueline Young. *The Natural Way: Cystitis* (Rockport, MA: Element Books, 1997), 15.

23 Ibid.

24 Ellen Michaud. *Total Health for Women* (Emmaus, PA: Rodale Press, 1995), 61.

25 Jacqueline Young. *The Natural Way: Cystitis* (Rockport, MA: Element Books, 1997), 16

26 Rebecca Chalker and Kristene Whitmore, M.D. *Overcoming Bladder Disorders* (New York: Harper and Row, 1990), 163.

27 Ibid., 162.

28 Andrew Lockie, M.D., and Nicola Geddes, M.D. *The Women's Guide to Homeopathy* (New York: St. Martin's Press, 1994), 87.

29 Rebecca Chalker and Kristene Whitmore, M.D. *Overcoming Bladder Disorders* (New York: Harper and Row, 1990), 162.

30 Carolyn Dean, M.D., N.D. *Menopause Naturally* (New Canaan, CT: Keats Publishing, 1995), 33.

31 Rebecca Chalker and Kristene Whitmore, M.D. *Overcoming Bladder Disorders* (New York: Harper and Row, 1990), 163.

32 Ibid.

33 Julian Scott, M.A., Ph.D., and Susan Scott. *Natural*

Medicine for Women (New York: Avon Books, 1991), 179.

34 Jacqueline Young. *The Natural Way: Cystitis* (Rockport, MA: Element Books, 1997), 19.

35 Christiane Northrup, M.D. *Women's Body, Women's Wisdom* (New York: Bantam Books, 1994), 237-238.

36 Andrew Lockie, M.D., and Nicola Geddes, M.D. *The Women's Guide to Homeopathy* (New York: St. Martin's Press, 1994), 89.

37 Joseph E. Pizzorno, N.D. "Natural Medicine Approach to the Treatment of Cystitis." *Alternative & Complementary Therapies* (October 1994), 32-34.

38 William G. Crook, M.D. *The Yeast Connection and the Woman* (Jackson, TN: Professional Books, 1995), 85-86.

39 Michael T. Murray, N.D. "Bladder Infections: Another Concern of Menopause." *American Journal of Natural Medicine* 2:9 (November 1995).

40 Jacqueline Young. *The Natural Way: Cystitis* (Rockport, MA: Element Books, 1997), 83.

41 J. Avorn et al. "Reduction of Bacteriuria and Pyuria After Ingestion of Cranberry Juice." *Journal of the American Medical Association* 271 (1994), 751-754.

42 "Nutrition Q and A." *Nutrition Science News* (August 1997), 406.

43 Jacqueline Young. *The Natural Way: Cystitis* (Rockport, MA: Element Books, 1997), 68.

44 Gary W. Elmer, Ph.D., et al. "Biotherapeutic Agents: A Neglected Modality for the Treatment and Prevention of Selected Intestinal and Vaginal Infections." *Journal of the American Medical Association* 275:11 (March 20, 1996), 870-876.

45 Judy Jacka. *The Complete A-Z of Common Ailments and Their Natural Remedies* (London, England: Foulsham), 128.

46 G. Reid et al. "Influence of Three-Day Antimicrobial Therapy and *Lactobacillus* Vaginal Suppositories on Recurrence of Urinary Tract Infections." *Clinical Therapies* 14 (1992), 11-16.

47 P.L. Chang. "Urodynamic Studies in Acupuncture for Women with Frequency, Urgency and Dysuria." *Journal of Urology* 140:3 (1988), 563-566.

48 Bill Gottlieb. *New Choices in Natural Healing* (Emmaus, PA: Rodale Press, 1995), 546.

49 Judith Lawless. *The Complete Illustrated Guide to Aromatherapy* (Rockport, MA: Element Books, 1997).

50 Ibid.

51 Susun S. Weed. *Menopausal Years: The Wise Woman Way* (Woodstock, NY: Ash Tree Publishing, 1992), 191.

52 Ralph Golan, M.D. *Optimal Wellness* (New York: Ballantine, 1995).

53 Glenn Geelhoed and Jean Barilla. "Urinary Tract Infections." *Natural Health Secrets From Around the World* (New Canaan, CT: Keats Publishing, 1997), 495-496.

54 Julian Scott, M.A., Ph.D., and Susan Scott. *Natural Medicine for Women* (New York: Avon Books, 1991), 180.

55 Andrew Lockie, M.D., and Nicola Geddes, M.D. *The Women's Guide to Homeopathy* (New York: St. Martin's Press, 1994), 88-89.

56 Carolyn Dean, M.D. *Menopause Naturally* (New Canaan, CT: Keats Publishing, 1995), 34.

57 Bill Gottlieb. *New Choices in Natural Healing* (Emmaus, PA: Rodale Press, 1995), 547

58 This bottle washing procedure first appeared in *Cystitis: How to Prevent Infection and Inflammation* by Angela Kilmartin (Thorsons, 1994) and is adapted from *The Women's Guide to Homeopathy* by Andrew Lockie, M.D., and Nicola Geddes, M.D. (New York: St. Martin's Press, 1994), 88.

59 Susun S. Weed. *Menopausal Years: The Wise Woman Way* (Woodstock, NY: Ash Tree Publishing, 1992), 190.

60 Marjory Spraycar. *Stedman's Medical Dictionary* 26th Ed. (Baltimore, MD: Williams & Wilkins, 1995), 1211.

61 Shannon D. Smith et al. "Improvement in Interstitial Cystitis Symptom Scores During Treatment with Oral L-Arginine." *Journal of Urology* 158:3 (September 1997).

Chapter 7
Vaginitis

1 D. Eschenbach. "Vaginal Infection." *Clinical Obstetrics and Gynecology* 26:1 (1983), 186-202.

2 National Vaginitis Association. "Women's Guide to Vaginal Infections." Internet: http://www.vaginal-infections.org. Julian Whitaker, M.D. *Dr. Whitaker's Guide to Natural Healing* (Rocklin, CA: Prima Publishing, 1995), 353.

3 *Johns Hopkins Medical Letter: Health After 50* (New York: Medletter Associates, 1995), 688.

4 Julian Whitaker, M.D. *Dr. Whitaker's Guide to Natural Healing* (Rocklin, CA: Prima Publishing, 1995), 353.

5 Paul Reilly, M.D. "Vaginitis and Vulvovaginitis." *A Textbook of Natural Medicine*, Vol. 2, Joseph E. Pizzorno Jr., N.D., and Michael T. Murray, N.D., eds. (Seattle, WA: John Bastyr College Publications, 1988), 1-8.

6 E.A. Fontaine et al. "*Lactobacilli* from Women With or Without Bacterial Vaginosis and Observations on the Significance of Hydrogen Peroxide." *Microbial Ecology in Health and Disease* 9 (1996), 135-141.

7 Enrique Hernandez, M.D., and Barbara F. Atkinson, M.D. *Clinical Gynecologic Pathology* (Philadelphia: W.B. Saunders, 1996), 98.

8 Paul Reilly, M.D. "Vaginitis and Vulvovaginitis." *A Textbook of Natural Medicine*, Vol. 2, Joseph E. Pizzorno Jr., N.D., and Michael T. Murray, N.D., eds. (Seattle, WA: John Bastyr College Publications, 1988), 1-8.

9 William G. Crook, M.D. *The Yeast Connection and the Woman* (Jackson, TN: Professional Books, 1995), 25-43.

10 Ralph Golan. *Optimal Wellness* (New York: Ballantine, 1995), 421.

11 Michael Murray, N.D. "Chronic Candidiasis: A Natural Approach." *American Journal of Natural Medicine* 4:4 (May 1997), 16-17.

12 Paul Reilly, M.D. "Vaginitis and Vulvovaginitis." *A Textbook of Natural Medicine*, Vol. 2, Joseph E. Pizzorno Jr., N.D., and Michael T. Murray N.D., eds. (Seattle, WA: John Bastyr College Publications, 1988), 1-8.

13 Sherry Boschert. "Drop of HxOx Can Help Diagnose Vaginitis." *Family Practice News* (July 15, 1997), 35.

14 From research done by Luis E. Todd, M.D., at the Universidad Autonoma de Nuevo Leon, Monterrey, Mexico. An abstract is available on the Internet: http://www.sover.net/~samallen/nutri.htm.

15 John R. Lee, M.D. *What Your Doctor May Not Tell You About Menopause* (New York: Warner Books, 1996), 237.

16 Paul Reilly, M.D. "Vaginitis and Vulvovaginitis." *A Textbook of Natural Medicine*, Vol. 2, Joseph E. Pizzorno Jr., N.D., and Michael T. Murray N.D., eds. (Seattle, WA: John Bastyr College Publications, 1988), 1-8.

17 Magdy S. Mickhail et al. "Decreased Beta-Carotene Levels in Exfoliated Vaginal Epithelial Cells in Women With Vaginal Candidiasis." *American Journal of Reproductive Immunology* 32 (1994), 221-225.

18 *Johns Hopkins Medical Letter: Health After 50* (New York: Medletter Associates, 1995), 688.

19 P. Nyirjesy et al. "Over-the-Counter and Alternative Medicines in the Treatment of Chronic Vaginal Symptoms." *Obstetrics and Gynecology* 90 (1997), 50-53.

20 Paul Reilly, M.D. "Vaginitis and Vulvovaginitis." *A Textbook of Natural Medicine*, Vol. 2, Joseph E. Pizzorno Jr., N.D., and Michael T. Murray, N.D., eds. (Seattle, WA: John Bastyr College Publications, 1988), 1-8.

21 Ibid.

22 Eliezer Shalev et al. "Ingestion Of Yogurt Containing *Lactobacillus acidophilus* Compared With Pasteurized Yogurt as Prophylaxis for Recurrent Candidal Vaginitis and Bacterial Vaginosis." *Archives of Family Medicine* 5 (November/December 1996), 593-596.

23 Paul Reilly, M.D. "Vaginitis and Vulvovaginitis." *A Textbook of Natural Medicine*, Vol. 2, Joseph E. Pizzorno Jr., N.D., and Michael T. Murray, N.D., eds. (Seattle, WA: John Bastyr College Publications, 1988), 1-8.

24 Ibid.

25 Gary W. Elmer, Ph.D., et al. "Biotherapeutic Agents: A Neglected Modality for the Treatment and Prevention of Selected Intestinal and Vaginal Infections." *Journal of the American Medical Association* 275:11 (1996), 870-876.

26 Andrew Lockie, M.D., and Nicola Geddes, M.D. *Women's Guide to Homeopathy* (New York: St. Martin's Press, 1994), 84.

27 Ralph Golan. *Optimal Wellness* (New York: Ballantine Books, 1995), 422.

28 Julian Whitaker, M.D. *Dr. Whitaker's Guide to Natural Healing* (Rocklin, CA: Prima Publishing, 1995), 353.

29 Paul Reilly, M.D. "Vaginitis and Vulvovaginitis." *A Textbook of Natural Medicine*, Vol. 2, Joseph E. Pizzorno Jr., N.D., and Michael T. Murray, N.D., eds. (Seattle, WA: John Bastyr College Publications, 1988), 1-8.

30 Julian Whitaker, M.D. *Dr. Whitaker's Guide to Natural Healing* (Rocklin, CA: Prima Publishing, 1995), 353.

Index

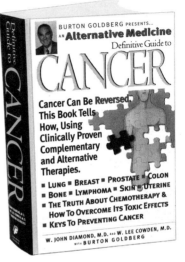
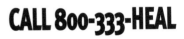

CURE YOUR HEADACHES...
USING NATURAL THERAPIES

If you suffer from headaches, this book could change your life. It is entirely possible that with this invaluable practical information, you may well put headaches behind you as something you once suffered from, but no more.

Robert Milne, M.D., and Blake More expertly guide you through the root causes and multiple treatment options for 11 major types of headaches, from sinus to migraine, cluster to tension.

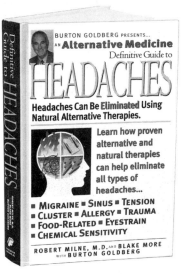

BURTON GOLDBERG PRESENTS...
AN **Alternative Medicine**
Definitive Guide to

HEADACHES

Headaches Can Be Eliminated Using Natural Alternative Therapies.

Learn how proven alternative and natural therapies can help eliminate all types of headaches...

- MIGRAINE ■ SINUS ■ TENSION
- CLUSTER ■ ALLERGY ■ TRAUMA
- FOOD-RELATED ■ EYESTRAIN
- CHEMICAL SENSITIVITY

ROBERT MILNE, M.D. AND BLAKE MORE
WITH BURTON GOLDBERG

We have made every effort possible to make this book practical and user-friendly for you. For a quick reference to headache types, symptoms, and treatment options, use our Master Symptom Chart. If you suffer from tension headaches, turn directly to Chapter 6; if migraines are your millstone, see Chapter 7; and if you're not sure what type of headache you have, study the symptoms list in the Master Symptom Chart until you find the clinical term that best matches your condition.

No matter what kind of headache you have, after reading this book your head may never pain you again.

Hardcover ■ ISBN 1-887299-03-3
■ 6" x 9" ■ 525 pages

TO ORDER, CALL 800-333-HEAL

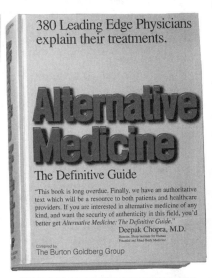

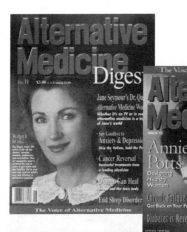

We digest it for you—*Alternative Medicine* tracks the entire field—all the doctor's journals, research, conferences, and newsletters. Then we summarize what is essential for you to know to get better and stay healthy. We're your one-stop read for what's new and effective in alternative medicine.

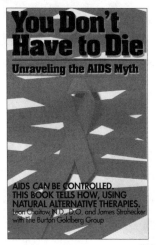
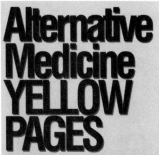

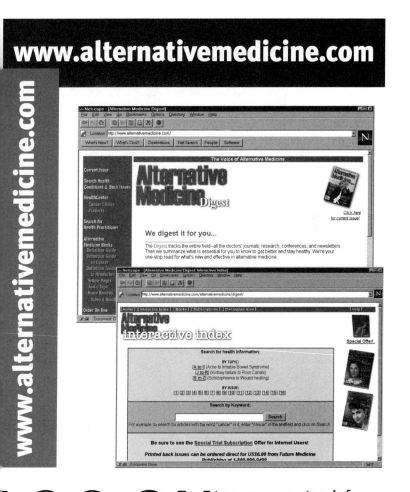

www.alternativemedicine.com

LOG ON to your one-stop information source for the best and boldest in alternative medicine. Find the answer to your health problem fast with our Interactive Index. Study the medical information you need to know by accessing our reference work, *Alternative Medicine: The Definitive Guide*. Browse all the back issues of *Alternative Medicine* or hyperlink to our newest issue—before it hits the newsstands. Network worldwide with other enthusiasts in our chat room.

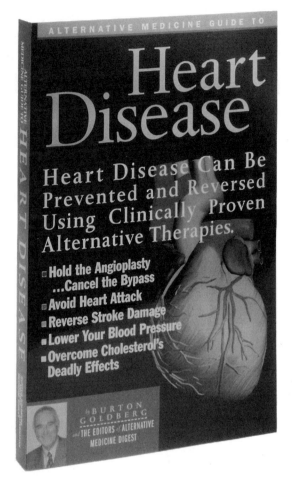

Save your heart from heart disease, attack, stroke, high blood pressure, and the dangers of angioplasty, bypass, and other invasive surgeries—12 top physicians explain their proven, safe, nontoxic, and successful heart-saving treatments.

Look for upcoming books in the Alternative Medicine Guide paperback series covering topics such as Women's Health, Supplements, Anti-aging, Weight Loss, and Enzymes.

TO ORDER, CALL 800-333-HEAL

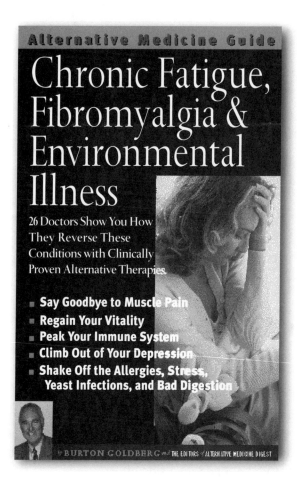

Chronic fatigue, fibromyalgia, and environmental illness can be permanently reversed using nontoxic alternative medicine treatments. In this book, 26 leading physicians explain the techniques and natural substances that brought complete recovery to their patients.

TO ORDER, CALL 800-333-HEAL

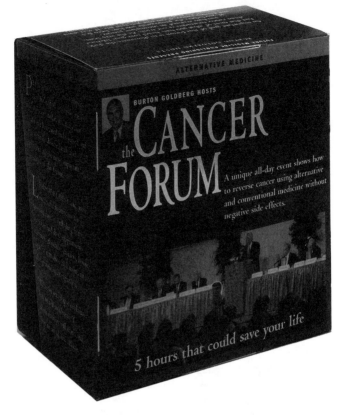

The Cancer Forum—five hours of lifesaving information from leading alternative medicine physicians who show you how to reverse cancer using alternative and conventional medicine without negative side effects.

Prevention is the most important and reliable cancer-fighting tool that exists today. The fact that cancer can be treated and reversed and that it can be detected early and prevented are the most important messages of this forum.

Learn the latest proven, safe, nontoxic, and successful treatments for reversing cancer, including herbs, nutrition and diet, supplements, enzymes, glandular extracts, home-opathic remedies, and more, in this groundbreaking video.

TO ORDER, CALL 800-333-HEAL